Caring for the Seriously Ill Patient

2004

Caring for the Seriously Ill Patient

EDITED BY

Christopher C. Bassett RGN, BA (Hons), RNT

Lecturer in Acute and Critical Care Nursing,
University of Sheffield, Sheffield, UK

and

Lesley Makin RGN

Clinical Effectiveness Advisor,
Chesterfield and North Derbyshire Royal Hospital, Derbyshire, UK

A member of the Hodder Headline Group
LONDON

First published in Great Britain in 2000 by
Arnold, a member of the Hodder Headline Group
338 Euston Road, London NW1 3BH

http://www.arnoldpublishers.com

© 2000 Chris Bassett and Lesley Makin

British Library Cataloguing in Publication Data
A catalogue record for this book is available from the British Library

ISBN 0 340 70582 5 (pb)

1 2 3 4 5 6 7 8 9 10

Commissioning Editor: Cathy Peck
Production Editor: Wendy Rooke
Production Controller: Iain McWilliams
Project Manager: Paula O'Connell

Composition in 9½/11½ Palatino by J&L Composition Ltd, Filey, North Yorkshire
Printed and bound in Great Britain by The Bath Press

What do you think about this book? Or any other Arnold title?
Please send your comments to feedback.arnold@hodder.co.uk

Contents

Contributors

Sarah Adams RGN, RM, MA(Nurse practitioner)
Nurse Practitioner – General Practice
32 The Linnets
Gateford
Nottinghamshire S81 8TX

Mr Chris Bassett RGN, BA(Hons), RNT
Lecturer in Acute and Critical Care Nursing
University of Sheffield
School of Nursing and Midwifery
Winter Street
Sheffield S3 7ND

Mr Robert Donald RN, BA(Hons), MA, Postgrad cert ED
Clinical Nurse Educator
8 Lomas Lea
Stannington
Sheffield S6 6EW

Ms Irene Gilsenan BA(Hons), RGN, EN(G), Cert Ed
Staff Nurse
Central Sheffield University
Hospital Trust
Sheffield S10 2JF

Mr Paul Harrison RGN, ONC, ENB 219, MA(Ed)
Clinical Development Officer
Princess Royal Spinal Injuries Unit
Northern General Hospital
Herries Road
Sheffield S5 7AU

Mr Michael J Macintosh RGN, ENB 124, ENB 100, Dip
Health and Community Studies, BA(Hons), RNT
Lecturer, Acute and Critical Care Nursing
University of Sheffield
School of Nursing and Midwifery
Winter Street
Sheffield S3 7ND

Ms Lesley Makin RGN
Clinical Effectiveness Adviser
Chesterfield and North Derbyshire Royal
Hospital
Derbyshire S44 5BL

Mr Robert McSherry RGN, Dip N(Lon), BSc(Hons),
MSC Social Research Methods, PGCE, RT, Doctoral Student,
University Tees-side, Middlesborough
Senior Lecturer, Adult Nursing
Centre for Practice Development
School of Health
University of Tees-side
Middlesborough

Ms Tracey Moore RGN, ENB 100, BSc(Hons), PG DipEd,
MSC
Nursing Lecturer/Diploma Leader (Acute and
Critical Care)
University of Sheffield
School of Nursing and Midwifery
Winter Street
Sheffield S3 7ND

Ms Jenny Muxlow MMedSci (Clinical Nursing),
BSc(Hons) Nursing, RNT, RCNT, RGN
Nursing Lecturer, Acute and Critical Care
Nursing
University of Sheffield
School of Nursing and Midwifery
Winter Street
Sheffield S3 7ND

Ms P Sutherland RGN, RM, RCNT, RNT, BA(Hons), MA,
TD
Nursing Lecturer
School of Nursing and Midwifery
Bartolome House
Winter Street
Sheffield S3 7ND

Mrs S A Zmarzty RGN, BSc Hons (Zoology), MMed Sci (Human Nutrition), Cert Ed, Doctoral Student, University of Sheffield
Lecturer in Nursing
Dept of Gerontological and Continuing Care Nursing

The University of Sheffield
School of Nursing and Midwifery
Samuel Fox House
Northern General Hospital
Herries Road
Sheffield S5 7AU

Setting the scene

Lesley Makin

Introduction

The care of seriously ill patients requires a high level of both medical and nursing skill. Close observation and early intervention when parameters change adversely are vital if there is to be a positive outcome for the patient. Advances in medical treatments and modalities, changes in patient populations and increased expectations mean that patients who were once considered too high a risk are now being operated on routinely.

In some areas, there has been a decrease in nursing support on the general wards, which, coupled with the decline in numbers of potential nurses entering training programmes (Liversley and Crosby, 1989), has only served to exacerbate the problem. Ward nurses are increasingly expected to cope with patients who require an intermediate level of care because their trusts may not have a high dependency unit, and intensive care facilities are stretched to capacity. High dependency care is, therefore, an evolving speciality that has been driven in part by the increasing demands made on intensive care.

The aim of this book is to provide the newly qualified practitioner, ward based nurses, or those embarking on a career in the field of high dependency care with background knowledge on which to base the care they deliver to patients.

Previous experience and knowledge is not essential to the reader, a series of reflective questions are used to test knowledge, and the practitioner is encouraged to reflect on the information given and to try to relate it to patients in their care. We hope that nurses wishing to specialize in this expanding field and those caring for the seriously ill patient on general wards will find it a useful resource.

Background

In 1990 Crosby and colleagues reported that less than 5 per cent of patients who were cared for in a high dependency unit which had been established adjacent to, but separate from the intensive care unit, needed their level of care upgrading to intensive care. Studies carried out in Sheffield (Sheffield Central University Hospital, 1993), following the development of their high dependency unit, showed a reduction in postponed operations and premature discharges.

Much work has been undertaken to try to establish the number of patients on general wards who would benefit from a higher level of care, and the cost of providing such care (Crosby *et al.*, 1995; Edbroke *et al.*, 1996). It is thought that between 0.5 per cent and 13 per cent of patients currently nursed on general wards would benefit from a higher level of care, dependent upon whether there are high dependency facilities within the hospital or not. A national survey carried out by Metcalf to determine the provision of high dependency care in England suggested that more than two-thirds of hospitals are not offering this level of care (Metcalf and Mcpherson, 1995). It was following this particular report that the working group which produced the Guidelines on Admission to and Discharge from Intensive Care and High Dependency Units was set up (DOH, 1996).

In January 1996, there was widespread publicity with regard to the acute shortage of intensive care beds during the winter months. This coincided with the Report of the Joint Working Party on Graduated Care (Royal College of Anaesthetists and Surgeons, 1996) and the Report of the Confidential Enquiry into Perioperative Deaths 1992–93, which stated that:

> Overall there is an inadequate provision of high dependency units across the country and this is something that should be addressed very urgently by both clinicians and managers. It is pointless to perform major surgery on patients who are physiologically compromised, unless there are facilities for these patients, to recover post-operatively.

With the evidence for the development of services for the seriously ill patient growing, and the mounting public concern in relation to the apparent increase in interhospital transfers, in the winter of 1996, further funding was made available to Regions for the provision of extra intensive and high dependency care (DOH, 1998).

What is high dependency care?

In the Guidelines on Admission to and Discharge from Intensive Care and High Dependency Units (DOH, 1996) high dependency care is defined as:

> providing a level of care intermediate between that on a general ward and intensive care. High dependency care monitors and supports patients with or likely to develop, acute (or acute-on-chronic) single organ failure. It should not manage patients

requiring multiple organ support nor patients requiring mechanical ventilation.

ACTIVITY 1.1

Take a few minutes now to reflect on the patients currently in your care. Do any of them meet the criteria?

Some examples of the types of patients who might be considered suitable for admission to a high dependency unit are listed in Table 1.1. This list is by no means exhaustive, but is intended to highlight just a few of the patients who should be considered in need of specialist care.

In a busy general ward, it is very difficult for the nursing staff to be able to spend the time required with the severely ill patient. This potentially leads to poorer outcomes for patients and may lead to dissatisfaction amongst relatives who feel that their loved ones are not receiving the care they deserve or require. High dependency facilities, where they exist as separate entities from intensive care, can be used as a step-down unit when patients no longer require the specialist skills of the intensivist but are not quite well enough to return to the general ward.

Where there are pressures on intensive care beds, patients are often transferred back to general wards with dependency scores that suggest a high dependency unit would have been more appropriate. Early intervention and provision of high dependency facilities may prevent an expensive admission to intensive care, and may favourably influence the patient's length of hospital stay and long-term prognosis (DOH, 1996).

The Guidelines on Admission to and Discharge from Intensive Care and High Dependency Units (DOH, 1996) states that:

> Research suggests that establishing an intermediate level of care reduces ward mortality by 25 per cent and cardiac arrests by 39 per cent.

The discharge of patients directly from theatre to a general ward at night, when staffing levels are

Table 1.1 Patients who may be suitable for admission to a high dependency unit

High dependency care should be considered in any of the cases listed below
1 Patients who require more than 40 per cent oxygen on a fixed concentration mask
2 Patients with unstable respiratory conditions which are likely to deteriorate
3 Patients requiring CPAP*
4 Patients with mini-tracheostomy requiring frequent suctioning and physiotherapy
5 Patients with unstable cardiovascular function from any cause, such as post-operative haemorrhage, or gastrointestinal haemorrhage with associated coagulopathy
6 Patients requiring inotropic support
7 Patients requiring epidural analgesia (except in obstetric analgesia)
8 Patients with impaired renal function and acutely abnormal fluid and electrolyte imbalance that does not require haemodialysis

*CPAP: continuous positive airway pressure

low, is not appropriate (Standards for Intensive Care, 1985). Pain control, management of fluids and regular observation all require a great deal of nursing time. One of the key recommendations of the NCEPOD report is that:

> Surgical operations should not be started unless critical care services are available.

In many hospitals where high dependency facilities do not exist as a separate entity, these patients are nursed in intensive care units if there is a bed available, or returned to the general ward, where their care may fall short of the required standard.

Unit design

It is generally considered that the most appropriate site for a high dependency unit is in close proximity, but physically separate from intensive care. This allows the intensivist easy access to the unit, to provide expert support and advice when it is required. The unit should also be within easy reach of the operating theatres and the medical wards, to facilitate the admission of both post-operative patients, and those requiring physical support for medical reasons.

There is currently no Building Note for high dependency units, but many of the facilities outlined in the Health Building Note 27 published by NHS Estates for intensive care units are relevant. Each bed space will require piped oxygen and suction as a minimum. There should also be enough electrical sockets to accommodate monitoring and infusion equipment. It is useful if this equipment is of the same or similar specification to that of the intensive care unit, in order to increase flexibility between beds on the two units in times of crisis.

Staffing

Nurse staffing

Nurses caring for the seriously ill patient require appropriate specialist training, and post-registration/post-graduate education is available for those nurses who wish to specialize in this field. The training will equip the nurses with the necessary skills to enable them to manage the physiologically unstable patient, and to manage the psychological needs of the patients and their relatives.

Nursing staff will often be required to make clinical decisions to institute treatment prescribed by medical staff when the patient's condition suddenly changes. Some of these changes will be potentially life-threatening, and it is vital that the nurse can react quickly and appropriately.

Qualified nursing staff new to the speciality require supervision from a more experienced and senior person, and there should be a comprehensive induction and continuing education package for them to follow.

The nursing skill mix should reflect the possibility that the patients may be physiologically unstable, and the average nurse:patient ratio should be 1:2 throughout the 24 hours. There should in addition be a nurse in charge, and extra staff available to assist with care according to the patient need.

Medical staffing

The ever-increasing workload of the staff caring for seriously ill and critically ill patients is daunting. Adequate consultant sessions are vital if the care of these patients is to be effective. The Intensive Care Society recommends that units of up to ten beds should have a minimum of 15 consultant sessions (ICS, 1990). Intensive care is now considered part of the basic surgical training for the FRCS, and in the Summer 1996 issue of the Intensive Care Society Newsletter, the recommendations of the Intercollegiate Committee on intensive care pertaining to training were outlined. The recommendations are that all junior medical staff in anaesthesia, medicine and surgery should receive 3 months' experience in intensive care within 2 years of registration. Senior House Officers are therefore perfectly capable of managing patients who require an intermediate level of care, under the close supervision of the intensivist.

Costs

The cost of caring for seriously ill patients in a high dependency unit will undoubtedly be higher than the cost of their care on a general ward. This can be attributed to the increase in nurse:patient ratio, the increased cost of consumables used in the close monitoring and observation of the patients, pharmacy costs and capital costs. However, the cost is much less than the cost of caring for these patients in the intensive care unit, being at least 50 per cent lower (Singer *et al.*, 1994).

Many hospital trusts have recently completed internal audits to determine their need for an intermediate level of care. Some have been fortunate in securing funding and the support of their trust board and local health authority to assist with the commissioning and implementation of such units.

There can be no doubt that this is a rapidly expanding field which, given time, will prove its value in improved patient outcomes.

Further reading

Anon 1985 Standards for intensive care units. *Care of the Critically Ill* **3**, 4–8.

Central Sheffield University Hospital 1993 *High dependency unit report. Sheffield 1992/3*.

Crosby, D.L. and Rees, G.A.D. 1994 Provision of post operative care in UK hospitals. *Annals of the RSCE* **76**, 14–18.

DOH 1995 *Report of the National Confidential Enquiry into Perioperative Deaths. 1992/3*. London: Department of Health.

DOH 1996 *Report on the Working Group on Guidelines on Admission to and Discharge from Intensive Care and High Dependency Units*. London: Department of Health.

DOH 1998 *El 96 106 109 – Funding for Priority Services 1996/7 and 1997/8*.

Edbrooke, D.L. 1996 *The provision of high dependency units in England – The cost and benefits of development and implementation*. ICM **22**, 303.

Gill, J. and Rees, G.A.D. 1990 The role of the high dependency unit in post-operative care: an update. *Annals of the RCSE* **72**, 309–12.

Intensive Care Society 1990 *The Intensive Care Service in the UK*. London: ICS.

Intensive Care Society 1996 *ICS Newsletter* Summer 1996.

Leeson–Payne, CG and Aitkenhead, AR 1995 A prospective study to assess the demand for a high dependency unit. *Anaesthesia* **50**, 383–7.

Liversley, B. and Crosby, D.L. 1989 Running out of staff for the NHS. *BMJ* **299**, 1–2.

Metcalf, A. and Mcpherson, K. 1995 *Study of intensive care in England 1993*. London: Department of Health.

Singer, M., Myers, S., Hall, G. et al. 1994 The cost of intensive care: a comparison of one unit between 1988 and 1991. *Intensive Care Medicine* **20**, 542–9.

The Royal College of Anaesthetists and Surgeons 1996 *Report of the joint working party on graduated patient care*. London: RCAS.

Wilson, A.J., Stevens, V.G. et al. 1996 *Intensive Care Medicine* **22**, 303(S).

2 Caring for the cardiovascular system

Michael Macintosh

Introduction

The cardiovascular system is a transport system with continuous responsibility for the delivery of oxygen and nutrients to the cells of the body, and for the removal of the waste products of metabolism. The quantity of oxygen that is supplied to the tissues is dependent upon three factors:

1 The arterial oxygen saturation.
2 The haemoglobin content of the blood.
3 The cardiac output.

That is, oxygen delivery (Do_2) = oxygen saturation (Sao_2) $\times$ haemoglobin (Hb) $\times$ cardiac output. In order to maintain adequate delivery of oxygen to all of the tissues of the body and to be able to increase this delivery when demands dictate, the cardiovascular system has to be able to adjust, that is, to increase the value of one or all of these physiological parameters. A very simple model of the cardiovascular system can be described that is conceptually useful despite its simplicity.

The cardiovascular system can be thought of as comprising three parts:

• A pump (the heart).
• Volume (the blood).
• Pipes (the veins and arteries).

Each of these three parts is constantly being adjusted in response to demand, and a problem with one of the three must be compensated for by one or both of the other two. When this compensation is not possible the consequences are disastrous and often fatal.

The aim of the cardiovascular system in continually making these adjustments is to maintain perfusion. In order to ensure the adequate delivery of oxygen to the cells there has to be adequate tissue perfusion. In other words, there needs to be an acceptable level of pressure maintained at the delivery end of the cardiovascular system to allow for internal respiration to take place. When this perfusion pressure falls, the delivery of oxygenated blood will fall.

Continuing with this simple model, the cardiovascular system can be likened to any system that delivers fluid under pressure, for example a garden hose. The purpose of a garden hose is to deliver a jet of water under sufficient pressure to supply the flowers with enough fluid to prevent them from dying.

Consider for a moment the pump (heart) to be represented by the tap. The tap can be turned up or down, or the hose-pipe (the blood vessels) can be made to have a narrower or larger diameter. Provided there is a sufficient and constant supply of water (the blood) then either of these measures will result in the jet of water at the end of the pipe increasing, that is, perfusion. If however the pump starts to fail by the tap being turned down, the jet of water will fall. Similarly, if the hose-pipe is changed for one that has a larger diameter, a fire hose for example, the jet of water will again fall. In each of these examples there must be compensation; either the tap is turned up to increase the pressure drop caused by the larger diameter hose, or the hose must be made smaller to increase the pressure drop caused by the turning down of the tap.

So it is with the cardiovascular system. However, this ability to compensate has limits. Just as the tap has a limit beyond which it cannot be increased so the heart has a limit to its output. Just as the hose has a limit to which it can be made to have a smaller diameter, so the blood vessels have a limit beyond which further constriction will not help. This then is the model of perfusion that will be used to describe the normal physiology and abnormal pathology, and to discuss logically, assessment and management of the individual with an actual or potential problem with the cardiovascular system.

Chapter 3 explains how the oxygen saturation of haemoglobin may be compromised and also how it can be optimized by appropriate nursing and medical intervention. The aim of this chapter is to help the nurse understand the factors that determine cardiac output and its role in oxygen delivery, to consider the possible situations that may contribute to failure of the cardiovascular system, and to help the nurse meet the needs of these seriously ill individuals.

SECTION 1: BASIC ANATOMY AND PHYSIOLOGY

The cardiovascular system is essentially a closed transport circuit, comprising a double pump and a network of blood vessels. The unidirectional flow of blood is ensured by valves, which are positioned at the entrance and exit to each ventricular chamber. To fully understand the assessment and management of cardiovascular disorders knowledge of the normal blood flow through this system is needed (Fig. 2.1).

- The right atrium receives deoxygenated blood from the inferior and superior vena cava that has drained from the systemic venous circulation and from the coronary sinus. (*See* coronary circulation (p. 15).)
- This blood then flows through the tricuspid valve and into the right ventricle.
- From here it is pumped up through the pulmonary valve and into the pulmonary artery which takes the blood to the lungs for oxygenation.
- The oxygenated blood then flows back to the heart via the four pulmonary veins that empty into the left atrium.
- The blood then passes through the mitral valve into the left ventricle, from where it is pumped out through the aortic valve into the aorta and so into the systemic arteries where it is distributed to the peripheral circulation.

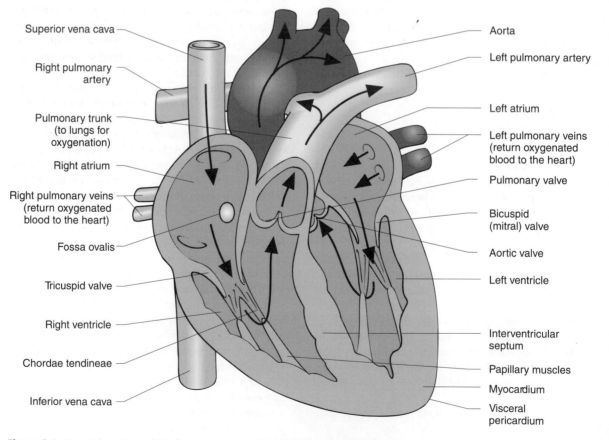

Figure 2.1 Frontal section of the heart, showing the direction of blood flow

This simple description followed the passage of blood around the system; it is also important to understand the events that comprise the cardiac cycle.

The cardiac cycle

The following description of the stages of the cardiac cycle begins at the point immediately following ventricular contraction, remember that the two sides of the heart operate simultaneously rather than in tandem.

The heart has just emptied its contents into the two arteries that leave the ventricles, on the left the aorta, taking oxygenated blood to the organs and peripheral circulation, and on the right the pulmonary artery, taking deoxygenated blood back to the lungs. The two ventricles then relax. This effectively begins the phase of diastole. During this phase blood flows into the atria and the ventricles, from the pulmonary veins on the left and the vena cava on the right; the atria now are resting and acting as passive conduits to the flow of blood. About 70 per cent of ventricular filling is achieved in this way, the blood flowing along its pressure gradient from the venous system into the relaxed ventricles.

Next is the phase of atrial contraction. Both atria contract and effectively 'top up' the ventricles. This 'topping up' by the atria contributes the final 25–30 per cent of the volume that is in the ventricle at the end of the diastolic phase, end-diastolic volume. This volume represents preload stress that is discussed below and plays an important part in the cardiac output. In the critically ill patient the loss of the atrial component can effectively reduce cardiac output by up to 20–30 per cent; this can be seen when patients lose the synchronized atrial contraction as in atrial fibrillation or ventricular pacing.

At the end of the atrial contraction the phase of ventricular contraction or systole begins. Tension increases in the muscular walls of the ventricles and pressure within the ventricular chambers rises rapidly. The valves of the heart are at this point all closed. The rising pressure in the ventricles causes the atrioventricular valves to close against the relatively low pressure in the atria. The aortic and pulmonary valves are still shut at this point, because the ventricle has yet to generate enough pressure to push them open against the pressure that is in the aorta and the pulmonary artery.

This phase is called isovolumetric contraction, that is, pressure is increasing but the volume has not yet changed. This phase consumes the most energy and therefore oxygen. It can be seen that the greater the pressure, particularly in the aorta, that has to be overcome the more work the heart must do. For example a hypertensive patient with a high diastolic pressure will have an increase in myocardial oxygen demand during this phase because of the extra pressure that must be generated.

Once the pressure in the ventricles overcomes the pressure in the aorta and pulmonary artery the valves will open and the contents of the ventricles will be ejected into the systemic and pulmonary circulation. This is the phase of ejection. About 70 per cent of the total end-diastolic volume will be ejected leaving the remainder in the ventricle. The term that is used to describe the amount of blood ejected is the ejection fraction, and it is normally 0.60–0.75. This represents about 70–80 mL of blood in the normal adult.

Once the ventricles have completed their contraction they relax to allow ventricular filling to begin again. Figure 2.2 shows the mechanical events of the cardiac cycle. An explanation of the electrical events will be given later.

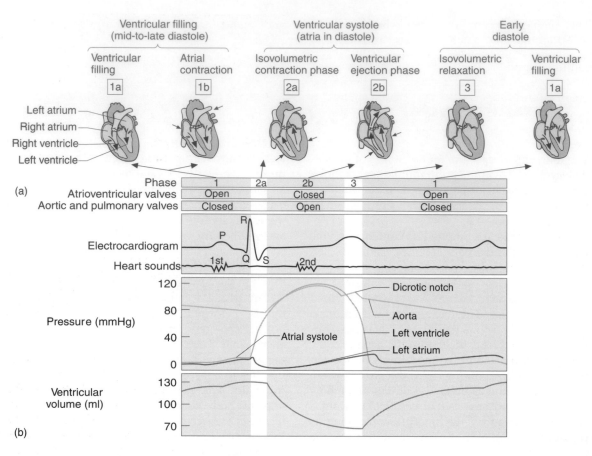

Figure 2.2   Mechanical events of the cardiac cycle

Cardiac output

To explore the cardiovascular system in more detail, consideration of the factors governing the output of the heart needs to be made. The heart is a demand-led pump. It will increase or decrease its output according to need. For example, when we exercise by running, the muscles of the legs require an increased supply of oxygen. This demand is met by increasing the output of the heart. Similarly in illness, such as sepsis, there will be an increased demand for oxygen delivery and therefore the output of the heart.

The output of the heart is called the *cardiac output*. Cardiac output can be defined as the volume of blood ejected by either ventricle per minute, and in a normal resting adult is approximately 5–6 L. This figure is an approximation. The true value for the output of the heart must be correlated with body mass. For clinical use body surface area is commonly used. In a normal healthy adult mean cardiac output is about 80 mL/kg/min or about 3.2 L/min/m². When output is adjusted for body surface area, the term *cardiac index* is used. Age influences cardiac output so that from its maximum at about 27 years of age output falls at the rate of 1 per cent per year; by the age of 65 it has dropped to approximately

60 per cent of its peak value (Smith and Kampine, 1990).

The figure of 5–6 L used above is arrived at by multiplying the *heart rate*, that is, the number of contractions per minute, by the *stroke volume*, the amount ejected per contraction. For example, at a heart rate of 70 beats per minute the stroke volume of a resting adult is approximately 80 mL, then:

Heart rate (70 bpm) × Stroke volume (80 mL)
= Cardiac output (5400 mL/min)

So, to understand cardiac output it is important to first understand the factors that will determine heart rate and stroke volume.

Heart rate

The rate at which the heart contracts is normally determined by the rate of impulse generation in the *sinoatrial node*, the 'pacemaker' of the heart. This in turn is regulated by autonomic control.

The regulatory centre for circulatory control via the autonomic nervous system lies in the medulla of the brain. It is the cardiac centre in the medulla that is concerned with heart rate. The cardiac centre is divided into two discrete centres: the cardioinhibitory centre, which slows down the heart rate via the vagus (parasympathetic) nerve; and the cardioacceleratory centre, which speeds up the heart rate via the sympathetic nerve.

The cardiac centre responds to feedback from baroreceptors situated in the aortic and carotid arteries. Stimulation of the receptors, as occurs when the pressure in these vessels changes, leads to a change in heart rate. The heart rate is also affected by direct chemical action. Adrenaline, produced by the adrenal medulla in response to sympathetic stimulation, will cause an increase in heart rate. An important reflex that affects the heart rate is the Bainbridge reflex. In this reflex the heart rate increases in response to increased atrial filling. This may be seen when administering a 'fluid challenge'.

Inappropriate heart rates may have a significant effect on the cardiac output in the seriously ill patient as will be discussed below.

ACTIVITY 2.1

Think of the patients that you have seen who have an altered heart rate. What possible causes of increased or decreased heart rate can you think of?

Stroke volume

Stroke volume is determined by three factors:

- Preload
- Afterload
- Contractility.

These are key concepts to understand when caring for the seriously ill patient. Each concept will be examined separately, but it is important to recognize that they are interrelated and will affect and be affected by, each other.

PRELOAD

Preload is related to the volume of blood in the ventricle at the end of diastole, namely, end-diastolic volume. The volume of blood in the ventricle is important because of a key property of cardiac muscle. The strength with which cardiac muscle contracts is related to the degree of pre-contraction stretch. The more it is stretched the greater the force of contraction. Much like an elastic band, the more you stretch it the harder it springs back. In the heart this stretch is gained as a result of the volume of blood, pouring into the ventricle during diastole, stretching the ventricular wall. This is 'Starling's law of the heart', which states:

As the end diastolic volume increases, so does the strength of contraction, within physiological limits.

Therefore, the greater the venous return, the greater the subsequent contraction, as long as it remains *within normal physiological parameters* (Fig. 2.3). However, it is possible to overload the heart with volume when the heart is failing; this will be discussed in more detail later when reviewing the impact of cardiac failure.

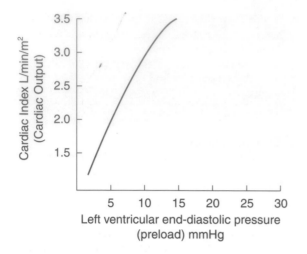

Figure 2.3   Left ventricular function curve

If the venous return is low, as in hypovolaemia, then preload will fall, the force of contraction will be reduced and subsequently cardiac output will drop.

ACTIVITY 2.2

Consider the factors that might affect the preload in the patients you have seen. You will probably find that they can be grouped together under the three headings given next.

Factors affecting preload are:

- Blood volume;
- The ability to pump blood back to the heart via the venous system;
- The vasomotor tone.

In the healthy heart increasing preload is one of the principle ways in which an increase in cardiac output is achieved. However the failing heart responds poorly to increasing preload, with little or no increase in output.

AFTERLOAD

Whilst preload is a major determinant of myocardial contractile power, afterload is mainly a mechanical factor that affects performance. Afterload may be described as *the resistance against which the ventricle must work*. In order to open the

aortic valve and eject the blood into the systemic circulation, the ventricle must generate enough pressure to overcome the pressure in the arterial system. Therefore alteration of systemic pressure, or resistance, will produce important effects on cardiac function because of the mechanical resistance it imposes on ventricular emptying. Sudden or chronic pressure changes will result in changes in strength, velocity and duration of left ventricular ejection and therefore stroke volume.

The healthy heart can overcome pressure increases reasonably well, but a significant increase in afterload in the failing heart can be devastating, as it can not overcome the added resistance. This resistance is determined largely by the vascular tone and is referred to as *systemic vascular resistance*.

Contractility

The contractile or *'inotropic'* state of the myocardium is the *ability of the myocardium to contract effectively*. The factors that influence and regulate myocardial contractility can be considered from two standpoints, *intrinsic* and *extrinsic* regulation.

Intrinsic regulation involves: (i) the response of the myocardium to preload stress, namely, myocardial fibre stretch; (ii) afterload stress, namely, increased aortic pressure; and (iii) heart rate. The effect of these factors on contractility is discussed under the relevant sections.

Extrinsic regulation involves outside factors that affect the contractility of the heart. These may be of three general types:

1 *Neurohormonal effects*: due to the influences of the sympathetic or parasympathetic nervous systems, either by direct innervation or through circulating catecholamines (adrenaline, noradrenaline).
2 *Chemical and pharmacological effects*: for example, contractile changes due to alterations in blood potassium, acid base balance or the affects of 'inotropic' drugs such as dobutamine.
3 *Pathological effects*: for example ischaemia or infarction of the myocardium, or the toxic effects of septicaemia.

Sympathetic stimulation will produce a positive effect; increased contractility will also result from injections of adrenaline, dobutamine or calcium ions. Conversely, myocardial ischaemia, toxic and anaesthetic agents and hypocalcaemia will produce a negative effect.

Blood vessels

The second part of the cardiovascular system to discuss is the *'pipes'*, that is, the blood vessels (Fig. 2.4). The network of blood vessels that are the conduits by which the transport system operates are not passive tubes that simply carry the blood around the body, but dynamic and interactive structures that are constantly responding to an ever changing environment.

The vessels are usually described as arteries, veins and capillaries. Each of these has a different function within the circulatory system. The large arteries that leave the heart are the pressure stores of the system. Their strong elastic walls allow them to recoil after expansion to aid the flow of blood and supplement the wave of pressure from the heart. The smaller arterioles are the pressure regulators. It is mainly these vessels that expand and contract to manipulate the total pressure within the system. In this way they are acting much like the nozzle on the end of the hose-pipe in our garden hose model. The capillaries are where the exchange of oxygen, nutrients and waste products takes place. The veins are the volume store of the system; if one were to pour a litre of fluid into the cardiovascular system, 90 per cent of it would be stored in the venous side, so acting as a reserve for ventricular filling.

The purpose of regulation of the blood vessels is to maintain the required perfusion pressure within the system (mean arterial pressure), and to provide local regulation for specific tissue needs; for example, to constrict vessels to an area that is haemorrhaging.

Central regulation lies predominately with the vasomotor centre in the medulla. The vasomotor centre is continually sending impulses to the arteriolar walls maintaining a degree of moderate vasoconstriction at all times. These impulses pass down the sympathetic nerves maintaining the sympathetic tone. To vasoconstrict, sympathetic impulses are increased; to dilate, they are de-creased. So if sympathetic impulses are lost, vasodilation will occur, as for example in a spinal cord transection where the loss of sympathetic tone leads to profound vasodilatation with the resulting drop of blood pressure.

The vasomotor centre responds to information received from the baroreceptors and chemoreceptors. The baroreceptors are situated in the carotid artery and the aorta and elicit a vasoconstrictive response to a fall in blood pressure.

e.g. ↓ BP   Arterial   Vasomotor
     → baroreceptor → centre
       stretch   (medulla)
                  ↓

                Vasomotor response
                  ↓
                Blood vessels
                  ↓
             ↑ Vasoconstriction
             ↑ Vasomotor tone →↑ BP

Chemoreceptors respond to biochemical changes in the blood and are sensitive to changes in P_{O_2}, P_{CO_2} and hydrogen ions.

As well as being under the influence of the medulla the vascular pressure is also affected by direct chemical action. For example:

1 Adrenaline and noradrenaline produced by the adrenal medulla cause dilation of cardiac and skeletal muscle arterioles and constriction of gut and skin arterioles in response to physiological stress.
2 Histamine produced in the inflammatory response causes local vasodilatation.
3 Antidiuretic hormone (ADH) causes vasoconstriction in response to severe bleeding.
4 Renin–angiotensin pathway leads to vasoconstriction and water retention.

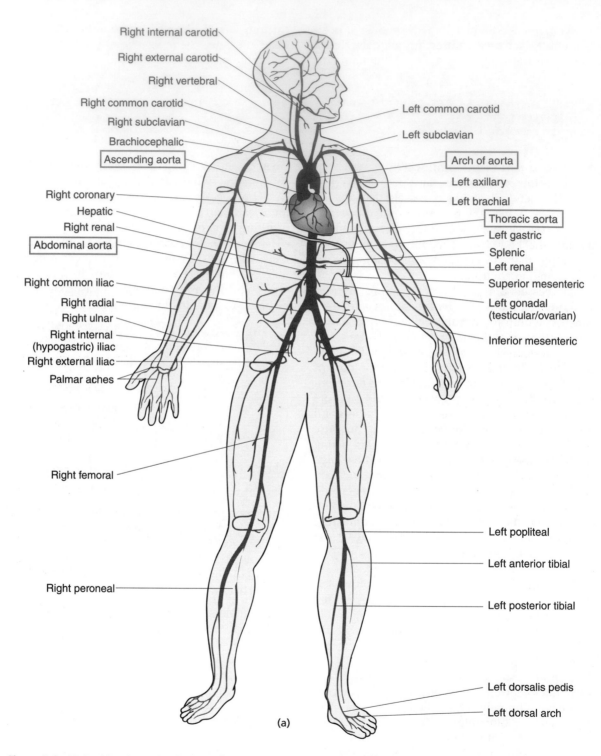

Right internal carotid
Right external carotid
Right vertebral
Right common carotid
Right subclavian
Brachiocephalic
Ascending aorta

Left common carotid
Left subclavian
Arch of aorta
Left axillary
Left brachial
Thoracic aorta
Left gastric
Splenic
Left renal
Superior mesenteric
Left gonadal
(testicular/ovarian)
Inferior mesenteric

Right coronary
Hepatic
Right renal
Abdominal aorta
Right common iliac
Right radial
Right ulnar
Right internal
(hypogastric) iliac
Right external iliac
Palmar aches

Right femoral

Right peroneal

Left popliteal
Left anterior tibial
Left posterior tibial

Left dorsalis pedis
Left dorsal arch

(a)

Figure 2.4 Major blood vessels of the systemic circulation. (a) Arteries. (b) Veins.

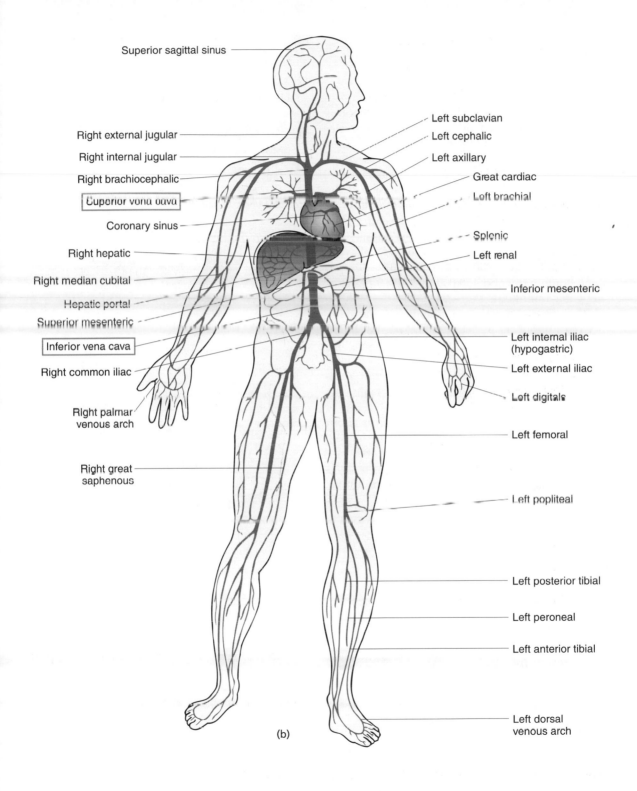

Superior sagittal sinus

Right external jugular

Right internal jugular

Right brachiocephalic

Superior vena cava

Coronary sinus

Right hepatic

Right median cubital

Hepatic portal

Superior mesenteric

Inferior vena cava

Right common iliac

Right palmar venous arch

Right great saphenous

Left subclavian

Left cephalic

Left axillary

Great cardiac

Left brachial

Splenic

Left renal

Inferior mesenteric

Left internal iliac (hypogastric)

Left external iliac

Left digitals

Left femoral

Left popliteal

Left posterior tibial

Left peroneal

Left anterior tibial

Left dorsal venous arch

(b)

Blood

The third component in our model of the cardiovascular system is the volume, the *blood*. Blood is essentially comprised of two parts: cellular elements and a liquid medium, the plasma.

The cellular elements are red cells (erythrocytes), white cells (leukocytes), and platelets.

Red cells occupy about 40–45 per cent of the total volume of the blood and give the blood its characteristic colour through the presence of the pigment haemoglobin. In the normal adult there are about 4.5 to 6.0 million red blood cells per cubic millimetre; 5000 to 10 000 white cells per cubic millimetre; and 150 000 to 300 000 platelets per cubic millimetre.

The plasma fraction of the blood normally occupies about 55 per cent of the normal blood volume and carries a variety of substances including plasma proteins, electrolytes, hormones, enzymes and blood gases. The normal concentrations of some of the most important constituents are given in Table 2.1.

Total blood volume in a normal adult is about 70 to 75 mL/kg of body weight; therefore a 70 kg adult may have a total blood volume of 5000 mL. The total amount of fluid in the human body is however much greater; about 40 L in our example.

Table 2.1 Normal ranges of various organic and inorganic substances in plasma

	Concentration
Organic substances	
Glucose	
fasting	3.3–5.5 mmol/L
after a meal	≤ 10.0 mmol/L
2 hours after glucose	< 5.5 mmol/L
Urea	2.7–8.5 mmol/L
Uric acid (urate)	150–580 µmol/L
Creatinine	40–110 µmol/L
Bilirubin	3–21 µmol/L
Aspartate aminotransferase (AST)	5–30 iu/L
Alanine aminotransferase (ALT)	5–30 iu/L
Hydroxybutyrate dehydrogenase (HBD)	150–325 iu/L
Creatine kinase	< 130 iu/L
Amylase (AMS)	150–340 iu/L
Alkaline phosphatase (ALP)	21–100 iu/L
Acid phosphatase (ACP)	< 8.2 iu/L
Inorganic substances (ions)	
Sodium (Na^+)	135–146 mmol/L
Potassium (K^+)	3.5–5.2 mmol/L
Total calcium (Ca^{2+})	2.10–2.70 mmol/L
Chloride (Cl^-)	98–108 mmol/L
Hydrogen carbonate (HCO_3^-)	23–31 mmol/L
Phosphate (PO_4^{2-})	0.7–1.4 mmol/L

The coronary circulation

The blood supply to the myocardium is via the coronary arteries (Fig. 2.5). The coronary areries arise from the root of the aorta just above the aortic valve. Anatomically there are two coronary arteries, the left and the right. However, in clinical usage, three arteries are described, the left being referred to by its two major divisions, the left anterior descending (LAD) and the circumflex (Cx). Disease may be present in one, two or all three of these vessels, referred to as single, double or triple vessel disease.

The left coronary artery arises from the posterior sinus of valsalva. The first part of the left coronary is called the left main stem and runs for several millimetres before bifurcating into the left anterior descending and the circumflex.

The left anterior descending supplies the:

- left atrium;
- septum;
- anterior wall of the left and the right ventricle.

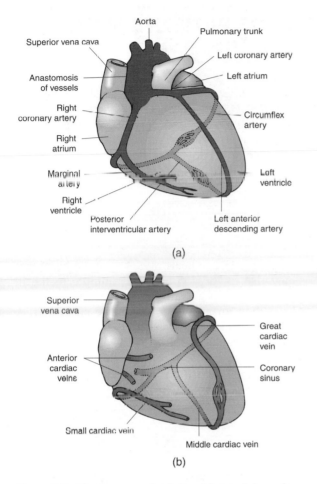

(a)

(b)

Figure 2.5 The coronary circulation (a) Arterial supply. (b) Venous drainage

The circumflex supplies the:

- left atrium;
- lateral wall of the left ventricle;
- the atrioventricular (AV) node and the sino-atrial (SA) node in some individuals.

The right coronary artery arises from the right anterior sinus and passes forwards and to the right before turning downwards to the lower border of the heart.

The right coronary artery supplies the:

- right atrium;
- inferior wall of the left ventricle;
- the right ventricle;
- the AV node and the SA node in the majority of individuals.

Coronary blood flow

As in other tissues the balance between oxygen supply and demand in the myocardium is crucial.

Myocardial oxygen demand (MVO$_2$) is determined by:

1 Myocardial contractility – the greater the strength of contraction, the greater the oxygen consumption.
2 Myocardial wall tension – which reflects the systolic blood pressure, the left ventricular end diastolic volume and the left ventricular wall thickness. Conditions such as hypertension and secondary hypertrophy will therefore increase oxygen demand.
3 Heart rate – which will increase MVO$_2$ as the rate increases.

Unlike skeletal muscle, the myocardium extracts 70–80 per cent of the available oxygen delivered. There is therefore little reserve and an increase in MVO$_2$ can only be met by an increase in coronary flow.

Coronary blood supply is dependent on:

1 Diastolic blood pressure:
    - Arterial diastolic pressure must be above 50 mmHg to maintain coronary artery perfusion.
2 Diastolic time:
    - Coronary filling occurs primarily during diastole, therefore diastolic time is important. There is an inverse relationship between diastolic time and the heart rate. As the heart rate increases, so the diastolic time (coronary filling time) reduces. This is one of the reasons that tachyarrhythmias are poorly tolerated in patients with coronary heart disease (CHD).

SECTION 2: ASSESSMENT OF PATIENTS WITH CARDIOVASCULAR DISEASE

Cardiovascular assessment of the seriously ill patient begins with recognition of the system's role in the adequate delivery of oxygen to the tissues. Survival in severe illness often depends on the ability of the body to respond to and meet the needs of adequate oxygen delivery (Shoemaker *et al.*, 1988). Having explored some of the factors that determine adequate cardiovascular function, this section will now consider how to apply this knowledge to patient assessment.

Heart rate

The heart rate is an important early warning sign of circulatory failure. As stroke volume falls heart rate must rise in order to compensate. In this way, a steadily rising heart rate is often the first objective sign of falling stroke volume and can presage more obvious and serious clinical features. Any situation that results in a fall in stroke volume will result in a rise in heart rate. At rest the heart rate may rise to 130–135 beats per minute in the ill patient. If the heart rate increases much above this level then an arrhythmia must be suspected. A falling heart rate will usually be either the result of increased vagal tone slowing the pacemaker of the heart, or some type of conduction problem.

Blood pressure

The systemic arterial blood pressure is a reflection of the relationship between the ventricular function and the degree of vasomotor tone. In this way it is not a true reflection of cardiac output alone.

There are wide variations in the normal range of blood pressure depending partly on age, gender and race. Systolic pressure may vary between 100 and 140 mmHg for example, whilst diastolic pressure may be between 60 and 90 mmHg. As with many aspects of monitoring and assessment it is the trend that is more important for an individual patient rather than absolute values, and each must be assessed in the light of the patient's clinical status and history. However, it is probably reasonable to suggest that a systolic blood pressure that is either less than 90 mmHg or is 60 mmHg below the normal for that individual, is indicative of cardiovascular failure, and suggests a situation in which tissue perfusion and therefore oxygen delivery will be compromised.

The diastolic pressure is also important, though it is harder to record when it is low by non-invasive means. Remember from the discussion on coronary blood flow that the coronary arteries will not properly perfuse if the diastolic pressure is less than 50 mmHg.

The pulse pressure is a useful tool in detecting falling cardiac output. Pulse pressure is the difference between the systolic pressure and the diastolic pressure. For example, if the systemic blood pressure were 120/70 then the pulse pressure would be 120 minus 70, that is 50 mmHg. When the cardiac output begins to fall we see a steady fall in pulse pressure. This is because the vasoconstriction that occurs in an attempt to maintain perfusion pressure in the system (remember the garden hose), keeps the diastolic pressure up whilst the systolic pressure, which is more an expression of cardiac ejection, is falling.

For example:

- 10pm, 120/70,
- 11pm, 110/70,
- 12pm, 100/65,
- 1am, 95/65,
- 2am, 90/65.

The pulse pressure has fallen thus: 50, 40, 35, 30, 25. This is a classic sign of falling cardiac output, whatever the cause. The point is that it is important to recognize this trend early, rather than wait until the pressure reaches the point at which we may feel the systolic is getting too low, for example 90/65.

The *mean arterial pressure* (MAP) is often used in critical care and is the arterial pressure averaged during one cardiac cycle. The MAP gives a rea-

sonable idea of perfusion pressure in the system and can be estimated by the following equation:

$$MAP = \frac{2 \times \text{diastolic pressure} + \text{systolic pressure}}{3}$$

A pulse pressure of 65 mmHg or less is indicative of severe circulatory failure. It must be noted that in situations of circulatory failure where there is significant peripheral vasoconstriction, non-invasive, or indirect, blood pressure monitoring may become inaccurate. In such circumstances direct (invasive) blood pressure measurement is more accurate and is usually higher than that recorded indirectly (Underhill *et al.*, 1992).

Skin colour/warmth

The patient's skin can give a good indication of the state of cardiovascular function and therefore perfusion. When perfusion falls, the response is to begin to vasoconstrict to maintain the pressure in the system. This will be manifest in the patient by cool and clammy skin due to the increase in sympathetic stimulation causing peripheral vasoconstriction.

One important exception to this picture is in

the early stages of septic shock where the inappropriate vasodilatation makes the skin feel warm and look flushed. Capillary refill provides an estimation of the rate of peripheral blood flow to the skin. When the tip of the fingernail is depressed the nail bed blanches, and on release, should regain its colour almost instantly. When perfusion is poor the colour returns much more slowly, giving an indication of the rate of perfusion.

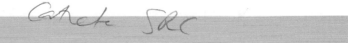

Urine output

Twenty per cent of cardiac output perfuses the kidneys, which are very sensitive to a fall in perfusion pressure. The urine output should be monitored hourly in situations of circulatory failure and gives a good indication of the extent of the failure of perfusion. A minimum of 0.5 mL/kg/h of urine should be produced; in a 70 kg person that would be 35 mL.

Again it is the trend that is as important as the absolute value of 35 mL, and a falling urine output should be addressed early rather than waiting for the output to reach any single figure. The 'quality' of the urine as well as the quantity is also an important factor that will be affected the longer that the cardiac failure is left untreated. (*See* Chapter 4.)

CVC *Ryst 15*
     insertion

Central venous pressure

Central venous pressure (CVP) is an expression of the pressure that is in the central venous system as it returns to the right side of the heart, and is therefore an expression of right-sided preload. The volume of fluid that is available to return, and the ability of the heart to deal with the fluid, that is, to pump it forward mainly determine this pressure. It may also be referred to as right atrial pressure or right ventricular end diastolic pressure. The importance of the relationship between this pressure and cardiac output has already been discussed. Central venous pressure is measured using a central venous catheter attached to either a fluid manometer or a pressure transducer.

Insertion of CVP catheters and associated complications

A central vein, usually the internal jugular or subclavian, is cannulated using a radio-opaque catheter to give access to the vena cava as it enters the right atrium. The catheter is sited with the patient in the head down (Trendelenburg) position, to minimize the risk of air embolus during insertion by ensuring a positive venous pressure. The catheter position must be checked by chest X-ray following insertion, as it is not uncommon for such catheters to double back on themselves, pass into the veins of the neck, or enter the right ventricle. As the dome of the pleura is close to the vessels being cannulated, the complication of a pneumothorax or haemothorax must also be eliminated.

Other complications associated with the insertion of these lines include:

1 Cardiac tamponade caused when the tip of the catheter pierces the wall of the right atrium and enters the pericardial sac.
2 Infection, either local around the site of entry or systemic due to organisms introduced through the catheter.
3 Venous thrombosis.
4 Blockage due to kinking of the catheter or obstruction by a blood clot.

Measurement of CVP

Where possible, the CVP should be measured in the mid-axillary line on a level with the 4th intercostal space (the phlebostatic axis), as this is on a level with the right atrium. In this position, when measured with a fluid manometer, the normal range of CVP is 3–10 cmH$_2$O, or 0–5 cmH$_2$O when measured from the sternal angle.

To read the CVP using a simple fluid manometer with a solution of either dextrose or saline, the following procedure is followed (Fig. 2.6).

1 Place the patient in a supine position, or if this is not possible, at a 45 per cent angle. All future readings should be made in the same position so that the trends can be monitored.
2 Check that the fluid is running freely.
3 Turn the three-way tap to allow the fluid to run into the manometer and so that it is closed to the patient.
4 Fill the manometer to a level above the expected pressure.
5 Close the three-way tap to the infusion source so that the manometer is open to the patient.
6 Watch the fluid level in the manometer. It will fall until the pressure from the column of fluid equalizes the pressure at the tip of the catheter. You should also see the fluid column rise and fall slightly when it has settled. This is due to changes in the intrathoracic pressure due to respiration.
7 When the fluid stops falling read the figure on the manometer. This is the central venous pressure (CVP).

Increasingly CVP is being measured via an electronic pressure transducer and displayed as a figure on the monitoring system. This is only possible if the equipment is available and at present will be confined to intensive care units (ITU), high dependency care units (HDU), coronary care units (CCU) and theatres. When measured in this way, the units are millimetres of mercury (mmHg) and the normal range is 3–8.

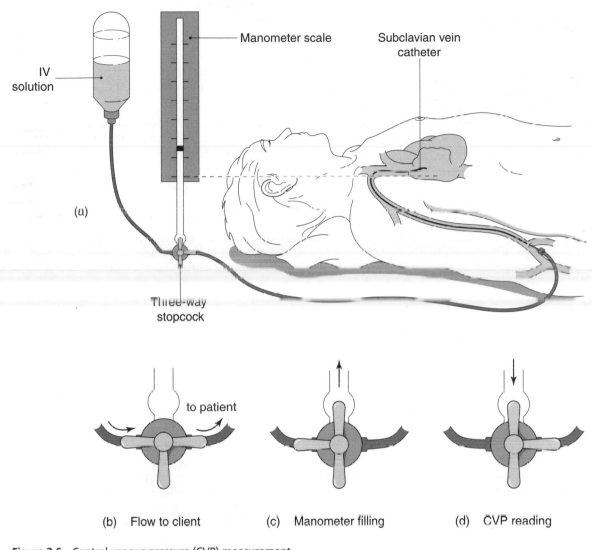

Manometer scale

Subclavian vein catheter

IV solution

(a)

Three-way stopcock

to patient

(b)   Flow to client   (c)   Manometer filling   (d)   CVP reading

Figure 2.6   Central venous pressure (CVP) measurement
(a) Placement of the manometer in relationship to the patient. The zero level of the manometer is at the phlebostatic axis. (b) Stopcock is turned for intravenous flow to the patient. (c) Stopcock is turned so that the manometer fills with fluid. (d) Stopcock is turned so that fluid in the manometer flows to the patient. A CVP reading is obtained when the fluid level stabilizes.

Clinical value of CVP

When the CVP is deviated from the normal range it may be due to a number of clinical scenarios. As already explained, the two main factors that determine CVP are the volume of fluid and the cardiac function. Therefore changes to the CVP are likely to be caused by situations that affect one of these two factors.

ACTIVITY 2.3

What situations do you think will be likely to result in:

- a high CVP?
- a low CVP?

HIGH CVP

The possible causes of a high or rising CVP are mainly related to either an excess volume of fluid or an inability of the right side of the heart to pump the available fluid forward, and may include:

- Over transfusion.
- Right heart failure. (In acute right sided failure it is important to recognize that the high CVP does not indicate a high volume of fluid.)
- Cardiac tamponade.
- Pulmonary embolism.

LOW CVP

The possible causes of a low or falling CVP are those that relate to a lack of fluid volume. Any significant cause of actual or relative hypovolaemia may lead to a fall in CVP, for example:

- Haemorrhage;
- Diuresis;
- A fluid shift out of the circulation such as in sepsis or following cardiopulmonary bypass.

When there is a loss of volume the compensatory vasoconstriction that is trying to maintain perfusion pressure keeps the CVP from falling significantly until quite late. So, for example, in a patient who is haemorrhaging a low CVP indicates a considerable blood loss.

Pulmonary artery flotation catheter (PA catheter)

Whilst primarily a critical/intensive care tool the PA catheter is increasingly used in assessment of the seriously ill patient in the high dependency unit (HDU) setting. The problem with CVP is that it gives only a very indirect assessment of left ventricular function and can consequently give misleading information. The pulmonary artery flotation catheter gives more direct information about the left side of the heart, specifically left ventricular filling pressures. These pressures are measured by attaching a transducer to the catheter, which allows both the pressure wave to be seen, and the pressure to be displayed as a digital readout.

The PA catheter is a flexible, radioopaque tube with a small inflatable balloon at its tip that is introduced via a large vein, usually the internal jugular vein. The catheter is advanced through the right atrium, right ventricle and then floated up into the pulmonary artery by inflating the balloon. As the tip advances the changing pressure wave can be observed on the monitor (Fig. 2.7).

The principal pressure that can be recorded with this equipment is the pulmonary capillary wedge pressure (PCWP). Once the tip of the catheter is in the pulmonary artery, the balloon is inflated and the catheter is then carried with the flow of blood until it 'wedges' in one of the

smaller pulmonary arterioles. The tip of the catheter then has an unobstructed 'view' across the pulmonary capillary system to the left side of the heart, specifically the left atrium. The influence of the right side of the heart is removed as the inflated balloon 'occludes' the vessel. The left atrial pressure is approximately the same as left ventricular end diastolic pressure, the pressure in the ventricle at the end of the diastolic phase. This can be interpreted as left ventricular preload. So, the PA catheter gives us an opportunity to measure this important aspect of cardiac performance.

> ### ACTIVITY 2.4
>
> Thinking back to the discussion on preload, what situations do you think will raise or lower the PCWP?

The normal pulmonary capillary wedge pressure when read from the mid-axillary line is 5–10 mmHg. This is the pressure that, in the normal heart, represents the preload that is required for a normal cardiac output.

Situations that will create a low PCWP are mainly those that are associated with volume depletion or vasodilatation. Both of these will

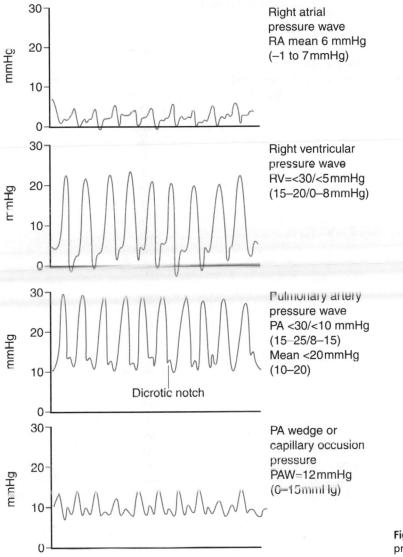

Right atrial
pressure wave
RA mean 6 mmHg
(−1 to 7 mmHg)

Right ventricular
pressure wave
RV=<30/<5 mmHg
(15–20/0–8 mmHg)

Pulmonary artery
pressure wave
PA <30/<10 mmHg
(15–25/8–15)
Mean <20 mmHg
(10–20)

Dicrotic notch

PA wedge or
capillary occlusion
pressure
PAW=12 mmHg
(0–15 mmHg)

Figure 2.7 Pulmonary artery catheter pressure waves

result in a reduced volume of blood returning to the left side of the heart. So, a PCWP of 2 mmHg in a patient who has been bleeding post-operatively will indicate that more volume is required to allow the ventricle to fill adequately.

A unique but important cause of low PCWP is acute right ventricular failure. Here the failed right ventricle cannot pump the blood round the pulmonary circulation to the left side, with the result that although the right side is adequately filled the left is 'dry'.

Situations that will raise the PCWP are mainly those that cause left ventricular failure and therefore suggest an inability of the left side of the heart to deal with the volume that is returning to it. The PCWP will also be raised in mitral stenosis and cardiac tamponade.

In the critical care environment, the pulmonary artery catheter will also allow a wide range of haemodynamic data to be collected, including the cardiac output and the systemic vascular resistance, and remains an important tool despite some recent controversy over its effects on mortality.

Mental state

If the patient has a low cardiac output then cerebral perfusion may be at risk. This will manifest itself as restlessness, confusion, agitation and sometimes aggression. If cerebral perfusion falls enough stupor and coma will eventually result. It must also be recognized that a patient with compromised cardiac output may also be exhibiting signs of anxiety and agitation that are not the result of low cardiac output, but are a result of the very real fear that may be present in a person who has in fact got a life-threatening condition. Objective assessment of the emotional/psychological status of the patient is difficult but some have advocated the use of the Hospital Anxiety and Depression Scale (HAD) as a useful tool.

Assessing the cardiac rhythm

As has been identified, the heart rate is a key factor in maintenance of adequate cardiac output. Therefore, a disturbance of cardiac rhythm has the potential to cause significant impact on the seriously ill patient and requires careful monitoring and assessment (Fig. 2.8).

A normal heart rhythm is called sinus rhythm because the natural pacemaker of the heart, the sinoatrial (SA) node, generates it. The impulse that is generated by the SA node spreads across the atria causing the atrial cells to depolarize. This wave of depolarization is detected by the electrocardiograph and shown as the *P wave*. The impulse then passes through the atrioventricular node into the ventricles. There is a slight delay here to allow for the atria to contract and start to relax before the ventricular activation begins. This period is called the *P-R interval*. The impulse then passes down the bundle branches and activates the ventricular muscle; this ventricular part is the *QRS complex*. This is the most important part of the ECG and can give the most information. The *S-T segment* immediately follows the QRS complex. The point at which it leaves the QRS complex is called the *J point*. The S-T segment should be isoelectric, that is, level with the base line of the ECG. The S-T segment should curve gently into the proximal limb of the *T wave* without forming sharp angles. The T wave represents ventricular repolarization, a return to the resting state. There is sometimes a small wave that follows the T wave called the *U wave*. This may represent repolarization of the papillary muscles. (*See* Fig. 2.9.)

The ECG criteria for normal sinus rhythm (Fig. 2.10) are as follows:

- *Rate*: 60 to 100 beats per minute (determined by the QRS complex).
- *Rhythm*: Regular (does not vary by more than 0.12 seconds).
- *P waves*: Normally < 0.11 second's duration, height < 2.5 mm.
- *PR interval*: Between 0.12 and 0.20 seconds.
- *QRS complex*: Between 0.06 and 0.11 seconds. (An intraventricular conduction defect will increase the duration of the QRS without necessarily affecting the rhythm.)

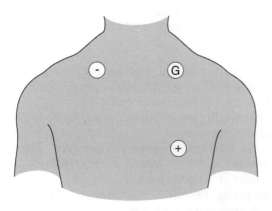

Figure 2.8   Monitor lead placements for three-lead monitoring (lead II)

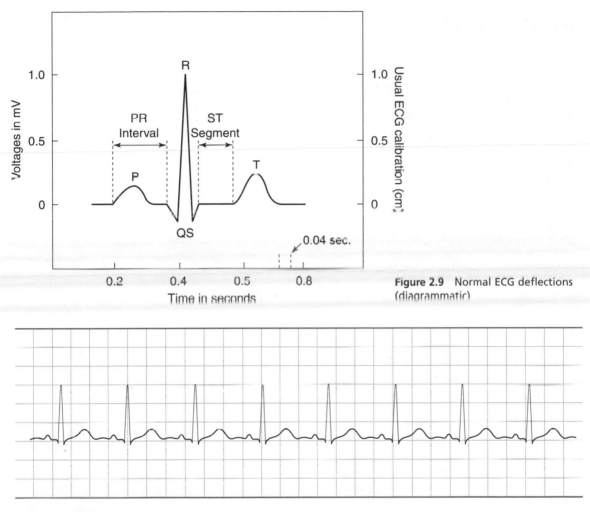

Figure 2.9 Normal ECG deflections (diagrammatic)

Figure 2.10 Sinus rhythm

Arrhythmias

Why is an abnormal heart rhythm bad for the cardiovascular system?

The two situations that are most concerning are when the cardiac rhythm is too slow and when it is too fast, bradycardia and tachycardia.

BRADYCARDIA

When the rhythm is bradycardic then one side of the equation:

heart rate $\times$ stroke volume = cardiac output

is compromised. For example if the heart rate is 35, then the stroke volume would have to compensate by increasing to about 140 mL to maintain a cardiac output of approximately 5 L. This is obviously unlikely, particularly in the seriously ill patient. The more likely scenario is that if the heart rate drops substantially then so will the cardiac output.

If the heart rate falls to a level that is thought incapable of maintaining an adequate cardiac output then attempts must be made to raise the rate. The approach to management of symptomatic bradycardia will be based on:

• The underlying cause

- The severity of the symptoms
- Whether acute or chronic.

The most common rhythm associated with a symptomatic bradycardia is sinus bradycardia. This is commonly due to an increase in parasympathetic stimulation such as in vomiting or whilst performing endotracheal suction. An important cause of sinus bradycardia is the effect of other drugs that the patient may be on, particularly beta blockers, or other antiarrhythmic drugs. Sinus bradycardia can also result from suppression of the SA node during myocardial ischaemia, myocardial infarction and in the sick sinus syndrome.

A more severe and prognostically more sinister cause of symptomatic bradycardia is when there is a problem with conduction of the electrical activity of the heart between the atrium and the ventricle, this is usually referred to as 'heart block'. There are many forms and many causes of heart block. Heart block can be used to describe slowing or blocking of the conduction in and around the SA node, the atrioventricular (AV) node, and the bundle branches. It is usually AV block that causes bradycardia which can be the result of myocardial infarction or ischaemia, drug overdose (particularly beta blockers and digoxin), or as a complication following accidental or surgical trauma of the heart.

The basic problem in 'heart block' is that the conduction from the atrium to the ventricle through the AV node is either slowed or blocked altogether. Three stages or 'degrees' of AV block are described:

1 *First degree* – where there is simply a delay in AV conduction.
2 *Second degree* – where some impulses are conducted through the AV node and some are not.
3 *Third degree* – where all the atrial impulses are blocked at the AV node and the slow ventricular escape rhythm takes over the ventricle.

It will usually be second and third degree AV block that may result in a bradycardia. As stated, management will depend on the cause and the symptoms. Reversible causes must be addressed such as sudden increases in vagal tone. In bradycardias that are symptomatic *atropine* is the first line therapy. This will be up to 0.5 mg given i.v. Care must be taken not to paradoxically create a tachycardia,

particularly in ischaemic heart disease, because the sudden increase in heart rate may cause a significant increase in myocardial oxygen demands. If the bradycardia is as a result of AV block it is quite probable that atropine will be ineffective. Second line drug therapy, often more likely to be effective in profound, symptomatic bradycardia during heart block, is *isoprenaline*, 100 µg i.v.

If the bradycardia is not a short-term, acute problem, or if it is unresponsive to atropine, then artificial cardiac pacing will be indicated. Cardiac pacing most commonly involves inserting a pacing electrode in the form of an invasive catheter into the right ventricle via one of the large veins, usually the subclavian or internal jugular and artificially stimulating the heart to initiate a contraction via pulse generator.

TACHYCARDIA

What about tachycardias? If a heart rate of 70 is good, then why is a heart rate of 170 not better? As explained previously in the explanation of cardiac output, the heart is dependent on an adequate preload to maintain stroke volume. The preload volume enters the left ventricle during diastole, and the diastolic period is inversely proportional to the heart rate. As the rate goes up the diastolic time decreases, therefore filling time and preload decreases. There is also an effect on myocardial oxygen supply and demand. As the coronary arteries fill during diastole, supply will fall and as the number of contractions per minute increases, demand will go up.

So, arrhythmias that are tachycardic result in:

- Reduced filling time.
- Reduced coronary blood flow.
- Increased myocardial oxygen demands.

As in bradycardia the management of tachycardia will depend on an assessment of the situation, particularly the condition of the patient. Typically three scenarios could arise:

1 The patient has a tachyarrhythmia but is haemodynamically stable.
2 The patient has a tachyarrhythmia and is haemodynamically compromised, with the clinical features of low cardiac output.
3 The patient has a tachycardia and no cardiac output.

The third situation is a cardiac arrest and therefore will require basic and advanced life support.

There are two choices for treating a tachyarrhythmia: drugs or cardioversion. If drugs are to be used two decisions will be made: firstly which is the right drug for this rhythm, and secondly will the drug be given orally or intravenously? In the acute situation where rapid haemodynamic stabilization is required, the intravenous route is the more appropriate.

There are many antiarrhythmic drugs available today and a detailed discussion of the various agents is outside the scope of this book. However the choice of antiarrhythmic drug is important and is dependent on the correct diagnosis of the arrhythmia. Giving the wrong drug because of misdiagnosis can be disastrous. The most important issue in choosing the right drug is whether the arrhythmia is ventricular or supraventricular. Supraventricular tachycardias (SVT) are those that arise 'above' the ventricles, that is, in the atrium or the AV node (therefore atrial fibrillation (AF), atrial tachycardia, and nodal tachycardia are all supraventricular). Ventricular rhythms are those that arise in the ventricle. The distinction is important, as it will affect the choice of drug therapy.

For supraventricular tachycardias the drugs currently recommended are:

1 *Adenosine*: 3–6 mg rapid intravenous bolus followed by 12 mg if no response in 2 minutes.
2 *Verapamil*: 5–10 mg intravenous bolus over 2 minutes.

For ventricular tachycardias (VT) the recommended drugs are:

1 *Lignocaine*: 100 mg intravenous bolus.
2 *Amiodarone*: 5 mg/kg over 20–120 minutes followed by 1 g over 24 hours, via centrally placed intravenous infusion (Opie, 1997).

If the patient is haemodynamically unstable, then direct current (DC) cardioversion is probably the most appropriate option. This is also the safest choice if there is any doubt about the correct diagnosis of the arrhythmia. In cardioversion, a DC shock is delivered to the patient's heart, the intention being to depolarize the myocardium, cancelling out the ectopic activity that is causing the arrhythmia. The first tissue to recover and to depolarize will recapture the rhythm, and this is usually the sinoatrial node, the heart's natural pacemaker.

Procedure for DC cardioversion

- Following explanation to the patient consent is obtained and a short-acting anaesthetic agent is given. Sometimes intravenous diazepam may be used, particularly in a situation that is becoming rapidly unstable and requires immediate intervention.
- The patient should be adequately oxygenated before and during the procedure.
- The cardioverter–defibrillator is switched on and the monitoring leads attached, ensuring that a tall R wave is present on the screen. (Some models will monitor through the defibrillator paddles, if so make sure that contact is good.)
- Make sure that the defibrillator is set to 'synchronize'. This will ensure that the charge is delivered on the R wave of the ECG so avoiding the vulnerable T wave.
- Cover the paddles with a conductive gel or alternatively use conducting pads.
- Select energy level:
  For SVT – start at 50 J
  For VT – start at 100 J
  For AF – start at 100 J.
- Place paddles firmly on the chest using 25 lb pressure. Position:
  One paddle to right of sternum below clavicle
  One paddle to left of nipple in anterior axillary line.
- Press charge button on paddle
- Check rhythm and ensure that everyone is clear of contact with the bed, equipment and patient.
- Press the 'shock' button and wait until the charge has been delivered. Note that with synchronized shocks there may be a short delay before the defibrillator delivers the shock as it waits for the next R wave.
- Assess patient, including rhythm and cardiac output.

SECTION 3: IDENTIFYING AND ANALYSING CARDIAC RHYTHMS

Learning ECG rhythms is not easy. The vast range of possible abnormalities combined with the considerable variation in the normal ECG conspire to make ECGs difficult for all but those who work with them every day. However it is important to be able to respond quickly in emergency situations when a potentially life-threatening arrhythmia arises.

It is possible to analyse the ECG rhythm without a detailed knowledge of electrocardiography. If a logical process is used then it will be possible to describe accurately the arrhythmia that you see on the monitor or rhythm strip. An adaptation of an approach suggested by Henry Marriott in Wagner (1994) is described as it gives us a way of logically analysing the rhythm using the information available to us.

Step one is to identify the type of disturbance that you see, that is, what disturbance would draw your attention to the rhythm. For example:

* There are early or unexpected beats;
* It is too fast – tachycardia;
* It is too slow – bradycardia;
* It is irregular;
* There are gaps or pauses.

Understanding the potential causes for each of the above allows you to identify the arrhythmia precisely once the features have been analysed. This first step starts you thinking about what type of problem you are facing.

Step two is to *examine the QRS complex*. The QRS complex gives the most information and represents the most important part of the cardiac cycle, namely, ventricular contraction. Also, it is the part of the ECG that you can guarantee to be there, unlike for example, the P wave. (If it is not then it is a cardiac arrest and you should not be engaged in rhythm analysis anyway.)

In tachyarrhythmias the QRS will tell you whether the origin of the arrhythmia is *ventricu-lar* or *supraventricular*; in bradyarrhythmias it will help you to work out whether it is a conduction problem or not. If it is of normal duration, that is, 2–3 small squares on the ECG paper, then the rhythm is supraventricular, namely, arising from the atria or around the AV node, not the ventricle. If the QRS is wide and bizarre it is most likely to be ventricular (it may also be supraventricular with aberrant conduction). Distinguishing between the two requires detailed knowledge of the possible morphology and is outside the scope of this book. Statistically it is more likely to be ventricular.

Step three is to *examine the P wave*. Finding the P wave may be difficult, particularly in the tachycardias, and may require you to examine several leads. Using a lead called S5 may be useful in amplifying the P wave. (Positive electrode – fifth right interspace by the sternum; negative electrode – on the manubrium.) The P waves may be completely absent as in atrial fibrillation.

Are the P waves:

* Present/absent?
* Normal/abnormal?
* Fast/slow?

Step four is to *establish the relationships* between the different complexes. Between the QRS complexes; and between the P waves and the QRS complexes. This may well be the key step in finally coming up with a diagnosis.

Step five is to identify the *primary disturbance*. For example, if the P waves stop then the primary disturbance is with the SA node. In other words, what is the root cause of the problem?

If the above steps are understood and applied consistently then most, if not all, rhythm disturbances should be correctly identified.

The above steps will now be applied to some of the common arrhythmias that may be encountered in the seriously ill patient.

Supraventricular arrhythmias

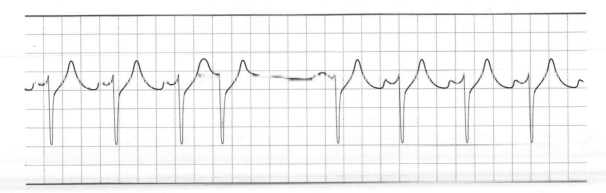

Figure 2.11   Ectopics (premature atrial contractions). Analysis. 1 There is an extra early/premature beat. 2 The QRS is narrow; therefore, supraventricular. 3 The extra beat has no P Wave. 4 The extra beat is followed by a non-fully compensatory pause.

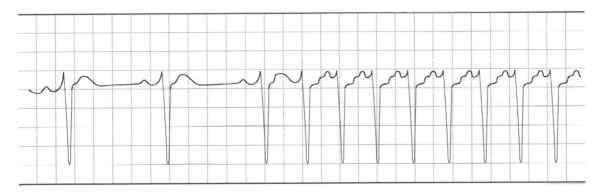

Figure 2.12   Atrial tachycardia. Analysis: 1 Sudden onset of tachycardia. 2 The QRS is narrow; therefore, supraventricular. 3 The P wave during the tachycardia is different to the sinus P wave. 4 The P is followed by QRS but the rate is too fast for sinus tachycardia. 5 This is a supraventricular rhythm with evidence of atrial contractions (P waves); therefore, atrial tachycardia.

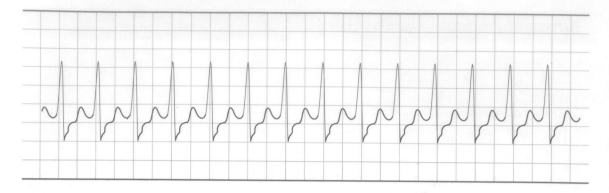

Figure 2.13   Nodal tachycardia. Analysis: 1 Fast rhythm – tachycardia. 2 The QRS is narrow; therefore, supraventricular. 3 No P wave can be seen. 4 The QRS rate is regular. 5 Because the QRS is narrow it is an SVT, and because there are no P waves, we can say it is nodal tachycardia. (Coming from the AV node.)

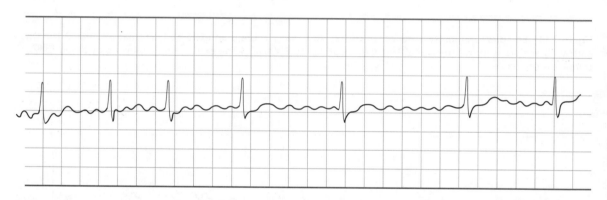

Figure 2.14   Atrial fibrillation. Analysis: 1 Rhythm is irregular. 2 The QRS is narrow; therefore, supraventricular. 3 No P waves – just 'chaotic' baseline. 4 The QRS are completely irregular – no pattern. 5 Therefore, atrial fiibrilation.

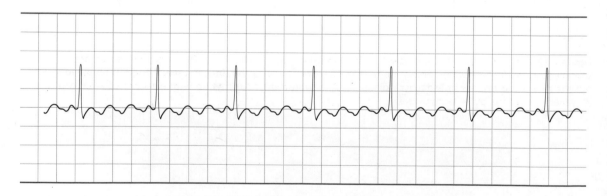

Figure 2.15   Atrial flutter. Analysis: 1 Normal QRS rate but rapid P waves. 2 The QRS is narrow; therefore, supraventricular. 3 Abnormal P waves – very rapid – 300 per minute. The atria are 'fluttering'. 4 There appears to be one QRS for every four 'F' (flutter) waves – 4:1. 5 Therefore, atrial fibrillation.

Ventricular arrhythmias

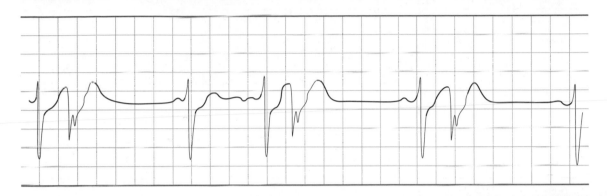

Figure 2.16 Ventricular ectopics. Analysis: 1 There are extra beats. 2 The extra beats (QRS) are wide; therefore, ventricular. 3 The extra beats have no P wave. 4 The extra beats are early – premature. 5 The extra beat is followed by fully compensatory pause.

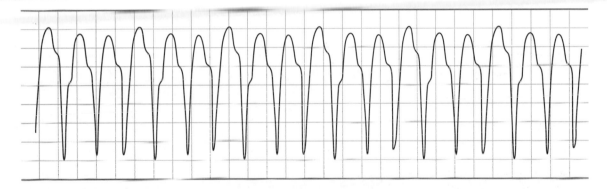

Figure 2.17 Ventricular tachycardia. Analysis: 1 There is a tachycardia. 2 The QRS are wide (3.5 small squares); therefore, ventricular. 3 There are no P waves. 4 The rhythm – QRS to QRS, is regular. 5 The broad complexes suggest ventricular tachycardia.

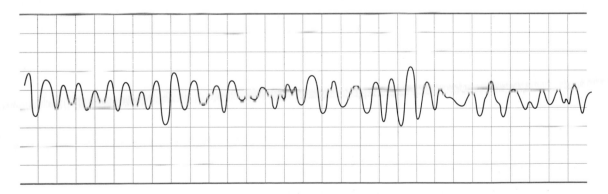

Figure 2.18 Ventricular fibrillation. Analysis: Chaos! No real complexes! Check pulse! Start cardiopulmonary resuscitation!

Disorders of conduction

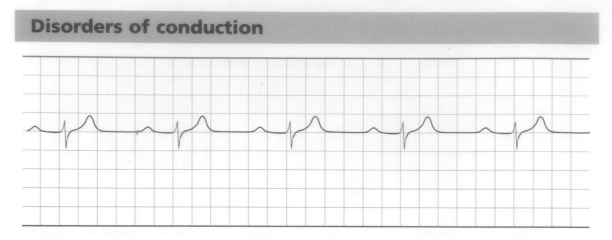

Figure 2.19 First degree heart block (delay in the AV node). Analysis: 1 The rate is a little slow (50) and there seems to be a pause between the P and QRS. 2 The QRS are narrow – supraventricular (normal). 3 P waves are regular and 1:1 with QRS. 4 The relationship between the P and QRS is wrong (the P-R interval). It should be no more than 0.2 seconds – 5 small squares; it is 8 small squares, 0.32 seconds, i.e. there is a P-R interval which is prolonged > 0.20 seconds.

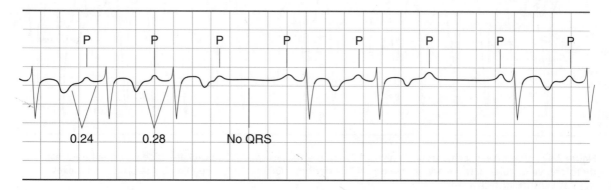

Figure 2.20 Second degree heart (AV) block – type 1. Analysis: 1 There appear to be pauses or gaps. 2 The QRS are narrow – supraventricular – normal. 3 The P waves – there are more P waves than QRS, so there must be some kind of block. 4 The relationship between the P and QRS is not constant. The P-R interval keeps changing. It gets wider and wider until a P wave is not followed by a QRS. The P-R interval then goes back to normal and the pattern starts again. 5 So – some conducted Ps and some not conducted indicates second degree heart block.

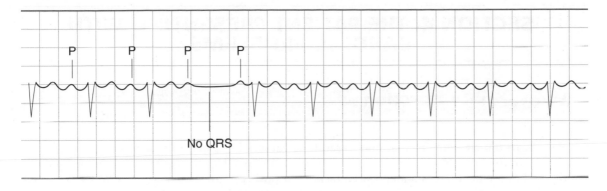

Figure 2.21 Second degree (A-V) heart block – Mobitz type 2. Analysis: 1 There is a pause or gap. 2 The QRS are narrow; therefore, normal. 3 The P waves are regular, but there is one more P than QRS. 4 The relationship between the P and QRS (the P-R interval) is constant. There is one 'dropped' beat. 5 There is a P wave that has not conducted through the ventricles (the dropped beat); therefore, there is AV block.

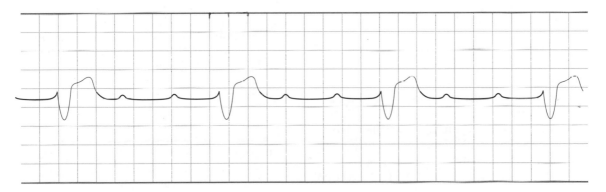

Figure 2.22 Third degree A-V (heart) block or complete block. Analysis: 1 The rate is slow. 2 The QRS are wide; therefore, ventricular. 3 The P waves – there are more Ps than QRS. The P wave rate seems about 120. 4 There is no relationship between the P waves and the QRS. They are separate – the QRS rate is 36. 5 Because there are more P waves than QRS complexes there is some kind of block. The wide slow QRS mean they are a ventricular 'escape' rhythm. The P and QRS are not related so it must be third (complete) heart block.

SECTION 4: THE PATIENT PRESENTING WITH CARDIAC PROBLEMS

Myocardial infarction

Coronary heart disease remains the single largest cause of death in Great Britain, and its most devastating and dramatic manifestation, heart attack, is currently experienced by one in five men of pre-retirement age.

The term myocardial infarction means the death of myocardium (heart muscle), due to a sudden cessation of blood supply. This represents an acute end-stage incident in the disease process of coronary atherosclerosis, CHD (coronary heart disease).

After several years of advancing disease resulting in narrowing of the lumen of one or more coronary vessels, the atheromatous plaque ruptures leading to a clot that occludes the coronary artery.

Once the artery is occluded the myocardial tissue will start to die, producing the clinical features that we recognize as acute myocardial infarction, a 'heart attack'. Whilst not all patients who experience a heart attack will be 'seriously ill', they will certainly be in an unstable condition with a 28-day mortality of 13–27 per cent (Lowel *et al.*, 1993) despite thrombolytics.

The typical presentation of acute myocardial infarction (AMI) is of sudden onset of severe, central chest pain. The features of this pain that are suggestive of acute myocardial infarction are that it is severe, crushing or heavy in nature, and has the classic feature of radiation to the left arm, lower jaw, neck and left shoulder. The pain will usually be continuous, last for longer than 15 minutes, and is not relieved by rest or anti-anginal medication. Extreme sweating, cold pale skin, tachycardia, and fear accompany the pain. Atypical presentations especially in the elderly, are syncope, dyspnoea, and fainting.

The diagnosis of AMI is confirmed by a positive 12 lead ECG. Currently the presence of ST elevation of > 2 mm in two adjacent chest leads, or > 1 mm in two adjacent limb leads combined with a positive patient history is considered sufficient evidence for a diagnosis of AMI. The patient's medical history and other investigations such as cardiac enzymes will also help to confirm the diagnosis.

Figure 2.23 shows the classic appearance of the ST segment in AMI. The site of the infarct, namely the part of the heart that is damaged, is determined by observing which of the 12 leads the ST elevation appears in. Whilst the ST elevation has a high specificity, about 90 per cent, for AMI it has a relatively low sensitivity, and in some studies has only been present in the first ECG in about 50 per cent of patients whose final diagnosis was AMI. Therefore patients who have convincing clinical features of AMI should have serial ECGs taken every 15–30 minutes (Littrell *et al.*, 1995).

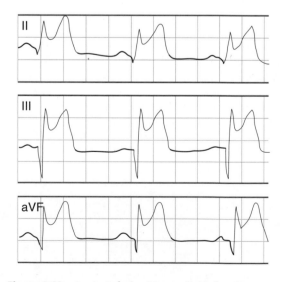

Figure 2.23   Acute Inferior Myocardial Infarction

The other main ECG indicator is bundle branch block (Fig. 2.24). Left or right bundle branch block may develop in the context of a new MI and is considered diagnostic when coupled with a positive history.

Principles of care

Management of the patient with AMI can be divided into three phases (Task Force on the Management of Acute Myocardial Infarction, 1996):

1 *Emergency care*. Main considerations – pain relief and prevention/treatment of cardiac arrest.
2 *Early care*. Main considerations – initiation of reperfusion therapy and to treat immediate complications such as pump failure and arrhythmia.

3 *Subsequent care*. Main considerations – later complications, preventing further infarction and death.

1 EMERGENCY CARE

The priorities in this stage are the relief of pain, breathlessness and anxiety, and the availability of basic and advanced life support.

Most people who die from a heart attack do so within the first hour of the onset of symptoms. Cause of death is usually due to ventricular fibrillation, and so having appropriately skilled personnel and equipment, particularly a defibrillator, is of major importance.

Pain relief should be given immediately, as prolonged pain and the fear accompanying it are associated with increased mortality and infarct size. Diamorphine is the drug of choice in AMI as it is both a potent analgesic and has positive

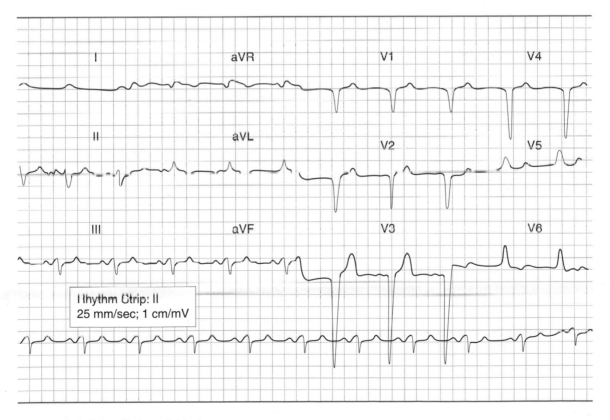

Figure 2.24 Left bundle branch block

haemodynamic effects, particularly vasodilatation, which reduces myocardial oxygen demand. This should be given intravenously in sufficient amounts to achieve pain relief. This dose will typically be between 5 and 10 mg, but will depend largely upon the size of the patient.

Oxygen should be given to patients suffering AMI. Whilst this will not deal with the main problem of obstructed flow, oxygen administration is important because optimizing the arterial oxygen content (Sao_2) will maintain the Sao_2 part of the oxygen delivery equation:

$$Sao_2 \times Hb \times CO = \text{oxygen delivery}$$

If Sao_2 falls, then the CO will have to increase to compensate thereby putting extra strain on the already damaged heart.

The patient will need constant reassurance at this time. Patients who experience AMI commonly report feelings of impending doom, a dreadful fear for their lives. What is required of the nurse is to ensure the patient knows you recognize their fear and are going to 'be there' for them. The patient needs to be sure that you can be relied upon to observe them constantly and that you will deal with their pain. Often, the unasked question is 'am I going to die?' and it is important to make the patient see that you acknowledge this fear and make them feel that they are in safe hands (Ashworth, 1984).

2 EARLY CARE

Reassurance and early information giving are important during this stage. The reason for this is the need to deal with the range of psychological responses and needs that may include:

- Fear
- Anxiety
- Hopelessness
- Knowledge deficit
- Denial
- Depression
- Anger.

If not recognized, these responses can have profound effects both psychologically and physiolog-ically. The immediate physiological effects are related to a high state of anxiety increasing myocardial oxygen demands through the release of catecholamines. There can also be long-term psychological problems caused by profound disturbing emotions experienced in the immediate aftermath of the AMI (Jowett and Thompson, 1995, p. 315).

- *Continued pain management.* The pain may not yet be under control or may return. Management includes further administration of diamorphine for continued infarct pain and nitrates (e.g. glycerine trinitrate), and beta blockers for ischaemic pain.
- *Monitoring for early complications.* Continuous ECG monitoring is essential during the early stages to allow for the early detection of arrhythmia, as is careful observation for the signs of possible cardiac failure (see below).

Thrombolytic therapy

The most significant development in the past 20 years in the management of AMI is thrombolytic therapy, that is, giving drugs to dissolve the clot in the coronary artery.

Thrombolytic drugs work by converting plasminogen to plasmin. Plasmin is fibrinolytic, therefore the clot is broken down, and the coronary vessel that is occluded has the potential to become patent once more, allowing re-perfusion of the affected myocardium. The earlier that this re-perfusion can occur the more significant the results, that is, increased myocardial salvage, preserved left ventricular function and lower mortality. Studies have shown that if given within 6 hours of the onset of symptoms, approximately 30 deaths are prevented for every 1000 patients treated (ISIS-2, 1988; ISIS-3, 1992).

The later the administration the less effective is the outcome. Currently most protocols advocate a time window of 6 hours from the onset of pain during which it is appropriate to give thrombolytics. After this time it is usually considered that the risks of the drugs outweigh the limited benefit to be gained.

The choice of agent for ward-based administration is currently between tissue-type plasminogen activator (rt-PA) and streptokinase, with the decision depending on individual assessment of risk, availability, and cost benefit. The most commonly used of these two is streptokinase, mainly because of the much greater cost of rt-PA.

> The principal differences between the two drugs are the increased incidence of hypotension and the possibility of allergic reactions with streptokinase, and the need for heparin as cotherapy when using rt-PA.

Side effects

For both agents bleeding represents a potential side effect that should be monitored. Stroke is a small but important risk with haemorrhagic stroke having a slightly higher incidence in rt-PA (GUSTO, 1993). Streptokinase carries a risk of allergic reactions (5.8 per cent) including rashes, pyrexia and anaphylaxis (rare 0.1 per cent), and of hypotension, particularly in those who have a low systolic blood pressure prior to administration (GUSTO, 1993).

Absolute contraindications are mainly those relating to increased potential for bleeding and include:

* Stroke;
* Recent major trauma/head injury (3 weeks);
* Gastrointestinal bleed in last month;
* Known bleeding disorder;
* Dissecting aneurysm.

Relative contraindications include:

* TIA in past 6 months;
* Warfarin therapy;
* Pregnancy;
* Non-compressible punctures;
* Traumatic resuscitation;
* Refractory hypertension (systolic > 180 mmHg);
* Recent retinal laser treatment.

In addition, streptokinase is contraindicated if there has been a recent streptococcal infection or if there has been previous administration of streptokinase because the bacterial toxins and antibodies reduce the effectiveness and because of an increased risk of allergy.

Ideally, unless clearly contraindicated all patients with clinical and ECG evidence of AMI should receive aspirin (150–160 mg, chewed) and thrombolysis within 90 minutes of call for medical assistance.

3 SUBSEQUENT CARE

The continuing management is aimed at monitoring and assessment of potential complications, particularly arrhythmia and heart failure. Other issues are the prevention of re-infarction and of sudden death. To this end the patient's heart rate and rhythm will be constantly monitored as will the blood pressure, urine output and pain. There is a good case for the use of early i.v. beta blocker as a preventative measure when there is tachycardia (with no failure), relative hypertension, or pain unresponsive to opioids.

Heart failure

Failure of the heart, the pump, is a common and important cause of circulatory problems and therefore will be explored in some depth. To fully understand the decision making in the management of pump failure it is essential to have an understanding of the physiological processes that are the response to the failing heart. The clinical consequences of cardiac failure have important differences in presentation, prognosis and management; these are dependent on the severity of the failure, whether it is acute or chronic, or whether the primary problem is with the left or the right side. The basic underlying physiology however is similar in each case.

Pathophysiological mechanisms in pump failure

If the heart fails to pump adequately, two key changes are seen:

- Firstly the heart dilates in response to the increasing pressure in the left ventricle caused by the volume that it is unable to pump forward.
- Secondly the forward pressure into the aorta begins to fall. These changes in pressure are detected by the baroreceptors discussed earlier.

The message that is given is that pressure within the system is falling. The response to this is less than helpful to the heart (Fig. 2.25).

First the sympathetic nervous system is activated; the result being that there is an increase in the production of adrenaline and noradrenaline. These produce a rise in heart rate and contractility; and in the degree of vasoconstriction respectively, this through the stimulation of alpha and beta receptors. The problem is that these responses, whilst creating an initial rise in perfusion pressure, have a negative effect on the myocardium in that they raise myocardial oxygen demands by the increase in heart rate and afterload.

The drop in pressure is also detected by the kidneys. The juxtaglomerular apparatus (Chapter 4) detects the pressure drop and stimulates the release of renin. Renin then increases the circulating levels of a substance called angiotensin I, which, although inactive in this state, is converted to the active angiotensin II in the lungs by angiotensin-converting enzyme.

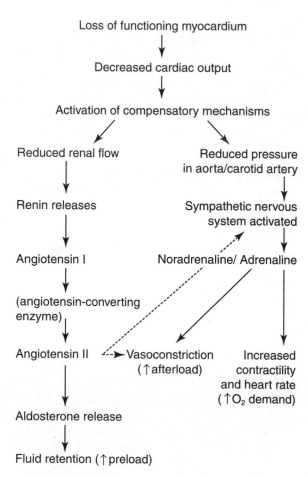

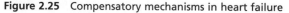

Figure 2.25 Compensatory mechanisms in heart failure

Angiotensin II has two key roles:

1 It is a powerful vasoconstrictor.
2 It stimulates the production of aldosterone, which leads to salt and water retention.

The net result of this activity is:

• Increase in heart rate, due to the sympathetic stimulation.

• Increase in afterload, due to vasoconstriction
• Increase in preload, due to the retention of Na$^+$ and water.
• Increase in contractility, due to the sympathetic stimulation.
• The increases in heart rate and contractility, whilst compensatory, significantly increase the myocardial oxygen demand and may lead to ischaemia, particularly if there is already IHD.
• The increase in afterload has a negative effect on the ventricular myocardium that cannot overcome the increased resistance. Figure 2.26 clearly shows this effect on a graph.
• The increase in preload, whilst beneficial in the normal heart leads to pulmonary and systemic venous congestion in the failing heart.

The circulatory response is trying to maintain perfusion pressure within the system, but in doing so places increasingly intolerable demands on the already compromised heart.

The failure of the heart as an effective pump can be referred to in a variety of ways and you will most likely have encountered the terms:

• Left ventricular failure (acute pulmonary oedema).
• Right ventricular failure.
• Chronic congestive cardiac failure.
• Cardiogenic shock (discussed under the section *Shock*) (p. 43).

Whilst the basic problem is one of an ineffective pump, these situations represent significantly different clinical scenarios and require different management.

Chronic congestive cardiac failure

Congestive cardiac failure (CCF) is a diagnostic term used to describe a complex clinical syndrome that arises from systemic and circulatory responses associated with heart failure. This condition is relatively common and carries a poor long-term prognosis.

Congestive cardiac failure is a syndrome characterized by signs and symptoms of:

• Reduced exercise tolerance
• Volume overload (congestion)
• Inadequate tissue perfusion.

Chronic congestive cardiac failure is usually secondary to CHD, hypertension, cardiomyopathy, or valve disease. Unlike the sudden, overwhelming failure of the left ventricle,

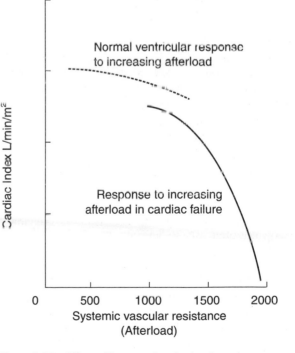

Figure 2.26 Effect of increase in afterload on the ventricular myocardium

chronic cardiac failure may present slowly and insidiously with the classic symptoms of fatigue, reduced exercise tolerance and oedema, eventually resulting in hospital admission. For the nurse in the acute ward or unit this condition represents a significant challenge. The possibility of a 'cure' is negligible in a condition in which half of the patients diagnosed with heart failure will die within 4 years. Of those with severe heart failure half will die within one year (Ho *et al.*, 1993).

The aims of management are:

1   To prolong survival.
2   To increase exercise tolerance.
3   To improve symptoms.

Dahlen and Roberts (1995) provide a useful approach to the management of the patient with CCF that seeks to address the range of patient problems that are likely to present. These are:

- Decreased cardiac output;
- Decreased tissue perfusion;
- Impaired gas exchange;
- Fluid volume overload;
- Ineffective breathing pattern;
- Reduced exercise tolerance;
- Hopelessness;
- Knowledge deficit.

Management is based around addressing these problems using the following nursing and pharmacological strategies.

ANGIOTENSIN-CONVERTING ENZYME INHIBITORS (ACE INHIBITORS)

ACE inhibitors, such as captopril, are now seen as the starting point for treatment of CCF. This group of drugs act by blocking the conversion of angiotensin I to angiotensin II. The effect of this is reduced vasoconstriction, and therefore afterload, and a decrease in sodium and water retention. The net therapeutic effects are of increased cardiac output and reduced volume overload.

DIURETICS

The use of loop diuretics such as frusemide will increase the excretion of sodium and water, which will reduce both systemic and pulmonary oedema.

HYDRALAZINE AND NITRATES

The combined effects of the arterial dilation of hydralazine and the venous dilation of nitrates (for example, glycerine trinitrate) has been shown to improve symptoms and prognosis, probably through the reduction of cardiac work that results.

DIGOXIN

Digoxin has the dual effect of controlling the ventricular rate in atrial fibrillation, which is common in cardiac failure, and increasing contractility.

SODIUM AND WATER RESTRICTION

Sodium restriction and water limitation are important associated measures in CCF. Monitoring of fluid intake and output, and daily weight, helps to assess the degree of fluid restriction required. A weight gain of 0.5 kg/day is significant and is associated with volume retention. The patient will need to understand the reason for these restrictions if they are to comply with what may be an uncomfortable aspect of their care. Ice cubes are a useful way of helping to reduce what can be the unpleasant sensation of not being able to take a drink whenever one wishes.

EXERCISE

Part of the approach to management is to reduce excessive demands for cardiac output that cannot be met. This usually means complete rest for the patient who has been hospitalized with CCF. However, the role of conditioning exercise has been increasingly recognized and this can begin with gentle exercises that maintain muscle tone but place little demand on the heart. Rehabilitative exercise may well play a part in the patients' subsequent management and has been shown to have positive effects on symptoms.

OXYGEN

Supplemental oxygen will need to be administered if the arterial oxygen saturation is not adequate.

PSYCHOLOGICAL SUPPORT

For the overwhelming majority of patients, the prognostic reality is one of slow deterioration marked by steadily reducing exercise tolerance and increasingly distressing symptoms. This picture is made more bleak by the high incidence of sudden death. Given this it is unsurprising that the nursing diagnosis of 'hopelessness' has been associated with this condition. The level of support needed by both patient and family will be considerable. The nature of this support should probably be centred on an optimistic but realistic outlook and the motivation associated with the attainment of achievable goals. This is related to self-esteem and is likely to be most positively encouraged by an improvement in exercise tolerance that will contribute to the patient's independence. It must also be recognized that this is, in effect, a terminal condition that the patient and family will need support to come to terms with. Part of this support will include education about the condition, dietary and exercise adjustments and drug regimes.

Acute left ventricular failure (acute pulmonary oedema)

As its name suggests this represents a situation in which the left ventricle has acutely failed and has become overwhelmed by the volume of fluid returning to it from the pulmonary circulation. This, resulting from the mechanisms described earlier, creates an acute rise in left ventricular diastolic pressure (preload) which is transmitted back through the pulmonary capillaries, giving rise to pulmonary oedema as the hydrostatic pressure in the vessels overcomes the osmotic pressure and fluid leaks out.

This leads to the all too familiar picture of acute LVF. The patient will be acutely and significantly breathless and distressed, tachycardic, possibly with systemic hypotension (although not always); there will be increased production of sputum that is classically 'frothy' in nature and is sometimes flecked with blood from small haemorrhages in the bronchial mucosa. There may be cyanosis and confusion. The diagnosis of acute LVF will be made on the basis of these signs, the presenting history, plus the objective evidence of pulmonary oedema that can be found on chest auscultation and examination of the chest X-ray and by the oxygen saturation, which may be as low as 87–88 per cent.

The underlying cause of acute LVF is most commonly related to ischaemic heart disease (IHD), but it may also be precipitated by tachyarrhythmia, chronic hypertension or mitral valve disease. It may also present as an acute exacerbation of CCF.

Management of this situation is aimed at improving the oxygen saturation by reducing the pulmonary capillary pressure. This is achieved by improving the myocardial oxygen supply/demand balance, reducing the amount of circulating fluid, and offloading the left ventricle. It is also important to consider the underlying cause. If tachyarrhythmia is the cause then the priority must be to control it.

NURSING INTERVENTION

The nursing role here will be central to the success of the therapeutic interventions.

The priorities are:

- *Position.* The patient should be sat upright in what is sometimes called the high Fowler's position. This will have the effect of increasing the lung capacity, reducing the venous return and reducing the work of breathing. If the patient is profoundly hypotensive however this position should be avoided or at least modified.
- *Oxygen administration.* Via a high percentage mask at a high flow rate, 8–10 L/min.

- *Diamorphine.* The dose prescribed will be between 2.5 and 5 mg depending on the size of the patient, and should be administered intravenously. This will have a sedative effect that is beneficial in this situation where the fear and agitation of the patient is increasing the oxygen demand. Diamorphine also has a mild vasodilatory effect which contributes to the lowering of preload.
- *Diuretic.* The loop diuretic frusemide is usually the drug of choice and will be prescribed in doses from 40 to 80 mg i.v. The effect of frusemide in this situation is probably first a vasodilatory effect and second a diuretic effect. The result is a reduction in the pulmonary capillary pressure and therefore pulmonary oedema.
- *Nitrates.* Unless the patient is profoundly hypotensive, a nitrate (nitroglycerine) will be prescribed, possibly sublingually, or by the intravenous route at a dose of 0.25 µg/kg/min increasing every 5 minutes until a fall in blood pressure of 15 mmHg or if the systolic pressure falls to 90 mmHg. This will vasodilate, mainly on the venous side and will reduce the volume of blood that is returning to the left ventricle and therefore reduce left ventricular and pulmonary capillary pressure.
- *Bronchodilator.* If there is bronchospasm that does not reverse with the initial strategies

above then a bronchodilator can be given, usually aminophyline 6 mg/kg i.v. over 30 minutes. This drug is a beta stimulant and so may cause tachycardia and arrhythmia, particularly in IHD and so caution should be exercised. It is probably best avoided in AMI.

If the above strategies fail to raise the Po_2 above 8 kPa, then the use of continuous positive airways pressure (CPAP) or intermittent positive pressure ventilation (IPPV) must be considered. The decision to instigate IPPV will probably depend on the underlying cause and the prognosis.

If the blood pressure fails to respond despite the compensatory mechanisms and above therapy then the clinical picture becomes one of cardiogenic shock (see below).

It should be recognized that the above scenario represents a medical emergency and is life-threatening. For the patient this is all too apparent and the distressing symptoms will create intense anxiety as they 'fight for breath'. Complicated explanations are not appropriate at this time but the patient will need simple assurances that you are doing something positive to relieve their distress. The mental state of the patient may change from anxiety and agitation to confusion and then to coma as the condition progresses. This can happen very quickly and is a poor prognostic sign.

Shock (circulatory failure)

In the seriously ill patient it is the complete failure of the cardiovascular system to meet the tissue demands that pose the greatest threat. When this failure begins to develop, a complex set of mechanisms are activated that attempt to compensate and to restore adequate perfusion. When these mechanisms fail then the term shock is often used. Shock is a complex clinical syndrome that occurs as a result of acute circulatory failure. The shock syndrome can be described as a state in which there is a significant reduction in cardiac output, effective tissue

perfusion and tissue oxygenation, resulting in multi-organ symptoms.

The unifying feature in all forms of shock is the critical reduction in the supply of oxygenated blood to the tissues.

The demand of the tissues for oxygen needs to be met by an adequate supply of oxygenated blood. Maintenance of an adequate blood supply is dependent on the ability of the cardiovascular system to meet this need. Catastrophic problems with the cardiovascular system may lead to a reduction in tissue perfusion sufficient to produce changes in cellular metabolism and a group of characteristic clinical features that we recognize as 'shock'.

- If the *pump* cannot maintain adequate perfusion despite the constriction of the pipes then the circulation has failed.
- If the *volume* is insufficient despite the attempt to increase the pump and to constrict the vessels then the circulation has failed.
- If the *pipes* are too dilated for the pump and the volume available to fill to an adequate pressure, then the circulation has failed.

Circulatory failure will arise because of a problem with either the pump, the pipes, or with the volume.

Shock is often classified on the basis of the causative pathophysiology, for example cardiogenic, hypovolaemic or septic. These three represent the most likely scenarios encountered when caring for a seriously ill patient. (Neurogenic shock encountered in patients with severe head injury is not covered here, as the condition of the patients is such that they usually require intensive therapy.)

Cardiogenic shock usually results from severe impairment of cardiac muscle contractility. Specific causes include myocardial infarction, valve disease, cardiomyopathy, and myocardial dysfunction after cardiac surgery. In cardiogenic shock secondary to myocardial infarction 40 per cent or more of the myocardium is necrotic or injured and as such does not contribute to contractility. By definition, therefore, cardiogenic shock usually implies the presence of extensive muscle damage. The prognosis for this shock state is extremely poor and the in-hospital mortality remains 70 to 90 per cent. Partial papillary muscle rupture and ventricular septal defects complicating MI may also result in cardiogenic shock.

In *Hypovolaemic shock* there is a decrease in the intravascular volume of 15–25 per cent, with haemorrhage being the most common cause. Clinical scenarios associated with hypovolaemic shock include surgical blood loss, burns, peritonitis, trauma and excessive diuresis.

The *Septic shock syndrome* is associated with the presence in the blood of microorganisms or their toxins. This leads to a complex syndrome in which there is an extremely low systemic vascular resistance leading to a reduction in preload and poor perfusion pressure, a decrease in myocardial contractility, and reduced cellular oxygen uptake.

The precise clinical picture of shock may vary. It is dependent on the cause of the disorder and on the stage of the shock. For the purposes of this chapter we will concentrate first on the failure of the pump that leads to cardiogenic shock and then look at hypovolaemia.

Cardiogenic shock

When there is a decrease in systemic blood pressure following, for example, extensive myocardial infarction, the series of compensatory mechanisms described in heart failure are initiated to maintain an adequate perfusion of the brain and the heart. The heart rate increases to assist in improving the cardiac output via the equation: $HR \times SV = CO$, and there is an increase in contractility in an attempt to augment the stroke volume.

Despite this the perfusion pressure is inadequate and so further extensive vasoconstriction occurs in the vessels supplying the skin, skeletal muscles, abdominal organs and the kidneys in an attempt to increase perfusion of the brain and heart. The systemic vascular resistance (SVR) increases as this vasoconstriction continues. At this stage blood pressure may remain within normal limits and symptoms may be minimal. An important early sign, a steadily rising heart rate with no apparent cause, should not be missed at this stage. Another early sign is the falling pulse pressure as the diastolic pressure is maintained due to the vasoconstriction whilst the falling cardiac output is reflected in the falling systolic pressure.

As the situation progresses the pump becomes unable to maintain adequate perfusion pressures in the vital organs despite the compensatory mechanisms of vasoconstriction and volume retention and we start to see the classic picture of the shock syndrome. The skin becomes cold, pale and clammy and the distal extremities become cyanotic. There is a significant drop in blood pressure accompanied by a critical drop in renal perfusion and urine output starts to fall and eventually stops. Poor cerebral perfusion will start to produce symptoms of confusion, agitation and reduced levels of consciousness.

Failure of tissue perfusion causes a change in cellular metabolism. The absence of oxygenated blood causes the cells to switch from aerobic to anaerobic metabolism, which results in the accumulation of the waste products of lactic acid leading to the development of metabolic acidosis.

By this stage the condition has usually become irreversible with profound hypoxia, and cellular acidosis leading to cell membrane destruction and cell death. As shock progresses, multisystem failure results with the ensuing complications of further myocardial ischaemia and depression; adult respiratory distress syndrome (ARDS); tubular necrosis in the kidneys and disseminated intravascular coagulation (DIC). The common scenario is that death will intervene before complications such as ARDS and DIC have become established. The multiorgan problems that occur as a result of the failing perfusion are summarized in the box below:

Brain – There is decreased cerebral blood flow and potential cerebral infarct.
Myocardium – The increasing mismatch of oxygen supply and demand leads to breakdown of cell membrane and cell death.
Kidney – Prolonged hypoperfusion leads to acute tubular necrosis and acute renal failure.
Gastrointestinal (GI) tract – There may be mucosal ischaemia, ileus and full thickness gangrene of the bowel with possible contamination with gut bacteria. There is also the possibility of GI bleeding.
Coagulation – Disseminated intravascular coagulation (DIC), with its characteristics of simultaneous coagulation and haemorrhage, may occur as the blood flow through the capillaries stagnates.
Lungs – Pulmonary oedema may occur. The toxic effects of fibrinogen degradation products from DIC, and serum complement depletion, lead to increased pulmonary capillary permeability and

adult respiratory distress syndrome.
Immune system – Immune system depression will leave the patient at heightened risk of serious infection.
Skin – Poor tissue perfusion and pooling within the interstitial space leave the skin vulnerable to breakdown.

MANAGEMENT OF CARDIOGENIC SHOCK

The aims of management in the patient with cardiogenic shock are:

- Improving and maintaining perfusion of the vital organs.
- Improving the myocardial oxygen supply/demand ratio.
- Early recognition of failure of treatment to allow a dignified and pain-free death.

The assessment and monitoring of the patient in cardiogenic shock are essential parts of the management. Decisions about therapeutic strategies will depend on the availability of accurate data on which to act.

The patient will require:

- Continuous ECG monitoring.
- Hourly urine output monitoring via an indwelling urinary catheter.
- Blood pressure monitoring, non-invasive or preferably intra-arterial monitoring as this is more accurate and also allows access for arterial blood gas analysis.
- Oxygen saturation monitoring via pulse oximetry.
- If available a pulmonary artery catheter will allow for a more direct indication of left ventricular function. The PCWP in cardiogenic shock is likely to be 25 mmHg +. If not available, then a central venous pressure line can give an assessment of the volume load on the right side of the heart.

The therapeutic strategies employed will depend on the precise clinical picture that presents. However in established cardiogenic shock where the decision has been taken to pursue active treatment the following specific treatment will be appropriate:

- Any arrhythmia is corrected in order to optimize cardiac output.
- Whilst the usual picture will be one of fluid overload there are occasions when the patient is relatively hypovolaemic, in that the left-sided preload is not adequate (reflected by a low PCWP) and should therefore be corrected.
- Arterial hypoxaemia is treated by giving supplemental oxygen via high concentration mask or, if required, CPAP. The patient's position is optimized by placing in the Fowler's position if the blood pressure allows.
- A metabolic acidosis may result from the impaired tissue perfusion, which should be treated with the judicious administration of sodium bicarbonate.
- Any electrolyte imbalance is corrected, particularly potassium as deranged potassium may predispose to cardiac arrhythmias.
- An attempt is made to optimize cardiac output by the use of agents that will have a direct effect on preload, afterload and contractility. Contractility is increased by the administration of a positive inotropic agent. Dobutamine was for many years the drug of choice in this context, however, its use in some areas is being reconsidered, and adrenaline and noradrenaline appear to be used increasingly as the drugs of choice. (See below for a further discussion of inotropic drugs.) Preload and afterload are reduced by the use of vasodilators such as nitrates and, if the blood pressure will allow, the arterial dilator sodium nitroprusside. The usual scenario however is that the mean arterial pressure is too low for arterial dilators like nitroprusside and so a nitrate is used with caution to reduce the preload pressure on the left ventricle. Vasodilators are unlikely to be used if the systolic blood pressure is less than 90 mmHg.
- Renal support is provided initially by giving diuretics to increase the urine output. If necessary this can be supplemented by giving dopamine that, at a low dose, may increase renal perfusion.
- Tissue oxygen demands are kept to a minimum by ensuring the patient is resting completely. This may require the administration of small doses of diamorphine as the distress caused by the low cardiac output and the dyspnoea may result in considerable agitation. Adequate explanations and reassurance must support this. The presence of family members at this time may serve to reassure the patient, particularly if they become confused.
- Nutritional requirements via enteral routes at this time are limited to maintaining comfort. It must be recognized that the poor tissue perfusion effects the gut that may be paralysed or even ischaemic.
- Prevention and management of any infection or inflammation is important as there will be suppression of the immune system.
- The skin is particularly vulnerable in this situation and the potential for pressure sore development is high. Moving the patient to a special low pressure bed or mattress must be considered.
- Consideration must be given to the patient's family who are facing a situation that carries a very high mortality rate. Social and emotional support is essential if the needs of the relatives of the critically ill individual are to be met. These needs have been identified as the need for hope, information and relief of anxiety and to feel useful.

Inotropic drugs

One of the mainstays of drug therapy in the seriously ill is the use of positive inotropic drugs and so a review of the currently used agents is included. Inotropic substances are those that have an effect on myocardial contractility. Positive inotropes therefore are those agents that increase myocardial contractility. The agents that we commonly refer to as inotropic drugs are also vasoactive. That is, their effect is more complex than simply increasing contractility. The clinical effects of increases in contractility combined with a vasoactive action are dependent upon a variety of factors including: the combination of agents used, the clinical scenario that is the indication for their use, the dose of the agent given, and the haemodynamic status of the patient. The selection of a particular agent depends on an understanding of the mechanism of action and indications for use.

Mechanism of action

The majority of inotropic drugs are catecholamines and therefore dependent on their interaction with sympathetic adrenergic receptors. These receptors are *alpha*, *beta₁*, *beta₂*, and *dopaminergic DA1*.

- Stimulation of the *alpha* receptors results in increased systemic and pulmonary vascular resistance.
- *Beta₁* stimulation results in increased contractility, heart rate and conduction.
- *Beta₂* stimulation results in mild vasodilation.
- *Dopaminergic* stimulation results in dilatation of the renal and mesenteric arteries.

Stimulation of the adrenergic receptor releases a second messenger within the cell; this substance is cyclic AMP. The role of cyclic AMP in this situation is to improve/increase the availability of calcium to the contractile units of the muscle cell (calcium is essential for muscle contraction), to speed up the velocity of the contraction and to improve/speed relaxation.

Non-catecholamine inotropes

Newer agents like milronone do not act via the adrenergic receptors. These agents are phosphodiesterase (PDE) inhibitors. Phosphodiesterase is a substance that breaks down cyclic AMP. PDE inhibitors therefore exert their inotropic and vasoactive effects by inhibiting the break down of cyclic AMP. In cardiac cells this leads to increased contractility and in vascular smooth muscle it leads to vasodilatation.

Action of individual agents

DOPAMINE

At doses of 2–3 μg/kg/min dopamine may have a unique effect on dopaminergic receptors and dilate the renal arteries. There is also a reported effect of selected vasodilatation of the intestinal mucosa.

At doses of 3–10 μg/kg/min there is a strong beta₁ effect that increases myocardial contractility. There will also be an unpredictable rise in heart rate and myocardial oxygen demand.

At doses of 10–20 μg/kg/min there are both increasing inotropic effects but also strong alpha effects resulting in vasoconstriction.

DOBUTAMINE

Dobutamine at doses of 2–20 μg/kg/min has a potent beta₁ effect producing a predominantly inotropic response. There is some beta₂ effect that will produce mild vasodilatation and may therefore lower left ventricular preload. The net result is increased contractility without severe increases in myocardial oxygen consumption.

ADRENALINE

Adrenaline is a potent beta₁ agonist that will increase contractility and heart rate significantly. At doses up to 2 μg/kg/min there is also a beta₂ effect that causes a mild vasodilatation.

At doses above 2 μg/kg/min the strong alpha effects will raise the SVR (afterload) and increase myocardial oxygen consumption.

NORADRENALINE

Noradrenaline is a powerful alpha agonist that also has some beta$_1$ effects. The predominant effect is to raise SVR which is positive in the appropriate circumstances, such as massive vasodilatation, but the profound vasoconstriction can lead to renal or gut ischaemia. Dose is from 1 µg/min.

MILRINONE

Milrinone is a phosphodiesterase inhibitor that will improve cardiac output in the right circumstances by reducing SVR and by a positive inotropic effect. It is commonly used in patients with end stage heart failure awaiting transplantation. Dose range is usually 50 µg/kg i.v. bolus over 10 minutes followed by 0.5 µg/kg/min.

Hypovolaemia

One of the key aspects of maintaining a satisfactory perfusion pressure in the system is the regulation of adequate volume. Hypovolaemia requires restoration of fluids and the circulating plasma volume, but the choice of fluid and the amount given will depend on assessment of the clinical situation presented. This section will examine the clinical management of fluid resuscitation in the seriously ill patient. First we will explore the normal distribution of fluid in order that we may better understand the approach to treatment.

Body fluid refers to body water and its dissolved constituents. About 75 per cent of total body weight is body fluid, for example about 40 L in a 70 kg person. This body water is distributed in three spaces, the intravascular space, the interstitial space and the intracellular space which, in our example of a 70 kg person, will have distribution of approximately 5 L intravascular, 13 L interstitial and 23 L intracellular. Fluid is able to move between each of these spaces at certain points and under certain conditions. The intravascular space is separated from the interstitial space by the semipermiable membrane of the capillary walls. The interstitial space is separated from the intracellular space by the complex structure that is the cell membrane.

In the patient with acute circulatory failure it is the volume in the intravascular space that is of immediate concern. Movement of fluid in and out of the intravascular space depends upon the opposing forces of hydrostatic and osmotic pressure. The capillary membrane is permeable to water and small ions, for example sodium, but impermeable to large protein molecules found in the plasma. There is normally a hydrostatic pressure gradient between the capillaries and the interstitial space that pushes fluid out of the intravascular space. The osmotic pressure gradient pulls fluid back into the intravascular space, this being generated by the plasma proteins and other large molecules. When intravenous fluid is given it initially goes into the intravascular space. How much of the fluid stays in this space and how it is ultimately distributed amongst the three spaces depends on the nature of the fluid given.

There are basically two types of fluid that can be administered to the patient, crystalloid and colloid:

- *Crystalloids* are electrolyte solutions that do not contain the oncotic particles that would restrict them to the intravascular space. Examples would be 0.9 per cent saline solution, Ringer's lactate, and 5 per cent dextrose. The distribution of crystalloids once infused is dependent mainly on the sodium concentration. As sodium is mainly extracellular (interstitial and intravascular), fluids with an isotonic concentration of sodium (e.g. 0.9 per cent saline) will be confined to the interstitial and intravascular spaces, with three-quarters of the fluid going to the interstitial space as this is much larger. The lower the sodium concentration the more fluid will go to the intracellular space. For example, 5 per cent dextrose contains no sodium and so is distributed proportionately over the three spaces; out of one litre infused 520 mL will go to the intracellular space, 360 mL will go to the interstitial space and only 120 mL will go to the intravascular space. This makes it inappropriate for an acutely hypovolaemic situation where the goal is to increase the intravascular volume.
- *Colloids* are fluids that contain particles that exert an oncotic pressure and are mainly confined to the intravascular space when given

because the capillary membrane is not permeable to the large molecules. Colloids can be classified as those that have an oncotic pressure that is the same as plasma, such as blood and blood products and those with a higher osmotic pressure. Whilst all colloids will pull fluid into the intravascular space, if the oncotic pressure of the colloid is higher than the natural oncotic pressure of plasma, then more fluid is pulled into the intravascular space. Such agents are called plasma expanders as they expand the plasma volume. Examples of plasma expanders are, Haemaccel and hydroxyethyl starch (HES), the latter having the potential to expand the plasma volume by up to 170 per cent of the infused volume.

When deciding upon fluid therapy the choice of fluid is dependent on the assessment of the fluid deficit in each space. In acute hypovolaemia, often secondary to haemorrhage, it is the volume in the intravascular space that is deficient. This can be estimated by the clinical picture that is presented. This is based on the degree of compensation undertaken by the pump and by the pipes, namely, the attempted increase in the output of the heart, and the degree of vasoconstriction. The following guidelines in Table 2.2 are from the American College of Surgeons and provide an attempt to give an objective assessment.

The guide in the table is useful in that it requires no invasive monitoring equipment and therefore can be used in any situation where there is a sphygmomanometer.

If invasive monitoring is available then the CVP and/or the PCWP are used to titrate the volume replacement to the filling pressures of the heart.

The choice of fluid, then, will first be between a colloid or a crystalloid. Crystalloids are cheap and have few side effects. However adequate management of significant hypovolaemia requires very large volumes of fluid as only 25 per cent of the infused volume remains in the intravascular space. This raises the question of what happens to the rest of the fluid, the answer being that it is distributed between the intracellular and interstitial spaces. The interstitial oedema that can result is associated with poor oxygen uptake because of the increased diffusion distance between the capillaries and the cells which, in the lungs, will lead to the hypoxaemia we see in pulmonary oedema.

Colloids are expensive and can lead to more adverse reactions but less fluid is required to increase the intravascular volume. Colloid also remains in the vascular compartment for longer. However, in the critically ill patient the capillary cells are often 'leaky' and may allow large molecules to pass through into the interstitial space. This is seen in the systemic inflammatory response syndrome and in adult respiratory distress syndrome and it may lead to increased inter-

Table 2.2   Assessment of fluid loss in intravascular spaces

| | Percentage blood loss | | | |
	<15 per cent	15–30 per cent	30–40 per cent	>40 per cent
Clinical effect:				
Systolic BP	Unchanged	Normal	Reduced	Very low
Diastolic BP	Unchanged	Raised	Reduced	Very low
Pulse pressure	Normal	Decreased	Decreased	Decreased
Heart rate	<100	>100	>120	140
Mental state	Alert	Anxious	Anxious and confused	Confused, unconscious
Capillary refill	Normal	>2 s	>2 s	Undetectable

stitial oedema as the colloid that has become trapped in the interstitial space attracts fluid.

Whilst controversy still exists about the choice of fluid that should be given to the critically ill patient, however, the following may represent an approach that is taken and would seem reasonable given current knowledge (Kavanagh *et al.*, 1995; Schierhout and Roberts, 1998).

- For patients who are previously healthy and who are young, but who need fluid, such as in the uncomplicated post-operative patient or in acute trauma, then large volumes of crystalloid can be given safely as they can easily cope with fluid overload. However blood is the best option in hypovolaemia that is due to haemorrhage.

- In patients who are critically ill or who may have cardiac impairment large volumes of crystalloid have been avoided, as the potential fluid overload may be a significant threat. However recent evidence suggests that the use of colloids has been associated with an increase risk of mortality and this, combined with the extra cost throws considerable doubt on their continued use (Schierhout and Roberts, 1998). The use of human albumin solution has recently been contraindicated in critically ill patients. Larger molecular weight synthetic colloids such as hespan are being recommended instead (Cochrane Injuries Group Albumin Reviewers, 1998).
- In patients who are dehydrated 5 per cent dextrose is used, as this will most successfully correct the intracellular deficit.

Further reading

Ashworth, P. 1984 Staff patient communication in coronary care units. *Journal of Advanced Nursing* **9**, 35–42.

Cochrane Injuries Group Albumin Reviewers 1998 Human albumin administration in critically ill patients: systematic reviews of randomised controlled trials. *BMJ* **317**, 235–40.

Dahlen, R. and Roberts, S. 1995 Nursing management of congestive heart failure, Part 1. *Intensive and Critical Care Nursing* **11**, 272–9.

GUSTO (Global Utilisation of Streptokinase and Tissue plasminogen activator for Occluded coronary arteries) 1993 An international randomised trial comparing four strategies for acute myocardial infarction. *New England Journal of Medicine* **329**, 673–82.

Ho, K.K., Anderson, K.M. *et al.* 1993 Survival after the onset of congestive heart failure in Heart Study subjects. *Circulation* **88**, 107–15.

ISIS-2 (Second International Study of Infarct Survival) 1988 Randomised trial of intravenous streptokinase, oral aspirin, both, or neither among 17 187 cases of suspected acute myocardial infarction: ISIS-2. *Lancet* **ii**, 349–60.

ISIS-3 (Third International Study of Infarct Survival) 1992 A randomised comparison of strep-

tokinase vs tissue plasminogen activator vs anistreplase and of aspirin plus heparin vs aspirin alone among 41 299 cases of suspected acute myocardial infarction. *Lancet* **339**, 753–70.

Jowett, N.I. and Thompson, D.R. 1995 *Comprehensive coronary care*, 2nd edn. London: Scutari.

Kavanagh, R.J., Radhakrishnan, D. and Park, G. 1995 Crystaloids and colloids in the critically ill patient. *Care of the Critically Ill* **11**(3), 114–19.

Littrel, K., Walker, D. and Worthy, C. 1995 Myocardial infarction and the non-diagnostic ECG: strategies to meet the challenges. *Journal of Emergency Nursing* **21**(3), 287–95.

Lowel, H., Dobson, A., Keil, U. *et al.* 1993 Coronary heart disease fatality in four countries. *Circulation* **88**, 698–706.

Opie, L.H. 1997 *Drugs for the heart*, 4th edn. London: W. B. Saunders.

Schierhout, G. and Roberts, I. 1998 Fluid resuscitation with colloid or crystalloid solutions in critically ill patients: a review of randomised trials. *BMJ* **316**, 961–4.

Shoemaker, W.C., Apple, P.L. and Kram, H.B. 1988 Prospective trial of supranormal values of survivors as therapeutic goals in high risk surgical patients. *Chest* **94**, 1187–95.

Smith, J. and Kampine, J. 1990 *Circulatory physiology: the essentials*, 3rd edn. London: Williams and Watkins

Task Force on the Management of Acute Myocardial Infarction of the European Society of Cardiology 1996 Acute Myocardial Infarction: pre-hospital and in hospital management. *European Heart Journal* **17**, 43–63.

Underhill, S., Woods, S. *et al.* 1992 History taking and physical examination. In Underhill, S. *Cardiac nursing*, 3rd edn. Philadelphia: Lippincott.

Wagner, G. 1994 *Marriott's practical electrocardiography*, 9th edn. Baltimore: Williams and Wilkins.

Supporting respiration

Tracey Moore

Introduction

The aim of this chapter is to examine the purpose of the respiratory system, how this system may fail and the nursing care and management of a patient with a failing respiratory system.

Patients needing high dependency care share the challenge of similar life threatening situations. Whether the cause is cardiogenic shock, acute pulmonary embolus, septic shock or another diagnosis these patients have altered cellular metabolism from inadequate uptake, delivery or use of oxygen. Nurses caring for these patients need to understand the principles of oxygen delivery, the conditions which will affect haemoglobin-oxygen affinity, the methods of assessing a patient's oxygenation status and interpretation of these results to be able to effectively intervene and attempt to correct tissue hypoxia.

Oxygenation of all body systems is essential to optimum functioning. Oxygen is needed to generate energy, which the cell uses for metabolism. If oxygen is not available then tissues may cease to function and ultimately die.

SECTION 1: PHYSIOLOGY OF THE RESPIRATORY SYSTEM

The role of oxygen in generating energy for cell metabolism

Oxygen aids energy generation by accepting electrons removed from hydrogen during the catabolism of substrates, especially fats and proteins. As the hydrogen is removed from the substrates (fats and proteins) the electron from the hydrogen is passed from one element to another through a series of chemical events in the *Krebs or tricarboxylic acid cycle and cytochrome pathway* (*see* Fig. 3.1). As the electron is passed from one element to another energy is generated. As the energy is produced some of it is captured by adenosine diphosphate (ADP), which is then converted to adenosine triphosphate (ATP). The conversion of ADP to ATP is termed oxidative phosphorylation because oxygen is needed for the process to continue. As the electron continues down the cytochrome pathway it is passed from one cytochrome to another cytochrome, as it does so energy is produced which is again captured by ADP and converted into ATP. When the electron reaches the last cytochrome in the pathway it is accepted by oxygen to finally form water. This process is known as *aerobic metabolism*, i.e. metabolism using oxygen.

If the amount of oxygen available for this process is inadequate then electron transfer is inhibited and oxidative phosphorylation stops. At this point *anaerobic metabolism*, i.e. metabolism without using oxygen, then becomes the primary source for energy production. Anaerobic metabolism produces energy through the catabolism of carbohydrates and use of creatinine phosphate. However both carbohydrates and creatinine phosphate are short-lived energy sources, and whilst they may be invaluable as an energy source during a clinical emergency such as a cardiac arrest they are unable to sustain cellular activities over time. This lack of energy will eventually result in a failure of all cellular functions and cell death.

Furthermore, as anaerobic metabolism increases so does the production of lactate. Systemic lactate accumulation correlates with the decreased survival of patients since it reflects the lack of oxygen available for aerobic metabolism.

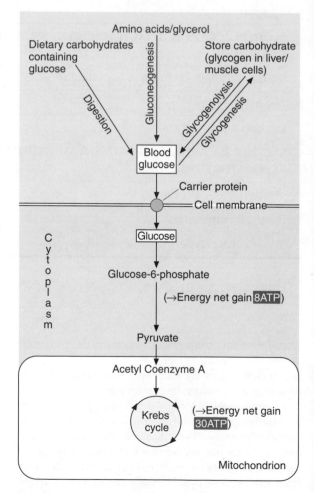

Figure 3.1 Glucose metabolism (cellular respiration)

So, since it is clearly shown that molecular oxygen must be continuously available to body tissues and cells in order to maintain aerobic metabolism, then monitoring oxygenation in patients has to be a primary nursing concern. Many interventions are directed towards this goal in the high dependency care setting where accurate assessment and treatment of oxygenation disturbances may determine a patient's survival. Therefore understanding the principles of oxygenation is crucial to the nurse's knowledge base.

The transport of oxygen and disposal of carbon dioxide to and from the organs and tissues of the body depends on effective pulmonary and cardiovascular functioning. This includes ventilation of the alveoli, diffusion of gases across the alveolar capillary membrane, perfusion of blood to the lungs and gas transport to the tissues.

Huber (1979) expresses these three sequential steps to oxygenation as:

1 *Oxygen uptake* – a means for extracting oxygen from the environment into the delivery system.
2 *Oxygen transportation* – a mechanism by which this uptake results in the delivery of oxygen to the cells.
3 *Oxygen utilization* – a metabolic need for molecular oxygen by the body cells.

For the sake of simplicity the oxygenation process is examined using the headings:

1 *Ventilation* – the movement of air from the atmosphere to the alveolus.
2 *External respiration* – the diffusion of oxygen in the air from the alveolus across the alveolar capillary membrane to the plasma, and its subsequent binding to the haemoglobin in the red blood cells.
3 *Internal respiration* – the diffusion of oxygen from the blood in the capillaries to the tissues and cells.

Ventilation

Alveolar ventilation consists of two phases: inspiration, the period when air is flowing into the lungs, and expiration, the period when gases are leaving the lungs. Alveolar ventilation is a mechanical process dependent on volume changes occurring in the thoracic cavity. When a change in volume occurs there is a corresponding change in pressure that in turn leads to a flow of gases to equalize the pressure. Boyle's Law, an ideal gas law, explains this relationship between volume and pressure of gases: in a large volume gas molecules will be far apart and pressure will be low, as the volume decreases the molecules are compressed and the pressure rises. This forms the basis for inspiration and expiration.

Numerous gases that make up the earth's atmosphere surround each of us. Each of these gases has its own molecular weight, and each gas is pulled down toward the centre of the earth by gravity. Atmospheric pressure is the collective pressure exerted by all these gases. This pressure equals 760 mmHg at sea level, i.e. the downward force of all these gases will support a column of mercury 760 mm high. Respiratory pressures are always described relative to atmospheric pressure. For example a negative pressure of −4 mmHg means that the pressure in that area of the lungs is 4 mmHg lower than atmospheric pressure (760 mmHg − 4 mmHg = 756 mmHg)

Remember that a respiratory pressure of zero is equal to atmospheric pressure, i.e. 760 mmHg. To examine the principles of breathing (ventilation) the nurse must firstly understand the role of lung pressures in this process.

Ventilation is the process by which gases are exchanged between the atmosphere and lung alveoli. This flow of air occurs as a direct result of a pressure gradient. When atmospheric pressure is greater than the pressure inside the lungs then we breathe in (inspiration) and when the pressure inside the lungs exceeds atmospheric pressure we breathe out (expiration).

The mechanics of ventilation

INSPIRATION

The diaphragm is the major muscle of ventilation but the accessory muscles of ventilation including the scalene, sternocleidomastoid, trapezius and pectoral muscles also provide a great reserve. As inspiration begins the diaphragm and the external intercostal muscles contract. Contraction of the diaphragm causes it to be pulled down, increasing the volume of the thoracic cavity. Contraction of the external intercostal muscles elevates the anterior end of each rib causing the rib to be pulled upward and outward. This causes an increase in the anteroposterior diameter of the thorax. This overall expansion of the thoracic cavity causes the pressure inside the lungs to fall from 760 mmHg to 758 mmHg.

During normal breathing the pressure between the two pleural layers of the lung is always sub-atmospheric (756 mmHg). This is known as intrapleural pressure. The overall increase in the volume of the thoracic cavity just before inspiration causes the intrapleural pressure to fall to 754 mmHg. This fall in pressure creates a partial vacuum that causes the lungs to be sucked outwards. Movement of the pleurae also aids expansion of the lung volume.

This overall increase in lung volume and consequent reduction of pressure within the thoracic cavity causes a pressure gradient to be set up between the lungs and the atmosphere. Air then rushes from the atmosphere into the lungs in an attempt to make the pressure both inside and outside the lungs equal (*see* Fig. 3.2).

EXPIRATION

Because inspiration is initiated by muscle contraction it is referred to as an active process. Expiration on the other hand is largely a passive process determined more by the natural elasticity of the lungs than by muscle contraction.

As the inspiratory muscles relax, the diaphragm and external intercostal muscles resume their initial resting length, the rib cage descends and the lungs recoil. This results in a reduction in thoracic and lung volume with subsequent compression of the alveoli. This causes intrapulmonary pressure to increase until it finally exceeds atmospheric pressure. Again this creates a pressure gradient between the lungs and the atmosphere which forces gases to flow out of the lungs. This causes a decrease in thoracic and lung volumes and a normal resting phase resumes where atmospheric and lung pressures are equal (*see* Fig. 3.2).

> To summarize, during inspiration the lungs are stretched to expand the thoracic cavity. This increases the lung volume with a subsequent fall in lung pressure, which causes air to flow from the atmosphere to the lungs. On expiration the lungs passively recoil which reduces lung volume and this results in gases being forced out of the lungs into the atmosphere.

However several factors such as *airway resistance*, *lung compliance* and *elasticity* and *alveolar surface tension*, may influence the passage of air between the lungs and the atmosphere and therefore the efficiency of pulmonary ventilation.

Airway resistance

As already identified, the amount of gas moving in and out of the alveoli is determined by changes in pressure gradients between the alveoli and the atmosphere. Indeed very small changes in pressure cause very large changes in the volume of gas flow. For example a change in pressure of only 4 mmHg can bring about a gas flow of 500 mL into the alveoli. However gas flow is not only influenced by changes in pressure gradient but also by airway resistance. The relationship is represented in the following equation:

$$\text{gas flow} = \frac{\text{pressure gradient}}{\text{resistance}}$$

Airway resistance is determined by the diameters of the airway. In the larger air passages where the diameter of the airways is greater airway resistance is minimal and has little affect on gas flow. However, in the smaller air passages, for example in the medium sized bronchi, airway resistance can influence air flow to a greater extent.

The smooth muscle cells of the bronchial walls are very sensitive to neural control and to certain chemicals. If we inhale irritant and inflammatory

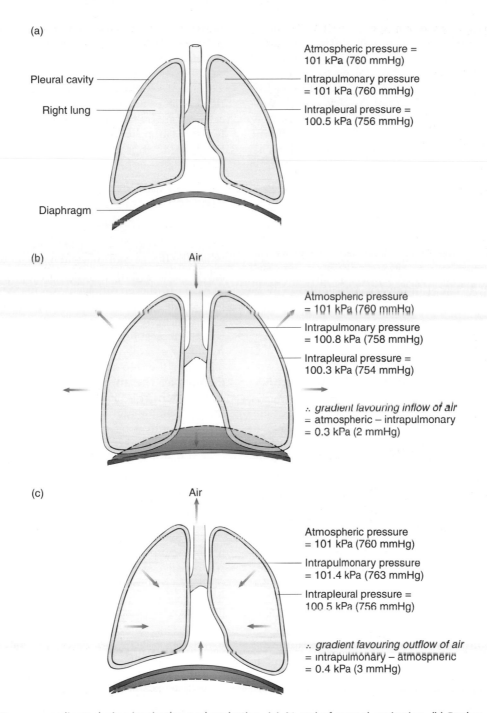

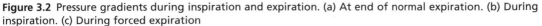

Figure 3.2 Pressure gradients during inspiration and expiration. (a) At end of normal expiration. (b) During inspiration. (c) During forced expiration

chemicals then our immune system responds by releasing histamine. Histamine release is part of the inflammatory response aimed at destroying the irritant. However histamine also causes the smooth muscle cells of the bronchi to constrict resulting in a narrowing of the airways. Narrowing of the airways increases resistance to air flow. This is the typical response of a person suffering an acute exacerbation of asthma where bronchial constriction is so great that pulmonary ventilation is inhibited despite the pressure gradients.

Mucus plugging of the airways in patients with bronchitis, pneumonia, asthma and bronchiectasis also increases airway resistance and in more severe cases pulmonary ventilation can be severely compromised.

Assessment and management of the patient with inefficient pulmonary ventilation will be examined in more detail later in this chapter.

Lung compliance and lung elasticity

Healthy lungs are very stretchy and the ease with which they can be expanded is defined as *lung compliance.*

More specifically, lung compliance is a measure of the change in lung associated with a change in intrapulmonary pressure where the more the lung expands for a given rise in pressure the greater its compliance. High compliance means that the lungs expand easily and low compliance means that the lungs resist expansion.

However, lung compliance is determined not only by how stretchy the lungs are but also by the size of the thoracic wall, and any condition affecting either of these factors will affect lung compliance. For example adult respiratory distress syndrome, a form of respiratory failure which results from direct or indirect pulmonary injury, is characterized by stiff lungs where the lung tissue loses its ability to expand resulting in decreased compliance. This in turn results in diminished pulmonary ventilation as a result of reduced tidal volumes. Similarly patients with emphysema characterized by fibrosed lung tissue suffer from inelastic lungs and therefore lowered tidal volumes.

Conditions affecting the thoracic cage will cause similar results. For example, paralysis of the intercostal muscles will reduce the outward movement of the rib cage prior to inspiration reducing the space for the lungs to stretch into and therefore lowering tidal volumes.

Lung elasticity will also affect lung recoil during expiration. Reduced elasticity will make this process less effective and the residual volume of air, i.e. the amount of air left in the lungs following expiration, will be increased. However, elasticity and thoracic size are not the only determinants of lung compliance.

Surface tension

Surface tension must also be considered to make the picture complete. Surface tension is created when the liquid molecules at a gas–liquid boundary are more strongly attracted to each other than they are to the gas molecules. This is what happens at the alveolar wall, which can be termed the gas–liquid boundary. Imagine the alveoli as air-filled bubbles lined with water. The attractive force between the water molecules lining the alveoli causes them to squeeze in upon the air within the bubble. The attractive force is known as surface tension. The surface tension makes the water lining resemble highly stretched rubber. This rubber constantly tries to shorten and resist further stretching. This cohesion and tension makes it very difficult to expand the alveoli and therefore the lungs during inspiration. Indeed were the lining made entirely of water the alveoli would collapse between breaths making ventilation largely ineffective.

However, the liquid film lining the alveoli is not made purely of water but also contains a substance called surfactant. Surfactant is a lipoprotein produced by type II alveolar cells. It acts to reduce the surface tension by lessening the cohesive bond between the water molecules on the alveolar surface. This increases total lung compliance enabling ventilation to be more effective, whilst also preventing total collapse of the alveoli on expiration.

Unfortunately problems occur when insufficient amounts of surfactant are present. Adult respiratory distress syndrome is characterized by limited surfactant production. This causes surface tension to rise and as a result a number of alveoli collapse. This requires that the collapsed alveoli be completely reinflated on inspiration. This demands increasing amounts of energy, which in an already compromised patient can lead to exhaustion and worsening pulmonary insufficiency.

This principle can be explained easily by examining what happens when you blow up a balloon. When the balloon is new out of the packet and is completely deflated, the effort required to inflate the balloon is great. Once the balloon starts to inflate, filling it with more air becomes easier. When the balloon deflates again it never collapses as fully as when new and reinflating it is always easier.

External respiration

Once inspiration is complete, oxygen diffuses from the alveoli into the blood for transport around the body. Using the same process, carbon dioxide is transferred from the blood into the alveoli for removal from the body during expiration. This stage is known as *external respiration*.

External respiration is optimized by several factors which are discussed below.

Fick's law, which describes diffusion through the tissues, states that the rate of transfer of a gas through a sheet of tissue is proportional to the tissue area and the difference in gas partial pressure between the two sides, and inversely proportional to the tissue thickness.

The area of the blood–gas barrier in the lung is large, measuring between 50 and 100 m^2. Equally important is the thickness of the blood–gas barrier, more commonly referred to as the alveolar-capillary membrane, which is only 3 nm thick in some parts. Together these form the ideal dimensions for diffusion.

The partial pressure of oxygen (Po_2) in a red blood cell entering a pulmonary capillary overlying an alveoli (deoxygenated blood) is 40 mmHg and alveolar Po_2 is 100 mmHg. This creates a steep oxygen partial pressure gradient, which causes oxygen to diffuse from the alveolus into the red blood cell. The Po_2 in the red blood cell rises quickly until equilibrium is reached.

Carbon dioxide moves in the opposite direction from the red blood cell into the alveolus, also as a result of a partial pressure gradient since the Pco_2 of pulmonary deoxygenated blood is 45 mmHg and that of the alveoli is only 40 mmHg. The carbon dioxide that diffuses into the alveolus is then eliminated during expiration.

For gas exchange to be most effective ventilation (the amount of gas reaching the alveoli) and perfusion (the blood flow in the capillaries) must match closely. In alveoli where ventilation is inadequate the Po_2 will be poor. In response to this arterioles constrict and blood flow is directed to alveoli where oxygen uptake may be more effective. Alternatively where alveolar ventilation is maximal pulmonary arterioles dilate increasing blood flow to the associated pulmonary capillaries. This autoregulatory mechanism exists to provide the most appropriate conditions for gas exchange.

Once oxygen has diffused across the alveolar-capillary membrane into the blood it is carried bound to the haemoglobin in the red blood cell and dissolved in plasma. Because oxygen is relatively insoluble in water only 1.5% is carried in the dissolved form with 98.5% being bound to haemoglobin.

Each molecule of haemoglobin can combine with four molecules of oxygen. The combination of haemoglobin and oxygen creates a substance called oxyhaemoglobin (HbO$_2$). When the first molecule of oxygen binds to the haemoglobin molecule, haemoglobin changes its shape. This change of shape makes it easier for the second oxygen molecule to attach itself to the haemoglobin molecule, which makes it even easier for the third to attach and easier still for the fourth.

When one, two or three sites are bound with oxygen the haemoglobin molecule is said to be partially saturated. Once all four sites are bound with oxygen the term changes to fully saturated.

In the same way that oxygen binding is enhanced as more sites become saturated with oxygen, so the removal of oxygen molecules at the tissues is made easier as more sites are unloaded with oxygen. The second oxygen molecule therefore is unloaded more easily than the first and the third even more easily and so on until all the oxygen has been unloaded.

Haemoglobin that has unloaded its oxygen molecule at tissue and cell level is referred to as reduced or deoxyhaemoglobin (HHb).

So it can be seen that tissue oxygenation depends in part on the ability of the oxygen to bind with and unload from haemoglobin. However, the rate at which oxygen binds with and unloads from haemoglobin is affected by several factors namely: *the partial pressure of oxygen* (P_{O_2}), *temperature, blood pH, partial pressure of carbon dioxide* (P_{CO_2}), and the presence of an intracellular compound called *2,3-diphosphoglycerate (2,3 DPG)*. 2,3 DPG directly affects the binding and dissociation of oxygen from haemoglobin as it competes with oxygen for the haemoglobin binding site.

These relationships are explained by the *oxyhaemoglobin dissociation curve*. This curve helps nurses to understand more fully how certain factors affect the oxygenation status of patients.

The oxyhaemoglobin dissociation curve

Two oxygen transfer sites exist within the body. The first of these is found in the lungs at the alveolar-capillary site where, following inspiration, oxygen diffuses across the alveolar-capillary membrane into the blood plasma and attaches itself to the haemoglobin molecule. The second transfer site, which will be discussed in more detail later, occurs at tissue level. Here, oxygen unloads from the haemoglobin molecule and diffuses across the capillary membrane into the cells.

The vertical axis of the oxyhaemoglobin dissociation curve represents haemoglobin oxygen saturation. The horizontal axis represents partial pressure of oxygen in the blood (P_{O_2}).

When plotting the normal oxyhaemoglobin

dissociation curve it is assumed that the patient's temperature is 37°C, pH is 7.4 and P_{CO_2} is 40 mmHg, i.e. within normal ranges. A change in any of these factors will cause a shift in the curve.

As you can see from Fig. 3.3, the oxyhaemoglobin dissociation curve is S-shaped with a steep curve between 10 and 60 mmHg P_{O_2}. This portion represents the dissociation of oxygen from haemoglobin and transfer into the tissues. The flatter part of the curve, which falls between 70 and 100 mmHg, reflects the alveolar-capillary transfer site where oxygen binds with haemoglobin for transfer to the tissues. Therefore you can see that the extent to which haemoglobin combines with oxygen increases very quickly between 10 and 60 mmHg P_{O_2}; at this point the haemoglobin is 90% saturated with oxygen. From this point on a further increase in P_{O_2} produces only a small change in haemoglobin oxygen saturation.

However, should one or more of the factors which affect the extent to which oxygen will bind with the haemoglobin molecule (P_{O_2}, temperature, blood pH or P_{CO_2}) increase or decrease, a shift in the curve either right or left will be seen.

A shift of the curve to the left causes increased affinity of the haemoglobin for oxygen. Therefore, for any P_{O_2} level oxygen saturation will be greater

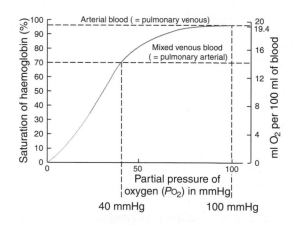

Figure 3.3 Oxyhaemoglobin dissociation curve

than is normally expected. At alveolar-capillary oxygen transfer sites this means that it is easier for oxygen to bind with the haemoglobin. However, the increased affinity of haemoglobin for oxygen can result in cellular hypoxia as the haemoglobin is also more reluctant to unload its oxygen.

Clinical situations which cause the curve to shift to the left include alkalosis, hypocapnia, hypothermia and decreased levels of 2,3 DPG which may occur following a massive blood transfusion.

For example, a patient admitted for surgery the following day is very afraid. In the middle of the night as their fear increases they start to hyperventilate. Hyperventilation increases the excretion of carbon dioxide and the patient becomes hypocapneic and alkalotic. As a result the oxyhaemoglobin curve will shift to the left. In this situation, haemoglobin has an increased affinity for oxygen. However, whilst this makes it easier for oxygen to attach to the haemoglobin in the lungs, when it reaches the tissues it is harder for oxygen to unload from the haemoglobin and unless the situation is rectified then tissue hypoxia may occur.

A shift of the curve to the right causes decreased affinity of the haemoglobin for oxygen. Therefore for any Po_2 level oxygen saturation will be less than is normally expected. This decreased affinity means that at alveolar-capillary oxygen transfer sites a high Po_2 is needed to saturate the haemoglobin. However, the oxygen that does bind with the haemoglobin dissociates easily at tissue level, so whilst it is more difficult for the oxygen to bind with the haemoglobin in the lungs, at cell level the oxygen readily unloads.

Acidosis, hypercapnia (an increase in the carbon dioxide tension of the blood), hyperthermia and increased levels of 2,3 DPG all cause the curve to shift to the right.

For example, a patient who has returned from theatre following a gastrectomy suddenly develops a fever the following day. His temperature is

39.5°C. This rise in temperature causes the oxyhaemoglobin dissociation curve to shift to the right. In this situation, whilst oxygen readily unloads at tissue level it is more difficult for it to bind with the haemoglobin in the lungs. If this situation continues then eventually most of the oxygen will have been used by the tissues where metabolism will have increased as a consequence of the fever and tissue hypoxia will eventually result.

It can be seen therefore, that certain disease processes and certain treatments will cause the oxyhaemoglobin curve to shift to the left or the right, which will result in either increased or decreased affinity of haemoglobin for oxygen. Insight into the factors and conditions causing these shifts will enable the nurse to assess and manage a critically ill patient's oxygenation status more effectively in an attempt to correct tissue hypoxia.

Having examined the importance of haemoglobin in oxygen delivery to the tissues, the next stage in external respiration, which will be examined in more detail in the following chapter, involves the pumping of the oxygenated blood to the tissues, i.e. the cardiac output.

For delivery to be effective the cardiac output defined as the volume of blood ejected by either ventricle per minute, must be able to meet the current metabolic demands of the body. For example, if you are running for a bus then your metabolic demand will increase to give you more energy to run. Cells producing greater amounts of energy will need more oxygen. To increase the supply of oxygen to the cells your cardiac output increases. It is this ability of the body to alter cardiac output to meet metabolic demand that is central to the maintenance of tissue oxygenation.

In certain clinical conditions such as hypovolaemia, acute myocardial infarction, cardiac tamponade, this function is impaired and metabolic demand for oxygen can no longer be met. This results in tissue hypoxia.

Internal respiration

The final stage in the process of respiration involves the exchange of oxygen and carbon dioxide between the blood in the systemic capillaries and the tissue cells. The exchange results from diffusion driven by the partial pressure gradients of oxygen and carbon dioxide on either side of the exchange membranes.

As tissue cells use oxygen for metabolic activity they also produce equal amounts of carbon dioxide. This creates a situation where the P_{O_2} in the tissue cells is 40 mmHg due to the use of oxygen during metabolic function, and the P_{O_2} of the blood in the systemic capillaries is 104 mmHg. This results in the rapid diffusion of oxygen from the capillaries into the tissue cell that continues until equilibrium is reached.

At the same time tissue cells are producing carbon dioxide as the end product of cell metabolism. This results in a situation where the level of CO_2 in the tissue cells is greater than that in the blood and therefore CO_2 diffuses from the tissues into the blood until equilibrium is achieved.

Carbon dioxide is then expelled from the lungs during passive expiration. In the healthy individual the amount of carbon dioxide produced during cell metabolism and the amount expelled during expiration are equal. This state of equilibrium is known as *acid–base balance*.

Acid–base balance

This part of the chapter examines the role of the respiratory system in acid–base balance.

All functional proteins such as enzymes, haemoglobin and cytochromes are influenced by the hydrogen-ion concentration of their environment. The hydrogen-ion concentration is frequently expressed in terms of the pH of a solution that is defined as a negative logarithm to the base of 10 of the hydrogen-ion concentration:

$$pH = - \log H^+$$

For example, a solution with a hydrogen-ion concentration of 10^{-7} mol/L will have a pH of 7. A more acid solution with a hydrogen-ion concentration of 10^{-6} mol/L will have a pH of 6. Therefore, as the acidity increases the pH decreases and the change in pH from 7 to 6 represents a 10-fold increase in hydrogen-ion concentration.

Water is neutral with a pH of 7.0. Solutions with a pH greater than 7.0, i.e. solutions with a lower hydrogen-ion concentration, are called alkaline.

Extracellular fluid is slightly alkaline with a pH 7.4. Intracellular fluid tends to be slightly more acid than extracellular fluid. At rates outside of these, functional proteins reduce their ability to function and so biochemical reactions relying on their influence become less effective. In fact, a pH of less than 6.8 or greater than 7.8 is incompatible with life.

Therefore, homeostasis of pH is essential to survival; indeed for many critically ill patients disturbance of this delicate balance can be life-threatening.

REGULATION OF BLOOD pH

Despite the continual production of acid as a by-product or end-product of cell metabolism the pH must be kept within normal limits. This balance is maintained through three systems:

- by chemical buffers in the blood;
- by the lungs;
- by the kidneys.

Chemical buffers are the immediate defence against acid–base abnormalities acting within seconds of the imbalance occurring. There are many systems in the body designed to buffer acids. These include:

- the bicarbonate and carbonic acid system;
- haemoglobins;
- plasma proteins;
- phosphates.

Basically, these buffers work by absorbing or releasing acid as required to maintain a normal pH. For example, if there is excess base or alkali in the blood the buffer system will release acid from buffering sites to mop up the excess alkali to a safe level. Alternatively, if there is excess acid in the blood then the buffer system will absorb the acid in an attempt to maintain pH homeostasis.

However, whilst an excellent short term answer to acid–base balance, chemical buffers can only maintain blood pH for as long as they are available so eventually other methods of restoring acid–base balance must be used. So within minutes of the imbalance occurring the lungs then attempt to resolve the imbalance followed by the kidneys hours or even days later. Therefore effective functioning of both these systems is vital to the maintenance of acid–base balance.

RESPIRATORY CONTROL OF ACID–BASE BALANCE

As already discussed, the respiratory system is responsible for eliminating carbon dioxide from the blood. Carbon dioxide, generated by cellular metabolism, enters the erythrocytes in the circulation and is converted to bicarbonate ions for transport in the plasma. This is shown by the following equation:

$$CO_2 + H_2O \rightleftharpoons H_2CO_3 \rightleftharpoons H^+ + HCO_3^-$$

This sign $\rightleftharpoons$ indicates a reversible equation. From the equation you will note that a reversible equation falls between dissolved $CO_2 + H_2O$ on one side and H_2CO_3 (carbonic acid) on the other, i.e.

$$CO_2 + H_2O \rightleftharpoons H_2CO_3$$

A reversible equation also falls between H_2CO_3 and $H^+ + HCO_3^-$ i.e.

$$H_2CO_3 \rightleftharpoons H^+ + HCO_3^-$$

As a result of the reversible equation, an increase in any of these chemical substances will push the reaction in the opposite direction. For example when CO_2 unloads in the lungs to be expelled during passive expiration then the equation will shift

to the left, and H^+ generated from H_2CO_3 will be reincorporated into H_2O. This means that hydrogen ions produced by carbon dioxide transport are not allowed to accumulate in the blood and therefore have little or no effect on the blood pH.

When a patient is unable to expel carbon dioxide, as a result of chronic obstructive airways disease for example, the high levels of retained CO_2 act as a stimulus on the medullary chemoreceptors in the brain stem. They respond by increasing both the respiration rate and depth of respiration in an attempt to try to 'blow off' the excess CO_2. In addition, a rising plasma hydrogen ion concentration resulting from any metabolic process, diabetes mellitus for example, will indirectly stimulate the respiratory centre, again causing respirations to become faster and deeper.

On the other hand, when the blood pH starts to rise (become more alkaline), then the respiratory centre will be depressed. As the respiration rate falls and breathing becomes shallower then CO_2 will be allowed to accumulate. As CO_2 accumulates the reaction will be pushed to the right causing hydrogen ion concentrations to rise once more. Again pH will be restored to within the normal range.

This method of maintaining an acid–base balance is an exceptional one and corrections to an abnormal balance are generally achieved within a minute or so. However, this method of control may be compromised by problems in the respiratory system. For example any conditions that cause a patient to hyperventilate, such as fear, anxiety, pain, will increase CO_2 elimination and the blood pH will rise. On the other hand, conditions such as chronic obstructive airways disease, pneumonia, asthma, will cause the patient to retain CO_2 and the blood pH will fall.

When the fall in blood pH is caused by an associated respiratory problem then the person is deemed to have a *respiratory acidosis*. When the blood pH rises this is termed *respiratory alkalosis*.

The role of the kidneys in the maintenance of acid base balance is examined more closely in Chapter 4.

SECTION 2: CARE AND MONITORING OF PATIENTS WITH RESPIRATORY DISORDERS

Respiratory induced acid–base imbalance

The next part of this chapter will examine causes, signs and symptoms and treatment of patients with a metabolic or respiratory acidosis or alkalosis.

Metabolic acidosis

This occurs when there is decreased bicarbonate either due to increased loss or increased use in attempting to mop up or neutralize excess acid. Loss of bicarbonate may occur in patients with a fistula or severe diarrhoea.

Metabolic acidosis may also occur in patients with impaired kidney function. Ineffective urine excretion causes acid levels in the blood to rise as hydrogen ions formed during tissue metabolism accumulate.

Diabetes ketoacidosis or an increased lactic acid production due to hypoxia, shock, heart failure or liver disease may also result in a metabolic acidosis due to the overproduction of acid.

Patients suffering from a metabolic acidosis may present with gasping respiration, lethargy, restlessness and disorientation, cardiac dysrhythmias, nausea and vomiting.

Treatment relies on being able to identify and reverse the metabolic acidosis. For example if the cause of the metabolic acidosis is acute renal failure then dialysis may be indicated. Sodium bicarbonate may also be prescribed.

Metabolic alkalosis

This occurs where there is an increase in bicarbonate either as a result of acid loss or excess alkali.

Potential causes of acid loss, resulting in an increase in the blood's pH include:

- Diarrhoea and vomiting.
- Prolonged, excessive nasogastric aspirations.
- Gastrocolic fistula.
- Prolonged use of diuretics causing potassium ion (K^+) depletion. (Low serum K^+ causes an increase in the excretion of H^+ ions instead of K^+ ions from the kidneys.)

Raised alkali levels may result from sodium bicarbonate administration and antacid abuse.

Patients suffering from a metabolic alkalosis may present with vomiting, restlessness, tremors, tingling of the extremities, tetany and convulsions.

Treatment is aimed at the primary cause. For example where alkalosis is caused by over-ingestion of antacids then bicarbonate intake must be discontinued and acid fluids such as citrus fruit juices may be given. Where alkalosis is due to vomiting and diarrhoea then the cause must be treated, antiemetics and antidiarrhoea drugs may be prescribed and appropriate fluid replacement treatment therapy maintained.

Respiratory acidosis

This is caused by carbon dioxide retention due to impaired ventilation resulting in an increase of carbonic acid in the blood. Impaired ventilation may result from conditions such as chronic obstructive airways disease, emphysema and asthma which compromise gaseous exchange. Drug or alcohol overdose, trauma and neurological disorders such as Guillain–Barré syndrome and myasthenia gravis may also cause it.

Respiratory acidosis may be characterized by a diminished mental state, drowsiness, muscle twitching, peripheral vasodilation and cardiac dysrhythmias.

Treatment is aimed at reversing the underlying cause of the acidosis. For example, using medication, correct patient positioning, chest physiotherapy and deep breathing. However, in more extreme cases it may be necessary to provide mechanical ventilatory support to help to 'blow off' the excess carbon dioxide.

Respiratory alkalosis

This occurs in patients who are hyperventilating, thus decreasing the level of carbon dioxide in the blood. Anxiety states, salicylate poisoning and pain are the more common causes of hyperventilation but neurological disorders such as strokes or a tumour, and breathing at high altitudes can also cause hyperventilation.

Symptoms of a respiratory alkalosis may include impaired consciousness, seizures, increased muscle tone, tetany and hypokalaemia which may cause irregular heart rhythms.

Treatment is again aimed at removing the underlying cause of the alkalosis. For example administering effective pain relief to reduce hyperventilation in patients with pain, or if the cause is anxiety, asking patients who can breathe spontaneously to re-breathe their own carbon dioxide by breathing into a paper bag.

To summarize then, both arterial blood gas analysis and pH measurements can be used to identify and suggest the cause of acid–base balance disturbances. They are also used to monitor the effects of oxygen therapy. Understanding and knowledge of these measurements is therefore crucial to both the nursing and medical management of the critically ill patient.

Obtaining arterial blood for analysis

Because the acid–base balance of body fluids is so vital to optimum functioning it is subject to strict monitoring in the acute setting by the analysis of arterial blood samples.

Samples of blood for arterial blood gas analysis can be obtained by either direct arterial puncture or from an indwelling arterial catheter. The most common site for catheter insertion is the radial artery. However, the brachial, femoral or dorsalis pedis artery may be used if necessary.

Arterial catheterization allows easy blood sampling for blood gas analysis, monitoring of acid–base status, and other serum investigations. An arterial catheter also enables more accurate, continual observation of the patient's blood pressure.

However, whilst its use is extremely valuable, arterial catheterization is not without its problems. As with any invasive technique, arterial catheterization can be a source of infection. Innoculation may occur during insertion or aftercare. To help to minimize this risk of introducing infection while blood sampling, an aseptic technique must always be used throughout the procedure.

Impeded blood flow along the cannulated artery also presents a risk. Blanching or discoloration of the area must be reported immediately. If the radial artery is used for catheterization performing an Allen's test before insertion may help to reduce this complication. This will ensure the presence of adequate collateral circulation to the hand by the ulnar artery.

To perform an Allen's test, both the ulnar and radial arteries are occluded. The patient then clenches and unclenches their fist until the hand is blanched. Pressure on the ulnar artery is then released. If ulnar circulation is efficient colour should return to the hand within 5 to 7 seconds. Extended filling time indicates inadequate ulnar circulation. If the hand remains blanched for 15 seconds or longer then the radial site should not be used for arterial catheterization.

The arterial cannulation site must be visible at all times where patient dignity allows, and secured well to prevent the catheter from being dislodged. Being placed in an artery, excessive haemorrhage will occur if the cannula is accidentally disconnected.

However, in spite of its complications arterial catheterization saves valuable time for the nurse, provides essential assessment data and saves the patient from the pain of repeated direct arterial puncture every time a blood sample is needed for arterial blood gas analysis.

Interpretation of arterial blood gases

Arterial blood gases (ABGs) include measurements of hydrogen-ion concentration or pH, base excess (BE), bicarbonate (HCO_3^-), partial pressure of carbon dioxide (PCO_2) and partial pressure of oxygen (PO_2).

Each of these will now be examined in more detail.

1 *Hydrogen-ion concentration* or *pH* has been defined earlier in the chapter.
2 *Base excess* measures the degree of metabolic acidosis and alkalosis. It refers to the amount of acid or base/alkali that is needed to restore the pH to 7.4 at a normal PCO_2. Negative base excess, for example BE -5, is referred to as a base deficit (acid surplus).
3 HCO_3 is an indicator of metabolic function. This measurement is sometimes measured by means of the standard bicarbonate measurement (SBC). Here the plasma concentration is measured in relation to a normal PCO_2 of 5.3 kPa with fully saturated haemoglobin and at a temperature of 37°C.
4 PCO_2 is an indicator of respiratory function and is a measure of acid secretion through respiration. A level of more than 6.0 kPa suggests too little ventilation resulting in the retention of carbon dioxide. A level of less than 4.5 kPa indicates too much ventilation resulting in carbon dioxide being 'blown off'.
5 PO_2 is not used in acid–base measurement but reflects the level of oxygenation in the blood.

Normal values of arterial blood gases

pH	7.34–7.44
PCO_2	4.4–5.8 kPa
PO_2	10.0–13.3 kPa
HCO_3	20–24 mmol/L
BE	$-2.0–+2.0$

Value of arterial blood gases in analysis of acid–base balance

Whilst pH does reflect the overall state of acidity or alkalinity of the blood, pH alone does not necessarily indicate the absence of an acid–base disturbance. To have the whole picture the pH, PCO_2 and HCO_3 must all be examined. If pH, PCO_2 and HCO_3 are all within the normal range then no acid–base disturbance exists. However, if any of these values is abnormal then both the primary disturbance and the degree to which the patient is compensating for this acid–base disturbance must be determined.

A simple checklist to use when analysing a patient's arterial blood gas is as follows:

1 Look at the pH – is it normal, acidic or alkaline?
2 Determine the primary cause of the imbalance by checking the values of the other parameters.
   The parameter that matches the pH is usually the primary disturbance. For example if the pH is acidic and the PCO_2 is elevated then the primary cause of the imbalance will be the respiratory system.
3 Determine if compensation has occurred.

COMPENSATION

Compensation can be described as total, partial or absent. It relates to the degree to which one system, i.e. the respiratory system or the renal system (metabolic system), is able to offset a change in the other and by so doing return the pH back to within normal limits.

When *total compensation* occurs the pH will fall within the normal range. However, theoretically total compensation is never complete because the pH will always fall closer to the side of normal that reflects the primary disturbance whilst still remaining between 7.34 and 7.44.

For example:

pH	7.35	(normal but close to the acid side of the normal range)
P_{CO_2}	3.0 kPa	(low – indicating respiratory alkalosis)
HCO_3	15 mmol/L	(low – indicating metabolic acidosis)

In this example the pH is normal but is closer to the acid end of the normal range (7.34–7.44) so, if a disturbance is present it must be acidic in nature. When assessing the other parameters it shows that the level of CO_2 corresponds to a respiratory alkalosis, whilst the level of HCO_3 is indicative of a metabolic acidosis. The metabolic parameter is the one that matches the pH value (acidity) and is therefore described as the primary disturbance.

The respiratory alkalosis seen in this example occurs as the respiratory system attempts to compensate for the metabolic acidosis by 'blowing off' more CO_2. In the patient this would be recognized as hyperventilating.

Since the pH has been returned back to normal by the efforts of the respiratory system then this is defined as *total compensation*.

Partial compensation occurs when, despite compensatory efforts, the pH still remains outside of the normal range.

For example:

pH	7.275	(acidic)
P_{CO_2}	12.98 kPa	(high – indicating respiratory acidosis)
HCO_3	44.0 mmol/L	(high – indicating metabolic alkalosis)

In this example the primary disturbance is a respiratory acidosis. There is a high bicarbonate indicating a compensatory alkalosis as the metabolic system attempts to return the pH back to a normal value. However this has not been completely successful because the pH value still lies outside the normal range, so compensation is described as *partial*.

Remember that it may take the kidneys hours or even days to resolve an acid–base disturbance (see page 61). As a consequence the attempted compensation by the metabolic system in this example would indicate that the respiratory disorder is chronic not acute.

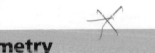

Pulse oximetry

Whilst arterial blood gas analysis provides us with valuable information relating to arterial oxygenation it is not without its disadvantages. The information is only available intermittently when ABGs are taken. At times this is not enough for in many critically ill patients the continual assessment of arterial oxygenation is needed. Other methods of monitoring the patient's oxygenation status are therefore required.

Pulse oximetry, first introduced a decade ago is a valuable, non-invasive monitoring device that provides data rapidly. If used appropriately it enables the nurse to estimate the patient's arterial oxygen saturation and to follow trends of arterial oxygen saturation to help in assessing for hypoxia.

However, pulse oximetry should not be applied to a patient unless the nurse is fully aware of both its uses and limitations.

It functions by positioning any pulsating vascular bed between a two wavelength light source and a detector. The pulsating vascular bed, by expanding and relaxing, creates a change in the light path that modifies the amount of light detected. This produces the familiar waveform. The amplitude of the varying detected light depends upon the size of the arterial pulse change, the wavelength of light used and the oxygen saturation of the arterial haemoglobin.

The accuracy of pulse oximetry is dependent on several issues:

1 The tissue being reasonably transparent to the wave lengths of light being used. For example

a finger, toe or ear lobe are the most common preferred sites. If the skin on the chosen area is thickened, for example on the fingers of a labourer, then the wavelengths of light may not be absorbed. In such instances a more suitable site must be selected.

2 The presence of pulsatile arterial blood within the tissues. If for example the patient is poorly perfused or hypotensive then the reading may be inaccurate.

3 Dark skin pigmentation, nail polish, nicotine stained fingers and patient movement may all affect the accuracy of the reading.

4 Arterial haemoglobin oxygen saturation levels of 85% and above are accurate within 1–2%. However, as saturation levels fall to below 85% then the oximeter reading becomes less reliable.

5 Delays can occur in the time it takes for the pulse oximeter to display any changes in arterial oxygen haemoglobin saturation. For example if a patient has a drop in inspired oxygen concentration it may take up to 30 seconds for this fall in concentration to be detected by the pulse oximeter. In a critically ill patient these 30 seconds could be vital.

6 Flooding or extreme light directed at the pulse oximeter, direct sunlight for example, can cause a false reading.

7 Using an incorrect sized probe such as a children's probe for an adult will give an inaccurate reading.

8 Abnormal haemoglobin will give a false reading. For example carboxyhaemoglobin (COHb). Very small amounts of COHb will make the arterial haemoglobin oxygen saturation equal to 100% (for every % COHb the saturation of the Sao_2 over reads by approximately 1%). COHb is caused by inhaling even small amounts of carbon monoxide. Therefore the use of a pulse oximeter is not recommended in patients who have been in or close to a fire, have attempted suicide using car exhaust fumes or those who are heavy tobacco smokers.

9 Other absorbants such as injected physiological dyes will cause inaccurate readings.

10 Bounding veins and venules as found in patients with tricuspid valve disease and hyperdynamic circulations.

Guidelines for patient selection and knowledge of the limitations of pulse oximetry are central to the provision of safe nursing care and management. Pulse oximetry is an invaluable monitoring device when the data it provides are interpreted accurately and correctly, but a false reading can also cause a false sense of patient wellbeing and lead to poor nursing and medical management.

For example, one common misconception in clinical practice is that maintaining arterial haemoglobin oxygen saturation above 90% is reassuring and can mean that the patient is clinically stable. However, an acceptable oxygen saturation does not necessarily imply adequate ventilation, tissue oxygenation, perfusion or oxygen transport. If you refer back to the oxyhaemoglobin dissociation curve earlier in the chapter (Fig. 3.3) you will note that a decrease in Po_2 from 84 to 59 mmHg causes only a small fall in oxygen saturation from 96% to 90%. Significant changes in saturation do not occur until the Po_2 falls to less than 60 mmHg.

So, in addition to monitoring devices nurses must also use their knowledge and skills to accurately assess a patient's clinical status. Objective measurements must be assessed in conjunction with other significant changes that may indicate ineffective ventilation and tissue hypoxia.

Indications of ineffective ventilation and tissue hypoxia

- Absent or diminished breath sounds.
- Decreased tidal volume and minute ventilation.
- Change in respiration rate, depth and pattern.
- Expiration time – in patients with any of the obstructive lung diseases expiration time is 1.5 times longer than the inspiration time.
- Tachypnoea – defined as greater than 24 breaths per minute.
- Dyspnoea.
- Air hunger.
- Position of trachea – is the trachea mid-line or is it deviated to one side or another? A pleural effusion or tension pneumothorax usually deviates the trachea away from the diseased side. Atelectasis pulls the trachea toward the diseased side.
- Cough – is it effective or shallow and ineffective?

- Cyanosis.
- Low urine output.
- Dysrhythmias.
- Clammy, cold, sweaty skin.
- Patient distress or anxiety.
- Confusion.
- Lethargy.
- Drowsiness.
- Coma.

Breath sounds can also be used as an indicator of abnormal or normal ventilation.

Abnormal breath sounds include:

- *Rales/crackles* – which are defined as fine or coarse short interrupted crackling or bubbling sounds heard during inspiration.
- *Rhonchi* – described as loud gurgling continuous noises in the larger airways. These are usually more prominent on expiration.
- *Wheezing* – described as whistling noises.
- *Expiratory grunt*.

The nurse may also use *chest percussion* when assessing a patient's ventilation state.

- In health the chest has a hollow percussion note.
- In diseases where there is air in the chest or lungs, in patients with a pneumothorax for example, the percussion note is hyperresonant (drum-like sound).
- A dull or flat sound will occur when an area with no air is percussed. Atelectasis, pneumonia, a pleural effusion, thickened pleura or a mass lesion will all cause a percussion note to be dull or flat.

Auscultation, i.e. listening with the diaphragm of the stethoscope pressed firmly against the chest wall, is a technique which allows the nurse to assess the intensity and loudness of the patient's breath sounds.

First listen to a patient's breath sounds when they are quietly breathing, then ask them to take a deep breath. When a maximum deep breath is taken this will normally cause a four-fold increase in breath sounds. In patients with airway obstruction, chronic obstructive airways disease or atelectasis for example, the breath sound will be diminished.

Restricting the movement of the diaphragm will also cause diminished breath sounds in the area of restriction. This happens in obese patients or in pregnancy.

Pleural thickening, pleural effusion, pneumothorax and obesity all insulate the breath sounds making them less loud.

When performing a respiratory assessment the nurse must also remember that patients with an underlying neurological disorder with characteristic muscle weakness may not necessarily exhibit the usual signs of respiratory distress associated with an increase in the work of breathing. In patients with such a neurological disorder the nurse must be able to observe for other indicators of ineffective ventilation.

So far, we have established how important it is for the nurse to understand the physiological mechanisms fundamental to the delivery of oxygen to the tissues. We have also examined how the nurse can use this knowledge to accurately assess the patient's clinical status and to interpret both objective and subjective measurements that may indicate a change in the patient's condition.

The next part of this chapter will examine the different methods available for administering oxygen therapy to the patient.

Oxygen administration

Oxygen can be delivered in a variety of ways. Whichever method is chosen it is essential that this is the most appropriate device. The oxygen delivery device should deliver a consistent concentration of oxygen, and as far as is possible, be comfortable for the patient.

Oxygen delivery systems can be divided into low-flow systems and high-flow systems.

Low-flow systems include nasal cannulae and the simple facemask. Whilst these devices tend to be the most comfortable for the patient they do not deliver a fixed concentration of oxygen. They work by allowing the patient to inhale room air. This mixes with the oxygen being administered via the mask. When the patient's breathing pattern changes then so does the concentration of oxygen they receive.

High-flow systems include venturi masks and non-rebreathing masks.

Venturi masks can deliver 24 to 40% oxygen. Oxygen enters the mask through a narrow jet opening. This increases the speed of the oxygen flow. Room air is inhaled and mixes with the flow of oxygen through ports cut into the mask. Oxygen concentration is changed by altering the size of the jet opening (the larger the jet the more room air is inhaled so oxygen concentration is lower).

Non-rebreathing masks have a bag attached to the base of the mask. This bag acts as a reservoir for the oxygen. As the patient breathes in, a one way valve between the bag and the mask opens and oxygen is inhaled. At the same time, one way valves over the exhalation ports close to stop entrainment of room air. This means that oxygen concentrations of between 90 and 100% can be delivered. When the patient breathes out, the exhalation ports open and the valve between the bag and the mask closes. This stops the reservoir bag filling with exhaled carbon dioxide.

Continuous positive airway pressure

For some patients supplemental oxygen delivered by nasal cannulae or mask is not sufficient to reduce hypoxaemia. In these patients the use of continuous positive airway pressure (CPAP) can be of benefit. CPAP increases a patient's functional residual capacity (i.e. the amount of air left in the lungs at the end of a normal expiration). This in turn improves lung compliance which helps to correct any mismatch in ventilation and perfusion.

The application of CPAP involves the use of a tight fitting mask. This can be uncomfortable and frightening for patients and is only suitable for patients who are alert, able to clear their own secretions and to protect their own airway (*see* Fig. 3.4).

CPAP can be delivered either by a continuous flow system or a demand-flow system.

Continuous-flow systems have gas flowing through the circuit throughout the whole of the respiratory cycle. These systems are noisy and use very large volumes of piped gases.

Demand-flow systems on the other hand, only deliver gas when the patient starts to breathe in. These systems are quieter and more economical. For them to work, however, the patient has to be able to make enough respiratory effort on inspiration to open a valve, which then allows the gas to flow. These systems therefore create additional respiratory work and the patient must be assessed to ensure they are able to provide the effort needed.

The type of valve attached to the mask determines the amount of CPAP administered. Valves which produce lower values of CPAP, i.e. 2.5 to 7.5 cmH$_2$O are more easily tolerated by the patient, but may not always sufficiently increase the patient's functional residual capacity. In these patients it may be necessary to change the valve to one capable of delivering higher degrees of CPAP, i.e. 10 to 15 cmH$_2$O. However, high degrees of CPAP can cause certain problems. The work of breathing will be increased and this may exaggerate the patient's respiratory distress. In such patients, diminishing ventilatory effort may offset the improvement in functional residual capacity.

The success of CPAP can be determined by observing certain factors:

- An improvement in oxygenation assessed through pulse oximetry or arterial blood gas analysis.
- A reduced respiratory rate with an increase in the patient's tidal volume.
- A reduced work of breathing with decreasing signs of respiratory failure.

Place (1997)

Nasal intermittent positive pressure ventilation

Nasal intermittent positive pressure ventilation (NIPPV) is another non-invasive form of ventila-

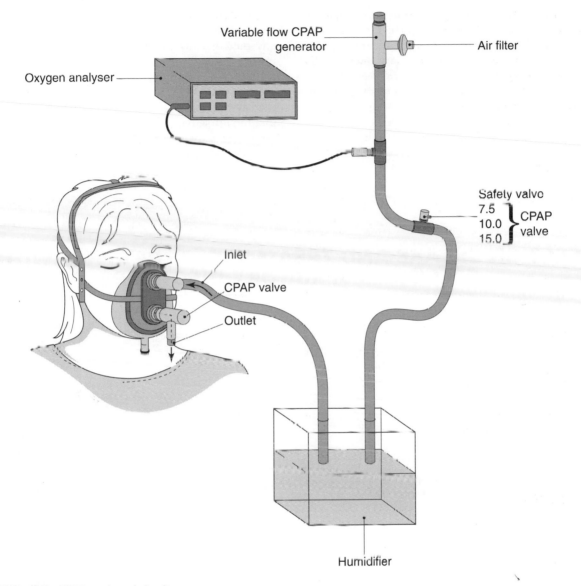

Figure 3.4 CPAP mask and circuit

tory support. Bott *et al.* (1992) advocate its use in the high dependency units, general wards and even in the patient's home.

This method of respiratory support is useful in the patient who can still spontaneously breathe at a reasonable rate but is too tired and weak to produce effective alveolar ventilation.

NIPPV has been shown to be especially useful in treating patients with both chronic and acute respiratory failure, especially those with restrictive chest wall and neuromuscular disorders. Its

use has also been advocated in patients with chronic obstructive airways disease (COAD), producing an improvement in arterial blood gases in both the chronic state and during a phase of acute exacerbation.

In NIPPV a respironics nasal mask attached to a small portable ventilator system administers ventilation. Machine ventilation is synchronized with the patient's own breaths, but if their rate or volume is inadequate the machine will 'top up' the patient's own efforts until it equates with the machine's preset tidal volume. Should the patient become hyponoeic or even apnoeic, the machine will deliver breaths at a predetermined rate set by the operator. Because of the safety back up, the synchronized pattern of breath delivery and the comfortable nasal mask, which is made of soft silicone this method of respiratory support is tolerated very well, often for long periods at a time.

The style of the mask also allows the patient to communicate more freely. Nurse–patient communication is vitally important; the nurse must gain the confidence of the patient, and should remem-ber that the patient being treated with NIPPV will be just as frightened, anxious or confused as any patient who is suffering from some form of respiratory failure. Competence and confidence relayed to the patient through the use of appropriate verbal and non-verbal techniques can help to allay the patient's fears. It is essential therefore that the nurse has a good understanding of respiratory physiology and of the equipment being used along with the skills and knowledge of patient positioning, the use of relaxation techniques and breathing control.

SECTION 3: CARE AND TREATMENT OF PATIENTS WITH SPECIFIC RESPIRATORY DISORDERS

The final part of this chapter will examine the pathophysiology, assessment and nursing management of patients suffering from specific conditions which compromise ventilation.

At the beginning of this chapter the three stages specific to oxygen delivery were discussed:

- Ventilation or breathing.

- External respiration.
- Internal respiration.

Each stage will now be considered in turn, and clinical conditions identified that will compromise that stage of ventilation.

Ventilation or breathing

- Consider patients you have cared for whose condition compromised their ventilation or breathing.
- Make a list of these conditions.

The list you have produced may look something like this:

- Asthma.
- Chronic obstructive airways disease.
- Chest wall injuries such as a flail chest segment, pneumothorax.
- Spinal cord injuries (*see* Chapter 7).
- Guillain–Barré syndrome.

- Head injuries (*see* Chapter 6).

One of these conditions will now be considered in more detail by examining the pathophysiology associated with the condition, why the condition causes ventilation problems and finally the nursing management of a patient with this specific condition.

Supporting the patient with acute asthma

The term asthma is derived from the Greek word for 'panting' which Hippocrates used to describe a condition in which:

paroxysms of difficult and distressing breathing were separated by periods of normal breathing.

The central feature of asthma is its spontaneous airflow obstruction variability. This causes the disease to present with different grades of severity and symptoms.

Asthma is not gender specific and its prevalence is around 5% to 10%, but once a person has been diagnosed as suffering from this disease the potential for it to recur at any time is always there.

The British Thoracic Society describes asthma as a common and chronic inflammatory condition of the airways (BTS, 1990). It is a condition characterized by widespread narrowing of the airways, as the airways become hyperresponsive and sensitive to stimuli. This is termed bronchial hyperresponsiveness and can be caused by many factors.

However, histological studies of the lungs of asthmatics that have died during an asthma attack have shown that asthma is much more than spasm of airway smooth muscle. Other pathological features have included oedematous airways filled with tenacious mucus and mucous plugs, inflammatory cells, i.e. eosinophils and T-cell lymphocytes, and shed epithelial cells.

The asthma inflammatory process can also cause a number of other physiological events to occur, including bronchospasm and hypertrophy of the smooth muscle. If managed well then such symptoms can be reversed and the inflammatory process can be controlled, leaving the patient free from symptoms whilst their lungs are being protected from long-term damage. If not managed properly the disease can cause irreversible damage of the airways. Consequently poor respiratory function accompanied by illness and hospitalization with long-term morbidity can result. Even patients with mild asthma can suffer long-term airway damage if their asthma inflammation is not treated properly (O'Byrne and Thompson, 1995, cited by Wooler and Piddock, 1996).

It is essential that the nurse caring for the patient with acute asthma understands the principles of the diagnosis, treatment and nursing management of this common disease, for, whilst asthma symptoms can be occasional and cause little impact on a person's life, at the other extreme it can be persistent and cause real debilitation.

Signs and symptoms of acute asthma

Acute severe asthma is diagnosed when a patient has had severe progressive asthmatic symptoms over a number of hours or days which remains despite adequate treatment with inhaled sympathomimetics.

The patient suffering with an acute, severe asthmatic attack will be distressed and dyspnoeic. Work of breathing will be increased and accessory respiratory muscle use exaggerated. Inspiratory and expiratory wheezing and chest hyperinflation also occurs. However, as the condition worsens air flow through the bronchi decreases further and the inspiratory and expiratory wheezes are replaced by silence. This may be misinterpreted by the health professional as an improvement in the patient's condition, but a silent chest is more suggestive of further deterioration.

As the condition becomes progressively worse, cyanosis, dehydration, exhaustion and ventilatory failure follow.

ASSESSMENT

Rate of progression of the disease can be estimated by the repeated measurement of specific indices. These include:

- Low peak expiratory flow rate (PEFR), i.e. less than 150 litres/minute.
- Poor bronchodilator response.

As well as these the patient will also present with one or more of the following symptoms:

- Disturbances in conscious level.
- Central cyanosis.
- Exaggerated use of accessory muscles.
- Tachycardia.
- Pulsus paradoxus.
- Pao_2 of less than 8 kPa.
- $Paco_2$ greater than 5.5 kPa.
- Gross lung over-inflation (seen on chest X-ray).
- ECG abnormalities.
- Pneumothorax.

Souhami and Moxham (1990)

These indices must be measured and documented accurately, since without these the severity of the asthma may not be appreciated.

The nursing care and management of a patient with acute severe asthma

The aims of management are to prevent death, to restore the patient's clinical condition and lung function to their best possible levels and to maintain optimal function and prevent early relapse.

OXYGENATION

Immediate treatment will involve the administration of supplemental oxygen and in most patients this can be liberally given without fear. Pulse oximetry and arterial blood gas analysis must be used to monitor its effect.

DRUG MANAGEMENT

High doses of inhaled beta$_2$ agonists are invaluable. Beta$_2$ agonists can be divided into a short-acting group and a long-acting group. The first group includes salbutamol and terbutaline. Given by a nebulizer salbutamol is often very effective in the patient with acute severe asthma. If necessary nebulized salbutamol can be repeated every 3 to 6 hours as prescribed. The longer lasting beta$_2$ agonists include salmeterol and eformoterol. These drugs have a slower onset of action and are most often used on a twice-daily basis in patients with mild to moderate, chronic or nocturnal asthma. In patients with very severe attacks it may also be necessary to administer bronchodilators intravenously.

Systemic corticosteroids are the most effective treatment for treating the underlying inflammation associated with bronchial asthma and should be prescribed and administered to any patient whose asthma is severe enough to warrant hospital admission.

Supportive measures are also important. Patients with severe asthma attacks may become dehydrated and this requires correction. Antibiotics may also be prescribed where there is evidence of an underlying bacterial infection. However, some patients may not respond to the treatment, resulting in worsening hypoxaemia.

When the attack first starts the patient will hyperventilate which will cause an acute respiratory alkalosis. As airway obstruction increases and the work of breathing becomes harder then the patient will become more exhausted. Alveolar ventilation will then fall as respiration declines. This causes retention of carbon dioxide and a corresponding acute respiratory acidosis. At this point transfer to an intensive care unit for mechanical ventilation is necessary.

PSYCHOLOGICAL CARE

Patients with an acute severe asthma attack will be very anxious, distressed, and frightened. Unless supported these symptoms can exacerbate the attack and increase hypoxaemia. Whilst often the best reassurance is improvement of the asthma, until this occurs several other supportive measures must be adopted.

A critical care nurse suffering an acute severe asthmatic attack spoke of the intensity of fear; fear of pain, of suffering, fear of the health professionals, fear of death. She spoke of panic, feelings of suffocating, not being able to take another breath. Her advice to the nurse caring for a patient with such an attack is to explain, give information, communicate in such a way as to convey warmth and confidence. She considers two different ways of behaviour of a nurse. Imagine their effect:

Nurse 1: 'you're nervous, calm down.'
Nurse 2: 'I know what's happening to you. Come on, fight it! A little more and you know it will all pass and you'll feel better. I'm watching you, although I may not be by your side.'

Ruiz (1993)

Summary

Around 30 per cent of patients who die from an acute asthmatic attack do so within 2 hours of onset of the attack. In such patients death is often difficult to prevent. However, many of the remaining 70 per cent of the 2000 deaths that occur in the UK from acute exacerbations of

asthma may be preventable. The use of appropriate long-term therapy, utilization of effective assessment skills which allow early detection of deteriorating asthma in a patient, and correct nursing care and management are all significant factors in improving mortality.

External respiration

For ease of reference, conditions that may compromise external respiration will be divided into:

1 Those which affect the diffusion of gases at the alveolar-capillary membrane.
2 Those which affect haemoglobin concentration and the ability of the blood to carry oxygen.
3 Conditions which affect the cardiac output.

ACTIVITY 3.1

- Consider patients you have cared for whose condition will have compromised the diffusion of gases across the alveolar-capillary membrane.
- Make a list of these conditions.

The list you have produced may look something like this:

- adult respiratory distress syndrome (ARDS);
- fluid aspiration;
- pulmonary oedema;
- pulmonary emboli;
- inhalation burns;
- pneumonia.

We will now consider one of these conditions in more detail by examining the pathophysiology associated with the condition, why the condition causes a disturbance in oxygenation and finally the nursing management of a patient with this specific condition.

Supporting the patient with adult respiratory distress syndrome

Adult respiratory distress syndrome (ARDS) is a form of respiratory failure that results from a variety of direct and indirect pulmonary injuries. It is defined as:

> a fulminant form of respiratory failure characterised by acute lung inflammation and diffuse alveolar-capillary injury.
> Davey et al. (1994) cited by Cutler (1996)

ARDS was first identified as a distinct clinical entity by Ashbaugh et al. (1967) who used it to describe a syndrome of respiratory failure in 12 adult patients with dyspnoea, hypoxia, decreased lung compliance and diffuse pulmonary infiltrates resembling pulmonary oedema. None of the patients had a history of lung disease or cardiac failure.

It is estimated that there are between 10 000 and 150 000 new cases of the syndrome in the UK each year (Cutler, 1996). Mortality rates for sufferers vary according to the severity of the syndrome and other accompanying factors but it is recognized as the major cause of death amongst trauma patients and patients with sepsis.

Causes of ARDS

ARDS is caused by an initiating condition that results in diffuse damage to the alveolar-capillary membrane. Conditions associated with ARDS are numerous but include:

- Shock — from any cause
- Infection — Gram-negative sepsis
  - viral, bacterial or fungal pneumonia
  - *Pneumocystis carinii*
- Trauma — lung contusion
  - blast injury
  - fat embolism
  - non-thoracic trauma
  - head injury
- Aspiration — near drowning
  - gastric acid
- Inhalation — smoke
  - corrosive gases
  - oxygen toxicity
- Haemotological – DIC*
  - massive blood transfusion
  - post cardiopulmonary bypass
- Metabolic — renal failure
  - pancreatitis
  - liver failure
- Drug overdose — heroin, barbiturates
- Miscellaneous — high altitude
  - radiation
  - eclampsia
  - increased intracranial pressure

*Disseminated intravascular coagulation.

Following injury certain pathologic conditions are initiated at cellular level. This includes the activation of macrophages, platelets, proteases, complement by-products, lysosomes, endotoxins, polymorphonuclear leucocytes (PMNs) and free oxygen radicals. Their release is part of the body's natural response to injury, more commonly referred to as the inflammatory response. Unfortunately, this response causes damage to the alveolar-capillary membrane which then becomes more permeable. This results in non-cardiac pulmonary oedema, which is often the first presenting sign of a patient with ARDS.

Pulmonary oedema results in poor gaseous exchange between the alveoli and the pulmonary capillary since it causes the thickness of the gas diffusion barrier and hence the distance that the gases have to diffuse across, to increase. Pulmonary oedema similarly causes small airway closure and microatelectasis which results in a reduced lung volume, reduced functional capacity and a stiff, non-compliant lung.

Secondary to atelectasis there is also a decrease in the production of surfactant which as discussed earlier is responsible for minimizing atelectasis by reducing surface tension. Hyaline membrane formation is also prominent in areas of severe epithelial damage. These membranes consist of necrotic type 1 alveolar cells and intraalveolar proteins, a product of inflammatory exudate. The type 1 alveolar cells, which cover 90 per cent of the gas-exchange surface, are particularly susceptible to injury and incapable of reproduction so as they are destroyed they are replaced by type 2 pneumocytes. These eventually line the alveolus with thick cuboidal epithelium and fibrosis.

The end result of these changes in physiological functioning is hyperventilation, followed by progressive dyspnoea and eventually *type 1* respiratory failure.

Type 1 respiratory failure is described as a PaO_2 of less than 8 kPa (60 mmHg) with a normal $PaCO_2$ in the absence of previous lung disease. Hypoxaemia and widespread cellular hypoxia exist as the patient's oxygen demands start to exceed oxygen intake. Anaerobic metabolism then results. As the patient's condition worsens then *type 2* failure develops.

Type 2 respiratory failure is characterized by a PaO_2 of less than 8 kPa (60 mmHg) with a $PaCO_2$ of greater than 7.0 kPa (53 mmHg), in the absence of previous lung disease. Hypoxaemia and retained carbon dioxide lead to acidaemia and eventually coma (Cutler, 1996).

However, whilst reduced lung volume, reduced functional capacity, reduced compliance, increasing atelectasis and an increased diffusion barrier are responsible for impaired gas exchange, the main cause of hypoxaemia is shunting.

Shunting occurs when ventilation and perfusion are not equally matched. As already established a fundamental characteristic of ARDS is alveolar collapse, which results in under-ventilation of the alveoli. However, the pulmonary capillaries are still perfusing these under-ventilated alveoli but, as the blood is shunted past them, no gaseous exchange can take place because of the collapse. This results in the blood remaining high in CO_2 and low in O_2, which causes a significant oxygenation problem for the patient. This is known as a ventilation/perfusion (V/Q) mismatch. When blood with a low Po_2 level is then mixed with the arterial blood of adequately ventilated capillaries then a total decrease in systemic arterial oxygen content will result which can then lead to tissue hypoxia.

Although the pattern of respiratory distress appears to be similar in all patients with ARDS, the onset of illness following the initial insult may differ considerably depending on the initial insult. For example, patients who have direct lung injury as in trauma, lung contusion or gastric aspiration may develop shallow, rapid breathing as soon as 1 hour after the insult. On the other hand, symptoms of tachypnoea may be delayed for up to 96 hours as in conditions of sepsis or serious pneumonia. However, most patients appear to manifest signs and symptoms of ARDS within 24 to 48 hours after the initial insult.

Indeed, according to how early in the course of the illness the patient is examined there will be certain clinical findings present that appear to be directly related to the physiological changes that occur in the respiratory system. Accordingly, four phases have been identified that correlate clinical findings as well as X-ray results to pathophysiologic changes in the progression of the disease.

The four phases of ARDS

The clinical path of ARDS can be divided into four phases:

Phase 1

Phase 1 is characterized by:

- an initial insult;
- an unexplained tachycardia;
- a mild respiratory alkalosis;
- a normal Po_2.

Phase 2

Phase 2 marks the beginning of respiratory failure and is characterized by:

- dyspnoea;
- fatigue;
- fine rales or crackles in the dependent lung regions;
- a decreasing Po_2;
- patchy infiltrates on the chest X-ray often described as resembling ground glass or white clouds.

Phase 3

Phase 3 is recognized by:

- progressive respiratory failure;
- diffuse rales or crackles;
- rhonchi or low-pitched wheezing;
- extensive infiltration on chest X-ray;
- presence of consolidation on chest X-ray;
- mechanical ventilation which is usually required by this phase to maintain adequate oxygenation.

Phase 4

The final phase usually occurs around 10 days after the onset of illness. At this stage the disease is almost always irreversible with a mortality rate of 80 per cent and is characterized by increasing hypoxaemia and hypercapnia (Brandstetter et al., 1997).

However, whilst these four phases may be clearly identified as the disease progresses, this is not always the case. When caring for a patient at risk of developing ARDS, the nurse must be aware that the patient can pass through these phases very quickly, and as such they may not always be clinically evident.

So, having identified the presenting signs and symptoms of a patient with adult respiratory distress syndrome it now seems appropriate to discuss the nursing care and management of a patient with this disease process.

The nursing care and management of a patient with ARDS

OXYGENATION

Nursing priorities are primarily aimed at maximizing respiratory function and oxygenation. Whilst in many patients, especially those in phases 3 and 4, admission to an intensive care unit for mechanical ventilation is needed to improve oxygenation, during the first two phases `of this disease patients may still be on the ward. In the early stages of the disease supplemental oxygen may be delivered using continuous positive airways pressure mask therapy (CPAP). In some instances, especially in patients with mild to moderate ARDS, facial CPAP has actually lessened the need for intubation and mechanical ventilation (Domigan-Wentz, 1985).

Positioning patients to optimize oxygenation must also be considered. Whilst turning and positioning patients is an important part of the patient's care, few nurses use it to improve their oxygenation. In patients with ARDS, the prone position has been shown to significantly improve their oxygenation. In some patients however, the practicality of turning them completely prone must be assessed. In patients where this position is not feasible the semi-prone position is a possible alternative.

Assisting the patient to cough can reduce retention of tracheobronchial secretions. Measures such as chest percussion, vibration, postural drainage and humidified air will also help to compensate for the decreased function of the cilia.

Serial haemoglobin must also be optimal. Most of the volume of oxygen is transported to the tissues in combination with haemoglobin so if anaemia is present then the oxygen content of the blood will be reduced. As a result the effects of supplemental oxygen would be minimized. Serial haemoglobin measurements are therefore necessary for calculation of the oxygen content, which will determine the need for transfusing red blood cells.

FLUID MANAGEMENT

Nursing care is also aimed at maintaining an adequate cardiac output to assist with oxygen delivery and organ perfusion. However, fluid management remains one of the most controversial debates in the discussion regarding the management of patients with ARDS.

Advocates of fluid restriction argue that by actively trying to lower pulmonary capillary pressures through the combined use of fluid restriction and diuretics the risk of pulmonary oedema is reduced. However, on the other hand fluid restriction may result in organ hypoperfusion. What does remain questionable is whether perfusion, when posing a threat, should be treated principally by adjustments in volume status or by the use of inotropes and vasodilators. However, what is important is that whatever treatment is prescribed, the nurse must be able to accurately assess and interpret its effects through the use of clinical and/or invasive monitoring of both organ function and haemodynamics. Therapy should then be manipulated as necessary to maintain adequate perfusion and oxygen delivery.

NUTRITIONAL SUPPORT

Adequate nutritional support in patients with ARDS is also strongly supported. Whilst nutritional manipulation to meet high metabolic rates and control inflammation is still in the early stages of understanding, it is suggested that antioxidant defences demand proteins, amino acids and certain trace elements and that the replacement of vitamins A, C and E is essential as large amounts are often lost especially if the patient is a burns or trauma victim.

Malnutrition also causes deterioration in a patient's pulmonary function. Wasting of respiratory muscles and the effects of malnutrition on the patient's central nervous system cause a reduction in the actual level of ventilation.

Where patients are too ill to meet their own nutritional needs, nutritional support by enteral feeding is suggested. Enteral feeding maintains the integrity of the gut wall, which may prevent systemic sepsis caused by the migration of enteric commensal microorganisms into the blood stream. If enteral feeding is not possible then parenteral feeding may be prescribed.

PHARMACOLOGICAL MANAGEMENT

Many pharmacological agents have also been tested to treat the inflammatory phase of the syndrome. Most recently it is the benefit of corticosteroids that has been described. These are thought to have the most effect if commenced early in the disease process. In fact Murch (1995), Tabor *et al.* (1992) cited in Cutler (1996), and Morris (1994), have indicated that with specific inflammatory inhibitors such as platelet-activating factor inhibitors and prostaglandin inhibitors only pre-treatment before inflammation is established will allow complete prevention of damage. This makes it even more important for the nurse to be on the look out for these signs in patients who may be at risk of developing ARDS.

However, there have been several advancements in the treatment of ARDS through the years. These range from corticosteroid administration which aims to modify the inflammatory response, inhaled surfactant and inhaled nitric oxide. Animal studies have demonstrated significant improvements in pulmonary mechanics and gaseous exchange following treatment with surfactant, and more recently the use of aerolized surfactant in patients with ARDS has been shown to improve oxygenation significantly. However, trials using surfactant in patients with ARDS remain in the early stages.

Inhalation of low concentrations of gaseous nitric oxide results in selective pulmonary vasodilation causing improvement in gaseous exchange and reduction of pulmonary hypertension. However, as a relatively new treatment, more evidence is needed before its effect on survival rates of patients with ARDS can be proven.

Pain assessment and management are also essential features in the nursing care of a patient with ARDS. Patients suffering with this syndrome are already struggling to meet their body's oxygen requirements. Anxiety, pain and restlessness can increase oxygen demands and shunting. Nursing measures must therefore aim to control pain and anxiety. Pharmacological approaches to pain control may be used, but non-invasive, alternative techniques such as relaxation, positioning, transcutaneous nerve stimulation and appropriate distraction strategies must also be considered.

PSYCHOLOGICAL CARE

Patients with ARDS may suffer from anxiety, confusion and irritability as a result of inadequate oxygenation. A strange, unfamiliar environment can also cause similar symptoms. As part of the management of the syndrome a multitude of diagnostic tests and treatments ranging from blood sampling, chest X-ray, postural drainage and physiotherapy will also be required. These can leave the patient feeling afraid and helpless.

Observation and management of such symptoms is a vital part of the nurse's role essential to the wellbeing of the patient and their family. Interventions should include the reinforcement of explanations and information giving at an appropriate level. Questioning should be encouraged and clarification provided where necessary. Communication, both verbal and non-verbal should be used to relay trust and confidence and the environment should be calm and restful. Nurses can also involve the patients' relatives in the relief of fears and anxieties by ensuring that they are also well-informed and reassured and by allowing them the freedom to visit their loved ones and participate in their care wherever possible.

Nurses can contribute a great deal to both the psychological and physical wellbeing of the patient. In fact, by attending to the psychological needs a reduction in anxiety and fear may be accompanied by an improvement in haemodynamic variables and reduced respiratory effort.

Summary

As work continues to find a cure for ARDS, patients suffering from this syndrome demand effective nursing care on all levels. At present the best therapeutic approach is to identify those patients most at risk of developing ARDS which allows early intervention and treatment (Brandstetter *et al.*, 1997). Treatment must also be aimed at correcting the primary disorder and any underlying disease. The unique position of the nurse, strengthened by the delivery of around the clock care, enables us to use our skills and knowledge to secure the best possible outcome for the patient with ARDS.

ACTIVITY 3.2

- Consider patients you have cared for whose condition caused a drop in their serial haemoglobin content and in the ability of the blood to carry oxygen.
- Make a list of these conditions.

The list you have produced may look something like this:

- haemorrhage;
- haematological disorders, e.g. leukaemia;
- inappropriate fluid replacement;
- carbon monoxide poisoning;

ACTIVITY 3.3

- Consider patients you have cared for whose condition compromised their cardiac output.
- Make a list of these conditions.

- haemoglobinopathies, e.g. sickle cell disease.

The list you have produced may look something like this:

- hypovolaemia;
- acute myocardial infarction;
- cardiac tomponade;
- dysrhythmias, e.g. atrial fibrillation, tachycardia;
- septic shock.

Internal respiration

Internal respiration describes the diffusion of oxygen from arterial blood into the tissues. Once inside the cells oxygen is used to produce energy required for cell metabolism. This process is known as aerobic metabolism.

ACTIVITY 3.4

- Consider patients you have cared for whose condition compromised this process.
- Make a list of these conditions.

The list you have produced may look something like this:

- hypovolaemia;
- disseminated intravascular coagulation;
- septic shock.

The reasons why these conditions affect the ability of the tissues to extract oxygen are discussed in Chapter 2 relating to the cardiovascular system.

Conclusion

Maintaining optimum oxygenation in high dependency care patients must be a primary nursing concern. This chapter provides the nurse with the necessary information needed to understand the physiological principles that underpin oxygen delivery, methods of assessing a patient's oxygenation status and the skills needed to interpret these results. By using this information effectively the nurse will be able to intervene more appropriately and attempt to correct tissue hypoxia.

Nurses caring for critically ill patients need to have the knowledge and skills that equip them to manage life and death situations. Appropriate nursing care can dramatically improve a patient's oxygenation and improve their outlook for recovery.

Further reading

Ashbaugh, D.G., Bigelow, D.B., Petty, T.L. and Levine, B.E. 1967 Acute respiratory distress syndrome in adults. *Lancet* 2319–23.

Bott, J., Keilty, S.E., Brown, A. and Ward, E.M. 1992 Nasal intermittent positive pressure ventilation. *Physiotherapy* **78**(2).

Brandstetter, R.D., Sharma, K.C., DellaBadia, M., Cabreros, L.J. and Kabinoff, G.S. 1997 Adult respiratory distress syndrome: A disorder in need of improved outcome. *Heart and Lung* **26**(1), 3–13.

British Thoracic Society 1990 Research Unit of the Royal College of Physicians of London King's Fund Centre, National Asthma Campaign. Guidelines for management of asthma in adults. I Chronic persistent asthma. *British Medical Journal* **301**, 797–800.

Cutler, L.R. 1996 Acute respiratory distress syndrome: an overview. *Intensive and Critical Care Nursing* **12**, 316–26.

Davey, S.S., McCance, K.L. and Cenzig Budd, M. 1994 cited by Cutler, L.R. 1996 Acute respiratory distress syndrome: an overview. *Intensive and Critical Care Nursing* **12**, 316–26.

Domigan-Wentz, J. 1985 The CPAP mask: A comfortable approach to ARDS. *American Journal of Nursing* 813–15.

Higgins, C. 1996 Principles and practice of blood gas measurement. *Nursing Times* **92**(46), 45–7.

Huber, G. 1979 *Arterial blood gas and acid–base physiology*. New York: Upjohn.

Marieb, E.N. 1992 *Human anatomy and physiology*, 3rd edn., Chapters 3 and 23. California: Benjamin/Cummings.

Morris, A.H. 1994 Adult respiratory distress syndrome and new modes of mechanical ventilation: reducing the complications of high volume and high pressure. *New Horizons* **2**, 219–33.

Murch, S.H. 1995 Cellular mediators of lung damage. *British Journal of Intensive Care* **5**(1), 27–32.

O'Byrne, P. and Thompson, N.C. 1995 cited by Wooler, E. and Piddock, C. 1996 Understanding asthma. *Nursing Standard* **11**(5), 41–7.

Place, B. 1997 Using airway pressure. *Nursing Times* **93**(37), 42–4.

Ruiz, P.A. 1993 The needs of a patient in severe status asthmaticus: experiences of a nurse-patient in an intensive care unit. *Intensive and Critical Care Nursing* **9**, 28–39.

Souhami, R.L. and Moxham, J. 1990 *Textbook of medicine*, Chapter 14. London: Churchill Livingstone.

Tabor, B.L., Lewis, J.F., Ikegami, M. and Jobe, A.H. 1992 cited by Cutler, L.R. 1996 Acute respiratory distress syndrome: an overview. *Intensive and Critical Care Nursing* **12**, 316–26.

Tortora G.J. and Anagnostakas, N.P. 1990 *Principles of anatomy and physiology*, 6th edn., Chapter 23. London: Harper and Row.

Walsh, M. 1997 *Watson's clinical nursing and related sciences*, 5th edn. London: Ballière Tindall.

Caring for the renal system

Bob Donald

Introduction

Renal failure, be it acute or chronic in nature, is not an uncommon problem, presenting a challenge to nurses in the assessment, planning, and implementation of care for patients requiring high dependency nursing. Acute renal failure (ARF) has been shown to prolong hospitalization for as long as 16 to 23 days and to produce a 6-fold rise in mortality (Toto, 1992). The number of patients presenting with chronic renal failure (CRF) continues to increase, and is often associated with age specific conditions and the increased survival rates in such conditions as diabetes.

The perception that renal dysfunction can only be treated by 'high tech' interventions carried out by specialist personnel is being questioned as rapid, conservative interventions have proved effective in the treatment of mild to moderate renal failure, while techniques such as haemofiltration has enabled intensive care and high dependency areas to instigate effective mechanical renal replacement therapy without recourse to renal units.

Those situations in which patients with existing CRF, receiving long-term renal replacement therapy, presenting in high dependency nursing areas for care, are increasing. This is due to the higher survival rates of CRF patients and also the increasing age of initial presentation and treatment. Such patients often have other pathologies requiring interventions from other specialities and the subsequent need for high dependency nursing care.

The aim of this chapter is to familiarize the nurse with the range of potential presentations of renal dysfunction, identify the conservative approach to the care of patients in renal failure, identify the potential mechanical renal replacement therapies available enabling care to be initiated as soon as possible, improving the ARF patients' survival rates and minimizing the complications to long standing CRF patients.

ACTIVITY 4.1

List the main functions of the kidney.

Basic anatomy

The role of the kidney is to provide a stable internal environment in the face of wide fluctuations in the intake of protein and its metabolism, the intake of water and electrolytes, and the body production of hydrogen. In addition the kidney has a major role in maintaining the body's homeostatic status in terms of calcium and phosphate, red blood cell production, and the active control of blood pressure.

The means by which the kidney achieves these functions lies in its highly vascular structure, its ability to control the movement of fluids through the semipermeable membranes of its nephrons and the way in which concentrations of substances stimulate the production of hormones produced directly by the kidney or from other sites which act on the kidney.

The kidneys are bean-shaped organs lying in the upper, posterior portion of the abdominal cavity, either side of the spinal column. The right kidney is situated slightly lower than the left due to the position of the liver.

Leaving the kidney at the inner aspect or pelvis is the fibromuscular tube of the ureter that extends downwards to the bladder, while at the point of the renal hilum are to be found the renal artery and renal vein. The branch of the aorta that gives rise to the renal artery, the fourth, gives some indication as to the vascular requirements of the kidney. The kidneys receive approximate 20 to 25 per cent of the cardiac output which accounts for a blood flow of about 1000 to 1200 mL per minute in a normal adult.

Visually, the kidney is divided into two distinct areas: the cortex and the more distinct medulla, which consists of a number of cone-shaped structures tapering towards the pelvis of the kidney (Fig 4.1).

The cortex is composed of the working units of the kidney, the nephrons, arranged along a series of collecting ducts leading to the calyces. These calyx structures are collecting tubules draining formed urine into the renal pelvis.

The nephrons, numbering approximately 2 million per kidney, have been described as 'blind ended' tubes, the ends being bulbous where arterioles enter the double walled chamber formed by the inversion of the tube, the Bowman's capsule, and where the arterioles form the even finer capillary network, the glomerulus (Fig. 4.2).

The three major processes in the production of urine by the nephron have been described as filtration, reabsorption and secretion. At the level of the Bowman's capsule and the glomerulus pressure is the main driving force in the production of a filtrate. The pressure in the efferent arteriole is high, due to its smaller diameter, compared to that in the afferent arteriole, while the pressure in the peritubular capillary network is considerably lower. The overall effect of this is to produce a far higher pressure within the glomerulus than

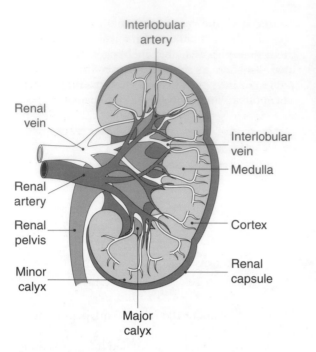

Figure 4.1   The kidney

would be expected in any other arteriole capillary bed elsewhere in the body. This gives rise to a filtration of fluid and other substances through the capillary wall and into the Bowman's capsule. This filtrate is biochemically similar to that of plasma but without the plasma proteins.

By the time the blood leaves the glomerulus and enters the efferent arteriole its composition has changed dramatically, having lost approximately one-fifth of its volume with a corresponding increase of its osmotic pressure from a normal value of 25 to 30 mmHg.

Reabsorption, the second stage of urine formation, takes place both actively and passively throughout the length of the tubule, however because of the osmotic strength of the blood leaving the glomerulus as opposed to the relative weakness of the filtrate in the proximal convoluted tubule then passage of water and nutrients takes place passively across the walls of the capillary and tubule by the action of osmosis. Sodium plays an important part in the creation and main-

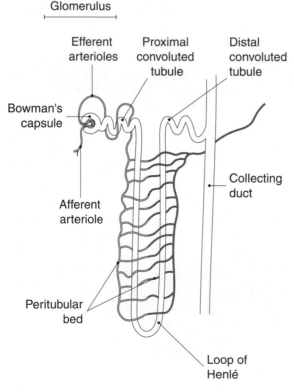

Figure 4.2   The nephron

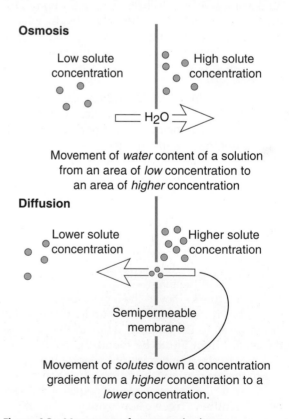

Figure 4.3   Movement of water and solutes

tenance of the osmotic gradients necessary for the movement of water back into the circulatory system. Active transport of sodium, and the co-transport of sodium and glucose and sodium and amino acids ensures that approximately 99 per cent of essential substances are reabsorbed from the filtrate while its volume has been reduced by approximately 65 per cent by the time it reaches the loop of Henlé.

Within the loop of Henlé the filtrate's concentration is altered, allowing the movement of sodium and chlorine ions from the filtrate to the interstitial spaces creating different osmotic gradients along the length of the loop. This process allows the conservation of body water (Fig. 4.3).

The distal convoluted tubule is where the 'fine tuning' of homeostasis takes place and the reabsorption of fluid and ions is under the control of antidiuretic hormone and aldosterone. The secretion of these hormones is instigated by increased blood osmolarity and changes to the blood pressure, resulting in the increased permeability of the distal convoluted tubule and the movement of water back into the circulation. In addition,

sodium and chlorine ions will be actively transported across the cell walls into the circulation, in exchange for potassium and hydrogen ions, with a resulting increase in the reabsorption of water.

Within the collecting duct the final movement of water occurs in response to the osmotic gradients created in the loop of Henlé. At this point the filtrate is finally urine, that is, water, salts, acids, and nitrogenous wastes.

The main functions of the kidney can be summarized as follows:

- Excretion of nitrogenous wastes: urea and creatinine
- Homeostatic control of water
- Homeostatic control of electrolytes
- Control of blood pressure
- Acid–base balance
- Erythropoiesis
- Vitamin D conversion to its activated form
- Calcium and phosphate homeostasis
- Excretion of drugs and toxins

Excretion of nitrogenous wastes: urea and creatinine

Urea and creatinine are waste products of protein metabolism. In the case of urea it is derived from the ingested proteins. These proteins are utilized in tissue protein metabolism which gives rise to amino acids, some of which are deaminated forming ammonia in the Krebs cycle. The liver then converts this ammonia into urea.

In the case of creatinine it is derived mainly from muscle metabolism and therefore is proportional to the individual's muscle mass.

The levels of urea and creatinine will be determined by the kidney glomerular filtration rate (GFR). Urea is readily filtered by the glomerulus

and some reabsorption occurs along the tubule dependent on the dietary intake of protein, the metabolic rate, and the speed at which urine is being formed. Therefore the levels of urea in the blood or urine are not accurate indicators of renal function over time, but can give a 'snapshot' of renal function which can prove useful. Creatinine, on the other hand is almost all excreted via the glomerulus with minimal amounts being reabsorbed; therefore, as muscle mass tends to stay constant, it is a good indicator of renal function over time.

Homeostatic control of water, electrolytes and control of blood pressure

The renal control of these functions are related forming two interrelated feedback cycles and so will be considered together.

The external influences of water and electrolyte balance are dependent on the dietary intake, while the non-renal loss is determined by loss of fluid and salt via sweat, respiration and gastric secretion. However the homeostatic control of the body's fluid and ionic concentration is determined by the kidney's response to osmotic pressures and hormonal influences.

Water balance is controlled by the filtration and reabsorption process within the nephron, under the influence of osmosis, in the proximal tubule, in which 90 per cent is reabsorbed passively, the loop of Henlé and selective reabsorption, under the influence of antidiuretic hormone (ADH) and aldosterone, in the distal convoluted tubule.

The passive reabsorpotion of water in the proximal convoluted tubule is determined by the volume filtered across the glomerulus and the retention, in the blood, of plasma proteins. Water obeys the drive from the area of low tonicity to the area of high tonicity. However the 'fine tuning' of the body is determined by the production of ADH and its activity on the distal convoluted tubule.

Osmoreceptors within the internal carotid artery respond to changes in the concentrations of sodium, and therefore the tonicity, of interstitial fluid. In the event of an increase in tonicity these cells stimulate the ADH-secreting cells of the posterior pituitary gland. ADH is released into the circulation and travels to the tubule where it alters the permeability of the tubule wall. This results in the increased movement, by osmosis, of water from the distal convoluted tubule and collecting duct into the circulating volume. The resulting reduction of tonicity removes the stimulus for the production of ADH resulting in a corresponding diuresis (Fig. 4.4).

The control of blood pressure, other than by the simple influence of circulatory volume, is also under the influence of a hormone, aldosterone, which is secreted in response to changes in blood pressure detected within the kidney.

As the kidney requires a blood flow of 20 to 25 per cent of the cardiac output to maintain function it is imperative that such a flow is guaranteed. This mechanism is controlled by the cells of the juxtaglomerular apparatus (JGA) which lie in the macula densa of the tubule which is formed by the conjunction of the initial portion of the distal tubule and the hilus of the glomerulus. This region touches the cells of the afferent arteriole and as the cell walls of the arteriole are shared with the macula densa they can 'communicate' information as to pressure and osmotic concentrations. In the event of a fall in pressure, thus threatening the glomerular filtration rate, the JGA secretes an enzyme, renin, directly into the blood. The renin then acts on the plasma protein angiotensinogen, produced by the liver, splitting off a fragment, angiotensin I. In the lungs this is converted into a smaller peptide angiotensin II by a converting enzyme which has a stimulating effect on the cortex of the adrenal gland which produces aldosterone. Aldosterone then acts on the distal convoluted tubule stimulating the reabsorption of sodium and with it chlorine. The resulting change in osmotic gradient ensures that water follows and so increases the circulatory volume. In addition angiotensin II also produces a vasoconstriction, thus pushing up the blood pressure. In this way the glomerular filtration rate is preserved by increasing the glomerular pressure and volume.

Where the two feedback systems interlink is at the level of the tonicity control. It can be seen that whatever influences the sodium concentration and fluid tonicity will produce the stimulus for the production of ADH.

Electrolyte concentration, especially of sodium and potassium, again, is fine tuned by these mechanisms. As sodium is absorbed so potassium is excreted by the activity of the active transport system of the sodium–potassium pump, actively moving sodium and potassium through cell walls in opposite directions; as sodium is stimulated to

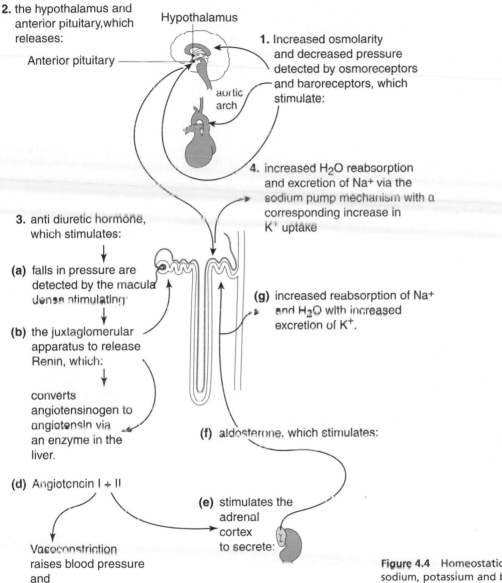

2. the hypothalamus and anterior pituitary,which releases:

Anterior pituitary

Hypothalamus

aortic arch

1. Increased osmolarity and decreased pressure detected by osmoreceptors and baroreceptors, which stimulate:

4. increased H_2O reabsorption and excretion of Na^+ via the sodium pump mechanism with a corresponding increase in K^+ uptake

3. anti diuretic hormone, which stimulates:

(a) falls in pressure are detected by the macula densa stimulating:

(b) the juxtaglomerular apparatus to release Renin, which:

converts angiotensinogen to angiotensin via an enzyme in the liver.

(g) increased reabsorption of Na^+ and H_2O with increased excretion of K^+.

(f) aldosterone, which stimulates:

(d) Angiotensin I + II

(e) stimulates the adrenal cortex to secrete:

Vasoconstriction raises blood pressure and

Figure 4.4 Homeostatic control of fluid, sodium, potassium and blood pressure

enter the blood stream, potassium is actively stimulated to leave via the walls of the tubule and enter the filtrate.

In these ways the homeostatic balances of blood pressure, electrolyte concentration and fluid are maintained in the face of wide fluctuation in the ingestion of water and salts, and variations in blood pressure.

Acid–base balance

The metabolic processes of the body result in the production of high concentrations of hydrogen ions, which not only require to be excreted in order to maintain a blood pH of 7.4, but also need to be transported safely through the body to where they can be excreted.

The hydrogen ions can be 'free', but there are many more that are bound to other substances, that is 'buffered' and it is this way that they are transported to their excretion site. Taking the example of carbonic acid, which is removed by the lungs in the form of CO_2 and water vapour, the carbon dioxide combines with the hydrogen ions to produce a stable blood pH until its removal. The buffering system of the body includes the plasma proteins, red cells, phosphate and sodium bicarbonate, all of which are influenced by the kidney. The kidney itself plays a major role in the maintenance of blood pH in its action of excretion of hydrogen in the urine, and the production of sodium bicarbonate, stimulation of the production of red blood cells, homeostatic control of phosphate and the preservation of plasma proteins. Homeostasis of the acid base balance depends on the three mechanisms of the buffering systems, respiration and kidney excretion of hydrogen.

The site for the active repletion of bicarbonate is the tubular cells, that is the actual walls of the nephron. This process, known as tubular secretion, has two effects, the acidification of urine and reabsorption of sodium bicarbonate by the elimination of hydrogen ions, and the elimination of ammonium which also is as a result of the acidification of urine and conservation of sodium bicarbonate. To do this carbon dioxide is absorbed from the peritubular blood into the tubule wall where it combines with water forming carbonic acid. The enzyme carbonic anhydrase then splits off a hydrogen ion, thus forming bicarbonate. The hydrogen ion enters the urine in exchange for another positively charged ion of sodium which moves into the tubule. This exchange ensures that the hydrogen ion is excreted while the sodium ion combines with the bicarbonate to form sodium bicarbonate which is absorbed back into the blood stream. Once the hydrogen is in the filtrate it is held there by being buffered by such substances as phosphate and creatinine which have been filtered via the glomerulus as part of the excretory function of the kidney. In this way new sodium bicarbonate is created in exchange for excess hydrogen ions.

The second method, which involves the removal of ammonium, also results in the formation of sodium bicarbonate. In the body, ammonium is formed by the deamination of amino acids which are converted by the liver into urea. This urea is normally removed by the glomerular filtration of the kidney. However the renal tubules themselves also deaminate amino acids thus forming ammonia. This ammonia then combines with hydrogen ions in the tubule to form ammonium which is exchanged across the tubule wall with sodium in the filtrate. Again, the sodium combines with bicarbonate to form sodium bicarbonate which is absorbed back into the circulation, while the ammonium is excreted in the urine.

The overall effect of these processes is to acidify urine, usually to a pH of 6, while maintaining blood pH. However, the maintenance of the blood buffers is also the main province of the kidney and so has a primary and secondary role in acid – base balance.

Erythropoiesis

Erythropoietin is the hormone responsible for the stimulation of the production of red blood cells in the bone marrow. It is produced mainly by the kidney although the liver is also capable of producing small amounts. Erythropoiesis is the activity of growth and differentiation of red blood cells in the bone marrow, from progenitor cells to proerythroblasts into reticulocytes which are saturated by haemoglobin. Sensors in the kidney are stimulated by falls in oxygen saturation and erythropoietin is produced, which in turn increases the production of red cells. These new red cells appear in the blood after approximately 2 days, reaching a peak at 5 days, and continue as long as the hypoxia remains. Once the hypoxia is reversed, erythropoietin production decreases immediately. It is thought that erythropoietin plays a role in the increased production of red blood cells by reducing the maturation time of the developing cells prior to leaving the bone marrow by its stimulation of red cell precursors. In this way there can be a relatively rapid response to hypoxia.

Vitamin D conversion and calcium and phosphate homeostasis

The two functions of Vitamin D conversion and the maintenance of calcium and phosphate homeostasis are intimately connected at the level of the control of the systems by the kidney. Calcium has many functions in the body, not just for the development of bone, but also in the regulation of the excitability of nerve fibres, the contraction of the heart, blood clotting, and the maintaining of normal membrane permeability. The body must have sources of calcium from both the diet and from internal 'stores', that is bones and teeth. It is the regulation of these sources of calcium that is the function of the kidney.

Vitamin D conversion is concerned with the ability of the body to absorb dietary calcium from the gut. Vitamin D itself is obtained both from the diet and the action of ultraviolet radiation on the skin.

In addition to this source of calcium from the diet, serum calcium levels are also maintained by the relationship of calcium in bone and the levels of phosphate. The stimulus produced by alterations in these levels are picked up by receptors in the parathyroid gland which is responsible for the hormonal control of calcium. Falls in the level of serum calcium stimulate the release of parathyroid hormone (parathormone) which acts directly on the bone to release calcium into the blood. In addition the parathormone stimulates the conversion of Vitamin D in the kidney and the tubular reabsorption of calcium from the filtrate, thus increasing the uptake of calcium. As the serum calcium level rises, so phosphate levels fall as it is actively excreted by the kidney and as bone cannot be laid down without the active participation of phosphate then serum levels of calcium will be elevated.

To return the calcium and phosphate levels to normal, calcitonin, another hormone secreted by the thyroid, responds to the increase in serum calcium levels by increasing urinary excretion of calcium. Phosphate levels increase and so enable calcium to move into the bone through the stimulation of osteoblasts and the suppression of osteoclast activity.

These complex 'negative feedback' systems ensure that calcium levels are maintained, but also that the skeletal structure is remodelled continuously.

Excretion of drugs and toxins

The kidney is perhaps the most important route for the excretion of most drugs and their metabolites. This in itself can cause potential problems for the kidney as not only drugs but also other potentially toxic substances can reach high concentrations in either the glomerulus or the renal tubule. Generally, drugs are lipid-soluble and therefore not rapidly excreted. Through the action of the liver which converts them to water soluble molecules, the kidney can readily excrete them. However, the process used is active transport via tubular secretion and so high intracellular concentration can occur in the renal tubular cells. To avoid the potential nephrotoxic effect of such concentrations adequate fluid intake to maintain a diuresis is advisable.

Acute renal failure requiring high dependency nursing

ACTIVITY 4.2

How might a patient present who is suffering from signs of renal failure?

In 1992 a survey of the management of acute renal failure (ARF) in the critically ill in England and Wales (Amoroso and Greenwood, 1992) indicated that a change had occurred in the transfer rates of patients in ARF to specialist renal centres over the past 10 years. Rather than transferring patients, they are more likely to be managed locally in intensive care or high dependency units. There is also a trend for treatment to be managed not by nephrologists or renal nurses but by ICU trained nurses and, in intensive care areas, by anaesthetists. This reflects the trend towards the use of continuous venovenous haemofiltration within high dependency areas as a means of controlling the patient's fluid and electrolyte balance. This change increases demands on nurses undertaking the care of such patients. The key to the effective planning and implementation of such care is an understanding of the causes and the effects of ARF.

Causes of ARF

The classic approach in identifying the causes of ARF is to identify whether it was due to factors affecting the whole body, *pre-renal causes*, those which effect the kidney itself, *renal causes*, or those which produce problems in the renal tract, *post-renal causes*.

PRE-RENAL CAUSES

- Severe reduction of renal perfusion due to hypovolaemia from loss of blood or plasma, therefore haemorrhage from trauma or surgery or burns.
- Severe reduction of renal perfusion due to impaired cardiac function due to congestive cardiac failure, myocardial infarction, arrhythmias, pulmonary embolism, pericardial tamponade or cardiogenic shock.
- Loss of glomerular perfusion pressure due to severe vasodilatation which may be secondary to septicaemia, use of vasodilatory drugs or ACE inhibitors. Alternatively, vasoconstrictive effects of non-steroidal anti-inflammatory drugs used for analgesia can result in the constriction of the afferent arteriole and therefore the hypoperfusion of the glomerulus.
- Fluid and electrolyte depletion due to extracellular fluid loss or dehydration, therefore bowel obstruction, severe vomiting and diarrhoea, gastric infections, fluid losses and volume shifts in pancreatitis and peritonitis etc.

RENAL CAUSES

- *'Acute on chronic'* presentation of a pre-existing renal condition, often undiagnosed, e.g. glomerulonephritis, pyelonephritis, diabetic nephropathy, or hypertensive nephrosclerosis.
- *Inflammatory causes*, such as the effects of infective agents such as streptococcus, or vasculitic causes such as an acute presentation of polyarteritis nodosa, or systemic lupus erythematosus.
- *Acute tubular necrosis* due to prolonged 'pre-renal' causes, including hypoperfusion, hypotension and hypovolaemia.
- *Effects of nephrotoxic substances* such as myoglobulinurea and haemoglobinuria from 'crush' injury and fractures. Also nephrotoxic damage from such drugs as antibiotics, particularly the penicillin derivatives, paracetamol and radiographic contrast medium.
- *Toxic poisons* from bacteriological sources such as *clostridium welchii*, and man made substances such as organic solvents, ethylene glycol and mercuric chloride.

POST-RENAL CAUSES

- Either mechanical or functional obstruction to the upper or lower renal tract including, ureteric strictures, calculi, blood clots, retroperitoneal fibrosis and tumours compressing the ureters, benign prostatic hypertrophy and urethral strictures or even obstruction of urinary catheters.
- Obstruction of the upper renal tract can be caused by intrarenal blockages brought about by such things as myeloma protein or uric acid crystals.
- Damage to the nerve supply to the bladder and ureter through spinal cord damage or disease preventing adequate micturition and promoting retention.

Principles of care

The care of a patient in ARF is based on three factors:

1 To treat the cause or causes.
2 To protect the patient from the consequences of the renal dysfunction in terms of the effects the ARF will have on the other body systems and ultimately the potential death of the patient from such problems as hyperkalaemia and cardiac overload.
3 To control the homeostatic functions in the face of very different demands as the ARF progresses through the stages to recovery.

What to look for

Initially the problem will be one of oliguria, that is a urine output less than 400 mL per day, which will be present in all three types of ARF, but will vary between anurea, urine output less than 100 mL per day, or even non-oliguria with an output greater than 400 mL per day dependent on the site and cause of the renal damage. In addition the ratio between the blood urea and the creatinine will vary also dependent on the site and cause.

Pre-renal failure, characterized by hypoperfusion, will result in a change in urea/creatinine ratio from the normal 10:1 to one greater than 20:1 due to the increased reabsorption of urea from slowly moving filtrate in the renal tubule.

The urine is characterized by having a high osmolarity and specific gravity while the urine sodium concentration is low and there are few, if any, sediments. This reflects the intact structure of the tubules which are attempting to respond to changes in the stimuli controlling their function.

Renal causes will be characterized by oliguria or anuria with a normal urea/creatinine ratio, both, however, being elevated. Urine osmolarity and specific gravity are low indicating the failure of the tubules to concentrate the urine, while urinary sediment will show the presence of renal epithelial cells, casts, and protein.

Post-renal causes will be typified by a normal urea/creatinine ration, both being elevated, and, like pre-renal failure, a urine osmolarity and specific gravity that is high. However as time passes the urine will become less concentrated and sodium content will rise. The oliguria may well fluctuate with polyuria with an output over 6 litres a day depending on the location and type of obstruction. Haematuria is a common feature in prostatic obstruction.

Following the oliguric stage, after a period ranging from hours to weeks, is the diuretic phase in which filtration increases but the tubules' ability to reabsorb remains compromised and so large volumes of dilute 'urine', which is more pure filtrate, is passed. It is during this phase that the principles of care appropriate to the oliguric stage are reversed in terms of fluid and electrolyte control and blood pressure regulation.

Finally the concentration or post-diuretic recovery phase is reached in which the tubule recovers the ability to reabsorb and to respond appropriately to hormone stimulation. This stage can last for anything up to a year before total control is re-established; however during this phase there is sufficient normal function to ensure health.

Assessing the patient

In assessing the patient attention must be paid to the cause of the renal insult and the needs generated by that cause. So, for example, a victim of trauma may well have haemorragic shock, have been subject to nephrotoxic drugs in the surgical stabilization of the injuries, received large doses of antibiotics and non-steroidal anti-inflammatory drugs post op, and as a consequence developed ARF. In addition to the care required with the original injuries, assessment of the effects of the ARF will generate very different requirements that must be taken into consideration if the patient is not to succumb to either permanent renal damage or death (Stark, 1994).

Urinalysis and the urea/creatinine ratio has already been discussed, however other haematological investigations will indicate potential problems associated with ARF (Driver, 1996).

Serum potassium (*normal range 3.5 to 5 mmol/L*) may well be raised due to the failure of the kidney to excrete the potassium load. There will also be a shift of intracellular potassium to the extracellular

space caused by the acidosis associated with ARF, hypoxia, infection and an increased metabolism resulting in a catabolic state. Potentially lethal hyperkalaemia can result in increased myocardial excitability and arrhythmias, ventricular tachycardia and eventual ventricular fibrillation where the potassium is greater than 7 mmol/L.

Serum sodium (*normal range 135 to 147 mmol/L*) can actually fall in ARF due to the diluting effects of fluid overload and water retention. However this may mask a total increase in total sodium within the body. The effects of such an increase will produce problems associated with the over-stimulation of anti-diuretic hormone (ADH) and the stimulation of thirst and the active reabsorption of water from the tubules even in the face of existing oedema.

Metabolic acidosis will be indicated by a fall in blood pH below 7.35 and a plasma bicarbonate below 22 mmol/L. This is due to failure to excrete hydrogen ions via the kidney and a failure of the kidney to conserve sodium bicarbonate.

Fluid balance

In considering the fluid balance of the patient attention must be given not only to volume but also to location.

Initially the problem with fluid balance could well be one of classic oedema affecting the tissues but progressing to left ventricular heart failure with pulmonary oedema. However, the problem could well be hypovolaemia due to dehydration or volume loss due to haemorrhage or dehydration. This will present with hypotension, which soon becomes a problem of fluid overload in the face of increased fluid intake in the presence of oliguria. This, in turn, will result in generalized tissue oedema as the kidney fails to regulate and excrete excess fluid leading to raised central venous pressure (CVP) and an increasing catabolism. Pulmonary oedema will result in dyspnoea and the associated cardiac failure will exacerbate the situation.

In terms of 'location', consideration must be given to the ability of the fluid to move between the intracellular and tissue compartments and the circulatory system. The problem here is the loss of serum protein (normal level 60 to 80 g/L) and therefore the loss of the osmotic 'pull' back to the circulation where the fluid would be available to the tubules. This reduced osmotic gradient means that fluid forced from the circulatory system to the tissues by the hydraulic pressure of the heart remains trapped in the tissues producing intractable tissue oedema.

In dehydration the picture is one of increased serum protein, however protein will be lost in such presentations as the nephrotic syndrome, malnutrition, liver disease, burns or haemorrhage and will be associated with a fall in serum albumin to below 35 to 55 g/L. Hypoproteinaemia presents the problem of tissue oedema that is unresponsive to diuretics or mechanical methods of removal and can occur either as a result of specific renal disease causing proteinuria, or as a result of the effects of secondary causes of ARF resulting in gross protein loss from routes other than the kidney.

The classic presentation of problems associated with protein loss in renal dysfunction in the face of non-oliguric output is that of the nephrotic syndrome, and the collection of symptoms that occur in this condition also casts light on the problems that occur in non-nephrotic causes of hypoproteinaemia.

Nephrotic syndrome is characterized by proteinuria with loss greater than 3.5 g per 24 hours resulting in hypoproteinaemia. The severe oedema resulting from loss of osmotic pressure is exacerbated by the loss of circulatory volume either to the tissues or from the osmotic diuresis that occurs resulting in polyuria. The corresponding hypotension stimulates the release of antidiuretic hormone and the subsequent reabsorption of water via those tubules still functioning. At the same time the glomerulus will have responded to the fall in pressure by increasing the production of renin, resulting in increased production of angiotensin and aldosterone and a subsequent increase of sodium uptake and retention. In this way the problems of fluid overload are not simply one of volume but of the disruption of the regulatory functions exacerbating the fluid overload problems causing additional complications to patients' treatment.

Cardiovascular problems

Cardiac problems occur which are closely related to the ability of the kidney to regulate fluid and sodium, as outlined above. They are also related to the kidney retaining sodium and water in response to the abnormal production of renin and angiotensin as a result of poor glomerular perfusion. The result is stimulation of active reabsorption of water and sodium from the tubules due to low arterial blood volume either through myocardial infarction, cardiac surgery etc. or cardiac failure due to overload itself. It is often a circular problem, the loss of glomerular pressure results in fluid retention, which results in cardiac failure, which results in loss of glomerular pressure, and so on until gross oedema occurs. The additional problems of initial hypertension associated with fluid overload, ventricular hypertrophy, left ventricular failure, pulmonary oedema, right ventricular failure, a fall in cardiac output and hypotension, will soon follow.

In addition, the efficiency of the myocardium will be compromised by the retention of potassium due to the inability of the kidney in ARF to excrete excess, and the failure to regulate its hormonal control via ADH. There is an additional potassium load as intracellular potassium is released through tissue damage, surgery or muscle trauma. This results in increased cardiac excitability presenting as ventricular tachycardia or ventricular fibrillation.

Finally, myocardial ischaemia can result from the low haemoglobin associated with either blood loss or the failure of the kidney in ARF to produce erythropoietin, resulting in a fall in oxygen carriage and generalized tissue hypoxia, exacerbation of acidosis, and angina.

Respiratory problems

Respiratory function is compromised in ARF due to fluid overload, pulmonary oedema and congestive cardiac failure resulting in, initially, hyperventilation, then progressively to respiratory distress and eventually collapse. Tissue hypoxia, confusion, dyspnoea are all potential symptoms.

'Air hunger', or 'Kussmaul' respiration, is a feature of metabolic acidosis in which the patient is blowing carbon dioxide and water vapour from the lungs in an attempt to lower blood pH. It is characterized by the smell of acetone on the breath.

Hiccoughing is a particularly distressing symptom for the patient in ARF. The cause is unknown, but is thought to be associated with a vasovagal stimulation and can continue for days at a time and is extremely debilitating.

Central nervous system problems

Central nervous system disturbances are due to excess of metabolites, electrolytes and acidosis. The manifestation of CNS disturbance in ARF are sometimes ascribed to uraemia. The specific manifestations are confusion, due to the high serum urea and creatinine, an increase in pH and also hypocalcaemia and hyperphosphataemia from the disturbance to the ability of the body to control calcium and phosphate homeostasis. In addition, hyperkalaemia can result in coarse muscle twitching and cardiac manifestations of ventricular arrhythmias or even fibrillation. Hypertension associated with fluid overload or an uncontrolled renin angiotensin cycle can exacerbate the muscular twitching and cognitive disturbance, while the hypernatraemia can cause fluid to be drawn away from the brain into the vascular system by an increased osmotic gradient resulting in minute brain haemorrhages and convulsions. Generalized neuromuscular weakness, lethargy and fatigue are symptoms of the overall toxic state of the patient often accompanied by a reduced tissue saturation of oxygen from such things as blood loss, septicaemia, respiratory failure, or a loss of erythropoietin production causing a drastically lowered red cell count.

Digestive and nutritional problems

Gastrointestinal effects of ulceration, nausea, vomiting, loss of taste and anorexia are due to a combination of factors, primarily the initial insult that results in ARF, but then the effects of the failure. Here the ammonia of hydrogen metabolism fails to be excreted by the kidney and so it is accumulated in the body where it attacks the gastrointestinal tract. In addition, the acetone on the patient's breath, also a symptom of acidosis, reduces taste, while pulmonary oedema leaves the patient severely restricted when it comes to eating. What makes these effects so dangerous in a patient in ARF is the effect on metabolism. The patient becomes hypercatabolic as they utilize their own muscle mass as a source of energy, the body's requirement having accelerated due to the initial insult and now also as a result of the effects of ARF. This in turn, accentuates the 'toxic background' of uraemia, driving up the levels of urea, creatinine and the hydrogen concentration, which in turn worsens the hypercatabolism.

Problems with the skin

Not only is the skin compromised by the presence of oedema, especially over bony prominences, but also due to the effects of acute disease processes resulting in ARF, and acidosis. Acute presentations of vascular disorders such as systemic lupus erythematosus (SLE) can result is purpuric rashes, while maculopapular rashes suggest either drug allergy or interstitial nephritis. Such rashes provide ample opportunity for skin breakdown, especially where there is severe itching and scratching. The reduced oxygenation of the tissues, which are waterlogged and with a background of toxins is a perfect recipe for opportunistic infection and breakdown. In addition, the effect of ARF on the immune response, with reduced macrophage activity, makes the treatment of such infections difficult, especially as antibiotics are nephrotoxic and could further compromise renal function.

ACTIVITY 4.3

Consider the kinds of problems your patient might be suffering from and devise a care plan to help you overcome the worst effects of renal failure

Nursing care considerations

In addition to the care requirements of the patient due to the initial insults to the renal function, specific care is required relating to the effects of the ARF.

Primarily the aim is to preserve and enhance any residual renal function in order to, potentially, shorten the oliguric phase and to maintain the homeostatic functions, avoiding the lethal consequences of ARF.

Hydration status

Maintain accurate assessment of fluid intake from all sources and output from all sources as far as is possible. Triangulate this information, which is notoriously inaccurate, with the patient's daily weight and weight gain over short time scales in order to increase its accuracy. As 1 kilo = 1 litre it is easy to identify fluid overload trends. The association of fluid and blood pressure is a further measurement that can give greater accuracy to the assessment, however this must be supported by assessment of the location of the fluid. In order to achieve this, examination of serum total protein and serum albumin, as well as the normalized catabolic rate, will be of use to identify loss of fluid to the tissues in hypoproteinaemia and therefore the unavailability of the fluid to removal via mechanical or pharmacological means. Assessment of breathing patterns will be of use as will the examination of sputum, white frothy sputum being evidence of pulmonary oedema. Ultimately the hydration status will be accurately established through the measurement of the patient's central venous pressure.

Conservative therapy to address problems associated with the patient's hydration status will depend on whether there is evidence of dehydration, in which case a fluid intake sufficient to maintain a CVP of between 5 and 8 cmH$_2$O will be required. The nature of the replacement fluid must be considered in relation to the evidence of the patient's serum protein, and human protein plasma fraction may well be in order, as well as the use of sodium chloride in relation to the patient's serum sodium.

Oral fluid intake has traditionally been based around the concept of a 500 mL loss through routes, such as respiration and sweat, requiring replacement, with the rest of the fluid allowance being made up of the volume of the previous 24 hours' output. However, this approach, while providing a starting point, should not be ritualistically adhered to. Rather, fluid modification to meet the individual patient's needs, responsive to the physiological changes occurring throughout the genesis of ARF is required. The problem with the 500 mL plus the volume of previous 24 hours is that it makes no concession to fluid overload or dehydration but can simply maintain a fluid overload state or dehydrated state.

Enhancement of whatever renal function remains is of prime importance, not only in relation to fluid balance, but also the maintenance of other homeostatic functions. Correcting circulatory imbalances in order to minimize the effects of hypertension or hypotension will assist in maintaining glomerular filtration rate, while the use of loop diuretics, particularly frusemide or bumetamide will enhance fluid removal. Potassium sparing diuretics should be avoided and the thiazide groups are relatively ineffective once the glomerular filtration rate falls below 25 mL/h and may accumulate causing side effects (Swanson, 1990; Harper, 1990).

In the case of pulmonary oedema, oxygen therapy will be of use as will rebreathing bags where there is evidence of falls in oxygen saturation, while chest physiotherapy will provide benefit.

In the case of poor renal perfusion due to the cardiovascular embarrassment, such as through left ventricular failure, hypovolaemia, cardiac ischaemia etc. then inotropic agents such as dopamine or dobutamine at 3–5 µg/kg/min can not only increase cardiac efficiency but also preserve renal function.

Tissue oedema is a particularly distressing feature of ARF, presenting problems in pressure area care and immobilization of the patient (Driver, 1996). Consideration must be made of where gravity puts tissue oedema; therefore in a prone patient it can be found along the legs, sacrum, back and shoulders and even in the scalp. More mobile patients will more likely present with the classic 'swollen legs'. To adequately address this problem attention must be paid not only to volume but also location of the fluid. As has been said, low serum protein levels will allow fluid loss to the tissues which will prove difficult to remove, therefore the patient's nutritional status must be addressed.

Electrolyte balance

The important electrolytes that require careful monitoring in ARF are sodium, potassium and hydrogen (via the serum bicarbonate level) as they produce some of the more dangerous effects on the body systems in their presentation of hypernatraemia, hyperkalaemia and acidosis respectively.

An assessment of the intake of sodium and potassium compared to the output via residual renal function is required in relation to the phase of the ARF, retention being the primary problem in the oliguric phase, and excess loss in the diuretic phase. The intake from all sources must be considered including i.v. infusions, drugs and nutrition, while in the case of potassium the level of tissue damage present or active physical disorder, such as congestive cardiac failure, will produce leakage of intracellular potassium to the extracellular fluid and circulation. The effect of hypernatraemia on fluid balance has been described, resulting in fluid retention and the stimulation of aldosterone and antidiuretic hormone resulting in escalation of the fluid reabsorption.

Hyperkalaemia will have a disturbing range of effects for the patient, including confusion, lethargy, coarse muscle twitching which can prove distressing, however, at levels in excess of 6 mmol/L there is a risk of cardiac irritability. Hypokalaemia, occurring possibly in the diuretic phase, where the excess loss of fluid 'washes out' electrolytes from the system, has similar effects, except that it will result in asystolic arrest.

The acidosis associated with ARF, due to the increased concentration of hydrogen ions resulting from the failure of the kidney to excrete hydrogen and the failure to conserve bicarbonate, also produces a range of systemic effects. Confusion due to acidosis accentuates the problem of cognitive disturbance due to other excess electrolytes and the patient's safety in the environment must be assessed and ensured.

The means of controlling these electrolytes is by preventing them getting into the system in the first place, so dietary modification and awareness of the sodium and potassium content of medication is essential. Again the stimulation of any residual renal function will assist in maintaining an adequate removal of excess sodium, and in doing so it will assist the patient to adhere to any oral fluid restriction by reducing the stimulus for the production of antidiuretic hormone and the associated thirst.

In the case of potassium it is sometimes difficult to control the hyperkalaemic state as potassium is leaking from damaged tissue. In this case the use of binding agents such as Resonium A or calcium resonium can be used to control the build up, however, where the potassium level is becoming critical then more drastic action is required and so the use of 50 per cent dextrose and soluble insulin i.v. will be called for. This will produce an osmotic shift of fluid from the circulation and tissues into the cells and as the fluid shifts so it carries the potassium into the intracellular compartment, thus lowering the serum potassium level which was causing the increased excitability of the myocardium.

Acidosis may be corrected through the use of i.v. or oral 'buffers' such as sodium bicarbonate or calcium carbonate if there is a problem with the retention of sodium, in conjunction with enhancement of residual renal function through the use of diuretics. In addition the availability of other buffers should be addressed by the improvement of haemoglobin levels, and the control of serum phosphate, as well as ensuring the maintenance or improvement of serum protein levels.

Nutritional requirements

The problems of poor nutritional status in the acutely ill has been well-documented (Arrowsmith,

1997; Dickerson, 1995) as has the consequences of such poor nutritional intake. Muscle loss and decreased body mass has been implicated in the development of depressed respiratory function, cardiac function and mobility. Subsequent impaired immune functioning associated with decreased nutritional intake has also been seen to contribute to chest infection, cardiac failure and increased risk of thrombosis and pressure sores, while the apathy, depression and fatigue forms the returning link of the cycle by further depressing nutritional intake. In patients with ARF the problem is accentuated by their hypercatabolic state brought about by the initial physiological insult and the systemic effects of the renal dysfunction such as cardiac failure, overload etc. In addition the problem of protein restriction used to reduce the workload on the renal system simply accelerates the hypercatabolic state. There is no benefit in protein restriction in catabolic ARF (Smith, 1997) and sufficient protein, nitrogen and carbohydrate sources must be maintained to compensate for catabolic loss.

Enteral feeding is the method of choice as it preserves the gastrointestinal barrier and so protects against bacterial infections. However in the unconscious or ventilated patient total parenteral nutrition may be the only available route. If so then great care must be taken to take account of electrolyte content and to avoid overload, the potential for suppression of the immune response, already suppressed by the ARF and the danger of septicaemia.

Efficient prevention and treatment of malnutrition will make a major contribution to the patient's survival as it not only avoids the potential complications of catabolism but also helps in the control of fluid balance by maintaining serum protein levels and so allows for the oncotic shift of fluid between the cellular, intracellular and circulatory compartments of the body (see Chapter 8). In this way tissue oedema can be corrected through the enhancement of renal function or by mechanical replacement therapy, while in the hypoproteinaemic patient the fluid is not available for removal, trapped in the intercellular compartments.

Control of infection

Infection is a leading cause of death in patients with ARF (Toto, 1992). Common presentations are pneumonia, urinary tract infections and wound sepsis, the progression of which are enhanced by the patient's immunosuppressed condition. Good nursing practice in the institution of central or peripheral venous lines and bladder catheters is essential. Any evidence of infection should be treated with a narrow-band antibiotic, care being taken as to the nephrotoxicity of such drugs and the appropriately modified dosage used. Broad-spectrum antibiotics, especially tetracycline, should be avoided due to their severe nephrotoxicity. Bladder catheters in the oliguric or anuric patient are contraindicated and serve only as an irritant and potential source of urinary tract infection. Frequent cultures of sputum, wound swabs and urine are required and any early signs of infection such as rises in temperature, fever, etc. should be acted on with speed. Early removal of lines (central venous pressure lines, venous cannulae, enteral feeding, etc.) is recommended, and early mobilization of the patient to alleviate the problems associated with bed rest and immobility undertaken.

Ultimately, the survival of the patient in ARF, using such conservative measures, may not be possible, even though the initial physiological insult may have been dealt with. The hypercatabolism, fluid overload, hyperkalaemia and acidosis can prove too great a stress on the body systems, resulting in multiple organ failure. In the face of such potential, mechanical renal replacement therapy will be the main treatment of choice to take over the main functions of excretion of nitrogenous waste, drugs and toxins, control of fluid balance, control of electrolyte balance and the correction of acidosis.

ACTIVITY 4.4
What factors will be included in your assessment of a patient in ARF? How will those factors affect your care plan for such a patient?

Mechanical renal replacement therapy in acute renal failure

Mechanical renal replacement therapy is indicated where the extent of the symptoms of ARF have produced uncontrolled fluid overload, catabolic production of high urea and creatinine, severe acidosis and hyperkalaemia requiring such interventions as dextrose and insulin to prevent cardiac arrhythmias. In addition, in the face of malnutrition and oliguria, 'space' needs to be created to allow for adequate feeding either orally with liquid supplements, or i.v. via total parenteral nutritional support (Stark, 1997).

ACTIVITY 4.5

Under what circumstances would a patient benefit from:

- Peritoneal dialysis
- Haemodialysis
- Haemofiltration

Temporary peritoneal dialysis

Temporary peritoneal dialysis, or 'stab PD', is an easy and effective method of treatment where there is evidence of mild to moderate severity, with associated electrolyte imbalances, fluid overload and metabolic acidosis. It is also the method of choice where haemodialysis is contra-indicated because of haemodynamic instability, lack of access to the patient's blood or intolerance of anticoagulation, or lack of specialist facilities. PD has the distinct advantages of being simple to institute and run, and affords swift control of fluid and electrolyte balance (Fig. 4.5). However, there are disadvantages.

Contraindications include recent abdominal surgery or trauma and hypercatabolic states as urea clearance is only approximately 25 mL/min (Gabriel, 1975).

The system is uncomfortable for patients and leakage of fluid from the entry site can excoriate skin. Protein is lost to the dialysate fluid and therefore hypoproteinaemia can be exacerbated with subsequent intractable oedema and potential circulatory collapse. In addition malnutrition can be precipitated or accelerated through this protein loss.

Respiratory problems can occur with the volume of fluid in the abdomen 'splinting' the diaphragm which can give rise to basal lung collapse or the retention of secretions and subsequent respiratory depression and chest infection.

Peritonitis is a likely complication due to the direct access PD provides to the abdominal cavity and will require swift and effective antibiotic treatment, usually via the dialysate fluid direct. While it is painful and distressing for the patient it does not represent the life threatening condition of peritonitis from other causes unrelated to PD.

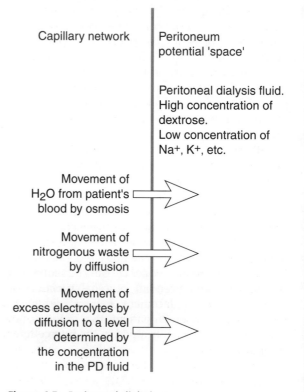

Capillary network

Peritoneum potential 'space'

Peritoneal dialysis fluid. High concentration of dextrose. Low concentration of Na^+, K^+, etc.

Movement of H_2O from patient's blood by osmosis

Movement of nitrogenous waste by diffusion

Movement of excess electrolytes by diffusion to a level determined by the concentration in the PD fluid

Figure 4.5 Peritoneal dialysis

However, if untreated or inadequately treated it can lead on to sepsis.

Despite these disadvantages, PD offers a gentle but efficient method of dialysis in the 'acute' situation in the relatively stable patient. It can be carried out by nursing staff as part of their routine care and requires no great specialist equipment or expertise, requiring only good nursing practice to manage the process.

TECHNIQUE

Temporary PD catheter insertion is a relatively simple process carried out under local anaesthetic as described by the 'abdominal paracentesis' procedure in manuals of clinical nursing procedures such as that produced by The Royal Marsden Hospital (Pritchard and David, 1990). A cannula is introduced through the abdominal wall approximately 2 inches below the umbilicus using a trocar. The position of the cannula is between the parietal and visceral layers of the peritoneum which forms an 'envelope' with a potential space between them. Once in position the cannula is held secure by the use of a purse string suture and keyhole dressings. The cannula can be further secured with the use of waterproof tape enclosing the insertion site and dressing.

Once the cannula is in place a closed delivery and drainage system is attached to the cannula consisting of a proprietary peritoneal dialysis fluid bag and associated giving set. Those systems which utilize a luer lock between the bag and giving set increase security of the system. Hypertonic fluid (up to 2 litres) is then instilled into the potential space between the peritoneal layers and then drained again. The bag is exchanged with a new one of fresh solution and the process is repeated. The speed at which these 'exchanges' are performed determines the efficiency of the dialysis.

The large surface area of the peritoneum and its semipermeable and highly vascular nature allows the transport of fluid, waste product and excess electrolyte across the membrane to the hypertonic solution. Water removal is under the influence of osmosis while substances of low molecular weight pass down a concentration gradient by the action of diffusion. The dialysis fluid is made hypertonic by its concentration of glucose or dextrose while its concentration of sodium, chloride, lactate, magnesium and calcium ensure that the patient can lose no more of these substances than the level in the dialysate fluid. A rapid exchange cycles will ensure the efficient removal of water, while the inclusion of a 'dwell time' of approximately 30 to 45 minutes will increase the removal of urea, creatinine and electrolytes. An even greater dwell time, in stabilized patients, of 3 to 4 hours may be effective in the removal of high molecular weight toxins. Therefore the exchanges can be modified to suit the individual needs of the patient.

Careful measurement of the drained fluid must be made, an easy method being to weigh the drained bag, and a running total of the fluid loss made. Blood results also require careful monitoring for evidence of hypokalaemia, as potassium removal is readily achieved in the non-catabolic patient.

Certain dialysate fluids can be obtained which contain bicarbonate in conjunction with lactate and so provide a total buffer level sufficient to correct metabolic acidosis.

Once the desired effect of PD has been achieved with the development of either the oliguric phase or recovery phase, or the need to move on to a more aggressive form of replacement therapy, then the cannula is easily removed and the site covered with an occluding, waterproof dressing.

Haemodialysis

In those centres where specialist renal personnel are available then haemodialysis may be the treatment of choice in both the moderate and the severe presentations of ARF. The treatment of the patient by haemodialysis utilizes machinery designed to drive the patient's blood through an artificial kidney or dialyser (Fig. 4.6). This dialyser is commonly made up of hollow fibres of a semipermeable material through which the blood will be pumped. Around the outside of these fibres will flow dialysate fluid, the hypertonic solution against which the blood will dialyse. Unlike PD, which is reliant simply on the forces of osmosis and diffusion for its effect, haemodialysis is far more aggressive, utilizing the positive pressure generated on the blood side of the dialyser and the negative pressure generated on the dialysate side by the action of drawing the dialysate fluid through the 'kidney' rather than pumping the fluid into it. In conjunction with the osmotic gradient created by the use of hypertonic dialysate, and a concentration gradient like that for PD fluid, the pressures generated across the membrane greatly increase the efficiency of fluid and solute removal.

Haemodialysis serves as a rapid method of correcting severe fluid and electrolyte imbalances (Stark, 1997) and is indicated where there is evidence of hypercatabolic 'uraemia', hyperkalaemia, hypernatraemia, volume overload and symptomatic metabolic acidosis. It can also prove useful in certain drug overdose situations.

The use of haemodialysis is generally restricted to situations where there is the necessary equipment and expertise to use it readily available and

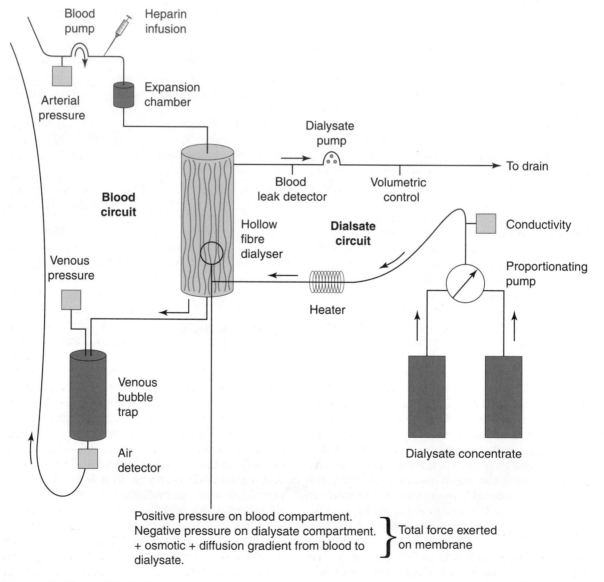

Positive pressure on blood compartment.
Negative pressure on dialysate compartment.
+ osmotic + diffusion gradient from blood to dialysate.
} Total force exerted on membrane

Figure 4.6 Haemodialysis circuit

so requires the infrastructure of a renal unit and specialist renal personnel. Treatment is usually delivered on an 'outreach' basis, consisting of daily haemodialysis of 4 hours' duration, with the care provided in the interdialactic period by the high dependency nursing staff.

The requirement for effective haemodialysis in the acute situation is a blood flow of 100–200 mL/min. Therefore the access line to the patient's circulation is of prime importance and it is vital that it be protected.

In recent years the method of gaining temporary access for haemodialysis has significantly improved with the development of the duel lumen central venous catheter which replaced the far less efficient and more dangerous external arteriovenous shunt. There are three potential sites for the insertion of the catheter: the subclavian vein, the internal jugular vein, both allowing the catheter tip to sit just above or inside the right atrium of the heart, and the femoral vein. The insertion is usually swift and can enable haemodialysis to be commenced within minutes of a check chest X-ray confirming the catheter position.

There are distinct advantages in the use of such catheters for the haemodialysis personnel, such as immediate availability with minimal patient discomfort; little danger of acute thrombosis and ease of removal. However the potential problems must be considered when planning the care of the patient. These include:

Infection

Localized infection of the catheter exit site, especially in the femoral site may occur, as may infection of the catheter tunnel with subsequent septicaemia or subacute bacterial endocarditis.

The use of occlusive dressings and strict aseptic technique will greatly reduce the incidence of infection; however any symptoms must be treated swiftly with narrow band, specific antibiotics, and possibly the removal and resiting of the catheter.

Thrombosis

Subclavian vein occlusion may occur due to the restriction of blood flow around the catheter and may result in swelling of the arm. Thrombosis

within the catheter and subsequent embolism is a very rare occurrence. Any occlusion of the blood flow must be treated by the removal of the catheter, elevation of the arm and possibly the use of systemic anticoagulation.

Patency

The catheter is literally the patient's 'life line' and so should be used only for the haemodialysis treatment and not for any other infusion purpose.

Between dialysis the catheter is 'heparin locked', that is a volume of heparin equal to the volume of each catheter lumen is inserted.

Air embolism

Any breach in the catheter integrity can result in air embolism owing to the 'vacuuming' effect of blood flow through the vein and heart.

The security of the connections, caps and line itself must be monitored. The catheter should be 'double clamped' at all times between dialysis, that is clamped by the in line clamps and by independent clips. The caps on each arm of the catheter must be luer locked and the restraining suture secure.

Cardiac and respiratory

Haemothorax and pneumothorax are potential problems during catheter insertion, however can occur at any time owing to the free movement of the catheter tip within the right atrium allowing potential perforation of the heart wall. Cardiac arrhythmias can occur as the catheter tip stimulates the heart muscle. Any symptoms of respiratory distress, cardiac tamponade or extrasystole must be investigated and catheter involvement ruled out. In the event of atrial perforation emergency procedures for severe respiratory distress must be instigated and an underwater sealed chest drain inserted. The catheter will be removed and repositioned, probably in the femoral vein, for continuation of haemodialysis.

The planning of care involving haemodialysis is very much a multidisciplinary exercise with discussion as to the volume of fluid to be removed considered against the volume to be replaced over the following 24 hours. Considerations of nutritional support and volume in the case of

TPN, as well as the volume of drugs and the cardiac effect of inotropic support will be made in order to tailor the dialysis to those needs. The patient's catabolic status and the effect of electrolyte imbalance will also form a major consideration as to the planned intervention, as will the effect of using bicarbonate-based dialysate fluid on acidosis. Clear aims and objectives of treatment are vital to ensure a seamless provision of care.

Haemofiltration

Increasingly, high dependency units and intensive care areas have developed their own expertise in the use of a continuous method of artificially replacing renal function in the ARF situation. These are:

- Continuous arteriovenous haemofiltration (CAVH).
- Continuous venovenous haemofiltration (CVVH).
- Continuous arteriovenous haemodiafiltration (CAVHD).
- Continuous venovenous haemodiafiltration (CVVHD).

Collectively they are known as continuous renal replacement therapy (Kramer *et al.*, 1982) and have enabled units to develop independent techniques that provide greater control of the patient's fluid and electrolyte balance, as well as mimicking glomerular filtration rate. Using a similar set up as for haemodialysis, haemofiltration uses a filter through which the patient's blood passes via lines. However, the membrane of the filter is far more permeable than that of the artificial kidney and relies on the pressure on the blood side of the membrane to achieve filtration (ultrafiltration) in conjunction with the 'dragging' effect of solutes and water through the movement of fluid by convection. The use of biocompatible membranes help to preserve blood cells and the less aggressive fluid and solute removal provides a far more 'gentle' effect than that of haemodialysis. The process is made efficient by its continuous use rather than the short bursts of treatment as with haemodialysis and therefore is suited to patients

who are critically ill with such complications as cardiovascular instability, sepsis or multiorgan failure (Smith, 1997).

ACCESS

Venous access will vary according to the type of haemofiltration used. CAVH will utilize an arterial and venous catheter, usually inserted into the femoral artery and vein, and will rely on the patient's own blood pressure to drive blood through the system. In this simple version of the process no pumps or plumbing is required and so it can prove highly effective in the initial stages of treatment where fluid removal may be a priority. The use of the femoral artery provides ready access and a 'core' blood pressure that will remain relatively stable even in the face of a falling blood pressure. However, there remain potential problems such as infection, displacement or occlusion of the cannula, thrombosis of the venous return with subsequent embolism and clotting of the entire system if blood flow or pressure is reduced.

CVVH, on the other hand, is far less subject to such problems as it relies on the pumping of blood through the system and so requires more sophisticated equipment including blood pump, venous pressure monitoring system, bubble trap with associated air bubble detector, anticoagulation delivery system, and possibly a filtrate volume monitoring system. As the blood is pump driven then access is achieved via a duel lumen venous catheter in those sites identified as suitable for haemodialysis. The same potential problems and care apply to such catheters as for haemodialysis.

TECHNIQUE

Once access has been achieved the lines and filter are primed with normal saline to exclude any air from the system. The connections to the cannula or the catheter are then made as a sterile procedure and in the case of CAVH, the clamps are removed and the blood flow through the filter commences. Anticoagulation via a pump delivery to the lines is commenced and regulated to give a clotting time of between 15 and 20 minutes using a Lee–White clotting time estimation or an activated clotting time (ACT) system. The anticoagulant used can vary between the heparins or the prosta-cycline groups and the balance between the anti-coagulant and any potential bleeding problems the patient may have must be monitored and adjustments made to prevent any potential haemorrhage.

Filtrate driven across the filter membrane drains into a measuring system and drainage bag at a rate determined by the pressure of blood in the system. A rate of approximately 1 litre per hour can be achieved and so, once the patient's over-hydration state has been corrected, a physio-logical electrolyte substitute solution must be returned to the patient to avoid dehydration. The rate at which this solution is returned to the patient will reproduce glomerular filtration rate and tubular reabsorption. The large volume of fil-trate produced will ensure the removal of water, excess electrolytes and nitrogenous waste prod-ucts, while the returned fluid will be at normal physiological concentration thus mimicking glomerular filtration and tubular reabsorption and maintaining the homeostatic balance.

Careful monitoring of the filtration rate and fluid removal in conjunction with the volume replacement is required and so makes this system rather labour-intensive. The alternative of CVVH, especially in a pump-assisted delivery system, reduces that workload considerably as the volume removed is matched automatically to the volume delivered back to the patient controlled by a microprocessor.

The major advantages of using such systems for patients in ARF are:

- Their simplicity, even in the cases of CAVHD and CVVHD.
- The continuous control of the patient's fluid and electrolyte balance.
- The ability to give adequate nourishment in the form of TPN without fear of fluid overload.
- No requirement for extensive plumbing modi-fications to the unit.
- The speed at which replacement therapy can commence thus reducing the potential side effects of ARF.
- The ease of training for high dependency nurs-ing staff to use such systems in comparison with haemodialysis.

The disadvantages, by comparison are few:

- CAVH and CAVHD are labour-intensive.
- Venous access can present particular nursing difficulties.
- Mobilization of the patient can be delayed.
- Expense and staff training will be required.

However in the face of the ability to take early action to preserve the life of patients in ARF and limit the systemic effects of renal dysfunction without recourse to renal personnel or the transfer of patients to other hospitals with renal units the systems can prove highly effective.

Care of patients with existing chronic renal failure

In the case of the high dependency nursing of patients with existing CRF requiring mechanical renal replacement therapy, attention will need to be paid to the care needs generated by the specific pathophysiology as well as the continuing care needs generated by the effects of CRF. In some cases these will be the same. What is important is the impact the CRF will have on their ability to recover and achieve the optimum healthcare goal. Continu-ity of treatment is the key, with modifications made to address specific problems in light of the effects of CRF, and so a multidisciplinary approach uti-lizing good communication is essential.

Within this section the causes and effects of CRF will be identified and the specific care requirements that are generated. Problems of assessment will be discussed in relation to the 'norms' associated with patients in CRF and finally the provision of continuing mechanical renal replacement therapy will be addressed in relation to possible 'outreach' programmes or the development of localized specialist expertise.

Chronic renal failure: causes

- Glomerulonephritis.
- Hypertension.
- Obstructive uropathy.
- Reflux nephropathy.
- Pyelonephritis: with structural abnormality.
- Toxic nephropathy.
- Drugs, including paracetamol and aspirin; antibiotics such as tetracycline the cephalosporins and amphotericin.
- Myeloma.
- Polycystic disease.
- Vasculitic disease.

Chronic renal failure: care

The patient in chronic renal failure requiring high dependency nursing for any reason will present certain difficulties associated with the long-term effects of their CRF. These effects will impact on the assessment and care planning and can present certain problems that need to be taken into consideration in addition to those associated with the pathophysiological conditions giving rise to their care needs.

First and foremost will be the continuing need for mechanical renal replacement therapy.

CONTINUOUS AMBULATORY PERITONEAL DIALYSIS (CAPD)

In the case of CAPD, the high dependency nurse's role may be confined to the care of the CAPD catheter, ensuring adequate nutritional support of the patient and control of the patient's fluid and electrolyte balance. However, as the system is designed to be carried out with ease, there is no reason for the nurse not to undertake the exchange procedure for the patient following the specific 'systems' procedure as outlined above. The specific procedure will be described by the system manufacturer, all being slightly different, but each following the principles of asepsis during the exchange.

In addition to the exchange procedure the nurse will need to monitor the patient for potential complications associated with the treatment. Peritonitis due to bacterial or fungal infection of the peritoneum will result in cloudy and turbid effluent and abdominal pain. A leukocyte count of greater than $100/mm^3$ in the dialysate will confirm the diagnosis and a culture of Gram-positive organisms or Gram-negative organisms will require the specific antibiotic to be administered via the dialysate fluid. In addition to the intraperitoneal route, i.v. antibiotics may also be administered, but care must be taken to allow for the requirement of a renally adjusted dosage. The other potential infection site is the exit of the catheter from the abdomen. These 'tunnel infections' are as a result of infection tracking back along the insertion site between the internal securing cuffs on the catheter and can prove extremely difficult to eradicate. Characteristics of exit site infection are tenderness, redness and inflammation with exudate, and care of the catheter will help prevent such infections. The catheter should be anchored at two sites to prevent pulling and potential exposure of the first 'cuff'. Cleaning of the site on a daily or two daily basis with soap and water as well as the use of a sterile non-occlusive dressing will also reduce potential infection. Treatment of infection varies, but will often include oral antibiotic therapy of a broad spectrum to cover both Gram-positive and Gram-negative bacteria until a specific organism can be identified, then continuing with the appropriate antibiotic for 14 days.

Nutrition is a particular problem with CAPD as the process 'flushes' protein from the patient's body. This can result in hypoproteinaemia with a corresponding hypercatabolic state as well as fluid loss to the tissues, intractable oedema and circulatory collapse as described earlier. Adequate nutritional support either orally, nasogastrically or via TPN will be required to supply sufficient protein and calories to prevent hypercatabolism. Accurate assessment of fluid balance is of paramount importance in the use of such feeds but is less critical than in other forms of mechanical replacement therapy, such as haemodialysis, as fluid balance is being controlled by the dialysate exchanges on such a regular basis. The use of stronger hypertonic fluids will assist in the removal of any excess fluid intake given that the serum protein level can be maintained. Another problem associated with the protein loss via the dialysate is the formation of fibrin in the fluid, appearing as either 'strings' of white fibres or as 'clouds' of milky white matter in the clear fluid. These collections of fibrin can block the catheter and so heparin 500 iu per exchange is added to the dialysate fluid to prevent this should they appear. Rapid exchanges of fluid will also assist in the removal of any potential blockages but in the event of non-draining fluid the specialist renal personnel will have to be called to carry out system flushing.

Finally, in the event of the patient becoming severely hypercatabolic it may be necessary to replace the CAPD treatment with the more aggressive haemodialysis or even CVVH or CAVH and to treat the patient as an 'acute' renal failure until stabilized.

HAEMODIALYSIS

The patient requiring regular haemodialysis as the means of mechanically replacing their renal function will need to continue this treatment at their usual or more regular dialysis times during their current pathophysiological problems. The high dependency nurse's role will usually be confined to the general care of the patient in the resting period, with the renal personnel providing the dialysis treatment as an 'outreach' service. However the success of the dialysis treatment will be dependent on the high dependency nursing that the patient receives, specifically consisting of care of the venous access, dietary and fluid modification and electrolyte control, as well as the specific care required due to the patient's specific condition.

VENOUS ACCESS

The venous access for a patient receiving long-term haemodialysis will usually consist of a Brescia–Cimino fistula, which consists of a permanent anastomosis of the patient's radial artery to the cephalic vein. The high pressure blood being 'shunted' across the fistula into the low pressure venous system results in the distension of the veins of the forearm and so provides sites for cann-ulation which will allow the rapid removal and replacement of blood during haemodialysis. The appearance of the patient's arm will be quite distinctive, having long areas of scar tissue along the distended veins from previous repeated canulation for treatment. In addition there will be a strong pulse at the fistula site and a buzzing sensation known as a bruit on palpation. This is the actual flow of arterialized blood into the venous system and on auscultation will give a whooshing sound. This fistula is literally the patient's 'life line' and so great care must be taken to ensure its survival. Blood pressures must not be taken on the fistulated arm, nor should tight strapping of any kind be applied as this will result in restriction of the blood flow through the fistula and the clotting of the anastomosis and veins. Venous cannulation for any purpose other than haemodialysis, such as i.v. drug administration, blood taking for investigations, or central pressure lines should not be allowed in the fistulated arm. In addition, in the care of the unconscious patient requiring regular turns, attention must be taken not to let them lie on the arm.

An alternative form of access, especially in those patients who have arterial disease, is the synthetic graft. These grafts form a loop in either the forearm or more usually in the thigh where the graft joins to the femoral vein. The major problem here is the danger of infection and secondary bleeding following treatment. Any evidence of infection, redness, inflammation or exudate from the puncture sites must be reported immediately. Evidence of secondary bleeding, with blood leakage or spurting from the needle sites, or swelling of the thigh, must also be reported immediately and pressure applied to the site until the bleeding ceases.

DIETARY AND FLUID MODIFICATION

Usually the patient in CRF cares for their own dietary and fluid; however, such patients requiring high dependency nursing will have very different requirements from those that they are used to, and so additional instruction and care should be given. The principle of ensuring a nutritional input sufficient to prevent catabolism remains the same, but as the patient may well be in a catabolic state due to their current condition then restriction of protein intake would be contraindicated. The approach already described in the section on acute renal failure applies.

Fluid intake would also have been modified according to the patient's residual renal function, incidental loss and the volume that can be comfortably removed mechanically via dialysis. In other words the mechanical renal replacement therapy creates 'space' which is filled during the intradialytic period. During acute episodes of illness the usual intakes and losses may well be disrupted and so will need careful monitoring and control. The 'standard' approach of a 500 mL fluid allowance to account for incidental losses, plus the volume of the output from the previous 24 hours with an additional allowance for volumes to be removed by dialysis should be supplemented by a more thorough assessment of the patient. This assessment should be based on a previous history of body weight changes in order to form a 'baseline' of normal fluid balance for comparison to their present status. If possible the patient should be weighed daily; however if the patient is too ill then accurate intake and output records, taking into account fluid from all sources, should be used, comparing them with evidence of fluid retention.

ELECTROLYTE CONTROL

As with fluid, dialysis creates 'space' which is then filled by dietary or metabolic production of electrolytes, the two of most concern being sodium and potassium. A familiarity with those foods containing high levels of these electrolytes will help the high dependency nurse to regulate their intake for the patient. Potassium, as identified earlier, is of particular concern as it poses a direct threat to life in levels exceeding 6 mEq/L due to its effect on the myocardial excitability. In patients with tissue damage potassium will be shifting from the intracellular compartment and so a restriction of dietary intake may be insufficient to control the hyperkalaemia. In such patients regular assessment of the serum electrolytes is required as well as attention to any arrhythmias such as elevated T waves, widened QRS complexes, flattened or absent P waves, or a pulse with extrasystoles, or tachycardia. In the presence of such irregularities intravenous glucose and insulin provides an emergency treatment, driving the potassium back into the cells and providing time for mechanical renal replacement therapy to commence.

In the general assessment of the patient there can be problems associated with CRF that can complicate the care planning for the patient's current condition and so will need to be taken into consideration. These include:

- *Hypertension*: dependent on renal artery disease, or salt and water retention.
- *Anaemia*: due to failure of erythropoietin production and complicated by blood losses due to dialysis, or surgery.
- *Acidosis*: associated with the failure of the kidney to excrete hydrogen ions and the failure to conserve bicarbonate.
- *Renal bone disease*: due to the failure of the kidney to convert Vitamin D into an activated form thus allowing the absorption of calcium from the gut and so activating the demineralization of bone.

As symptoms associated with CRF will be present it can be expected that the patient's current condition will exacerbate them. Infection, respiratory disorders, surgery, fractures, or any condition may give rise to the need for high dependency nursing. In such a case the effects of treatment and potential outcomes must be assessed in the light of what would be 'normal' for a renal patient; what can be achieved through direct intervention for the current illness and what via mechanical renal replacement therapy. It is therefore essential that good communication exists between the high dependency nurse, renal nurse and dietician in the care planning for the patient.

Ultimately the aim of the care is to return the patient to a level of independence that was previously experienced by them within their long-term treatment regimen. As more nurses become aware of the special needs of such patients then a favourable outcome of treatment becomes more likely. The sophistication of treatment offered to renal patients requiring high dependency nursing is an example of two specialist branches of nursing working in harmony to produce the best possible care goals.

Further reading

Amoroso, P. and Greenwood, R. 1992 Acute renal failure. *British Journal of Intensive Care* **8**(9).

Arrowsmith, H. 1997 Malnutrition in hospital: detection and consequences. *British Journal of Nursing* **6**(19), 1131–5.

Barton, I. and Thomas, P.A. 1997 Decision making in surgery: acute postoperative renal failure. *British Journal of Hospital Medicine* **57**(3).

Chmielewski, C. 1992 Renal anatomy and overview of nephron function. *ANNA Journal* **19**(1).

Dickerson, J. 1995 The problems of hospital-induced malnutrition. *Nursing Times* **91**(4).

Driver, D.S. 1996 Renal assessment: back to basics. *ANNA Journal* **23**(4).

Fox, S.I. 1996 *Human physiology*, 5th edn. London: Times Mirror Group.

Gabriel, R. 1975. *Postgraduate nephrology*. London: Butterworths.

Goodison, M. and Holmes, S. 1985 *Acute renal failure: aetiology and emergency treatment*. London: Baillière Tindall.

Gutch, C.F., Stoner, M.H. and Corea, A.L. 1993 *Review of haemodialysis for nurses and dialysis personnel*. London: Mosby.

Harper, A. 1990 Drug treatment in patients with renal impairment. *Pharmaceutical Journal* **244**(6576), 327–9.

Kapit, W., Macey, R.I. and Meisami, E. 1987 *The physiology colouring book*. London: Harper Collins.

Kelly, M. 1997 Acute renal failure. *American Journal of Nursing* **97**(3).

Kramer, P., Bohler, J., Kehr, A. *et al.* 1982 Intensive care potential of CAVH. *Transactions of the American Society of Artificial Organs* **28**(8), 26–31.

McHugh, M.I. 1997 Acute renal failure. *Care of the Critically Ill* **13**(2).

Pritchard, A.P. and David, J.A. 1990 *The Royal Marsden Hospital manual of clinical nursing procedures*. London: Harper and Row.

Smith, T. 1997 *Renal nursing*. London: Baillière Tindall.

Springett, J. and Murray, C. 1994 Direct input. *Nursing Times* **90**(17), 48–52.

Stark, J. 1994 Interpreting BUN? Creatinine levels. *Nursing* **2**(9), 59–61.

Stark, J. 1997 Dialysis choices. Turning the tide in acute renal failure. *Nursing* **27**(2), 1–47.

Summerton, H. 1995 End stage renal failure: the challenge to the nurse. *Nursing Times* **91**(6).

Swanson, P. 1990 Drug treatment of chronic renal failure. *Pharmaceutical Journal* March 24th.

Thibodeau, G. and Patton, K.T. 1996 *Anatomy and physiology*, 3rd edn. London: Mosby.

Toto, K.H. 1992 Acute renal failure: a question of location. *American Journal of Nursing* **92**(11), 44–53.

Tortora, G.J. 1994 *Introduction to the human body*, 3rd edn. London: Harper Collins.

Tortora, G.J. and Grabowski, S.R. 1996 *Principles of anatomy and physiology*, 8th edn. London: Harper Collins.

Van Stone, J. 1996 Controlling thirst in dialysis patients. *Seminars in Dialysis* **9**(1), 47–50.

Will, E.J. and Johnson, J.P. 1994 Options in the medical management of end stage renal failure. In: McGee, H. *et al.* (eds). *Quality of life following renal failure*. Boston: Academic Publishers.

5 Caring for the endocrine system

Sarah Adams and Christopher C. Bassett

Introduction

This chapter will consider patients who are suffering from a disorder of the endocrine system. It will consider the following conditions which are most commonly seen in the high dependency unit:

- Diabetes mellitus (type 1 diabetes).
- Diabetes insipidus.
- Acute pancreatitis.
- Thyroid dysfunction.

Its aim is to provide the reader with a clear knowledge and understanding of the system's function and will explore the pathophysiology of these diseases. Following reading the chapter the nurse will be able to recognize each serious condition and its signs and symptoms. The chapter's overall aim is to provide the reader with the underpinning knowledge and confidence to care and treat their patients in the most effective way possible. By using this knowledge it is hoped that the patient will be prevented from a worsening of their condition and admission to the intensive care unit.

The endocrine system comprises a series of organs or parts of organs that release chemicals (hormones) into the blood stream which regulate metabolic functions within the body. The organs that comprise the endocrine system are described below (Fig. 5.1).

The hypothalamus

The hypothalamus is positioned just above the pituitary gland at the base of the brain. The hormone secreted by this small organ stimulates or inhibits secretion of pituitary hormones.

The pituitary gland

The pituitary gland or hypophysis is the controlling or master gland. It secretes hormones that in

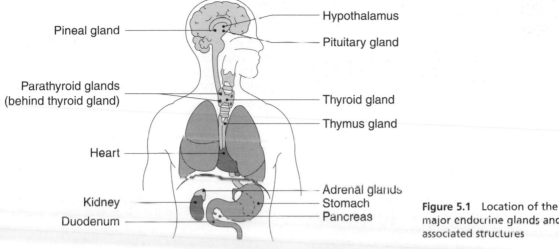

Pineal gland

Parathyroid glands
(behind thyroid gland)

Heart

Kidney
Duodenum

Hypothalamus
Pituitary gland

Thyroid gland
Thymus gland

Adrenal glands
Stomach
Pancreas

Figure 5.1 Location of the
major endocrine glands and
associated structures

turn control the secretion of hormones by the other endocrine glands. This gland is divided into three lobes. The anterior, intermediate and posterior lobes.

The hormones secreted from the posterior lobe are:

- Antidiuretic hormone; vasopressin. This controls excretion of urine via the kidney and will be covered later on.
- Oxytocin. This hormone increases the force of uterine contractions during childbirth.

The hormones secreted from the anterior lobe are:

- Follicle-stimulating hormone, luteinizing hormone and prolactin; these control fertility.
- Adrenocorticotrophic hormone stimulates corticosteroid production.
- Growth hormone controls growth and certain metabolic processes

- Thyroid-stimulating hormone will be discussed later in the chapter.

The pancreas

The pancreas secretes insulin and also has an exocrine function, as well as endocrine function and is dealt with later.

The thyroid and parathyroid glands

The thyroid gland and the parathyroid glands, which will also be considered later, regulate metabolic rate and maintain calcium levels in the blood.

Diabetes mellitus

Diabetes mellitus is the most common metabolic disease (Leibovitz, 1991). Presently it is estimated there are some 100 million patients with diabetes world-wide, and there may be as many again undiagnosed. It is certain that the nurse working in acute medicine or the high dependency unit will encounter the diabetic patient whose condition has become seriously unstable. When controlled, diabetes mellitus is not a life-threatening disease, in fact many sufferers feel well, even at the time of diagnosis. However, because of the very nature of the disease there may be need for hospitalization for a period of stabilization. Occasionally everyday normal illnesses can turn into serious medical emergencies for those with diabetes.

Who are we considering when we talk about diabetes?

Abnormal glucose tolerance (the term used to encompass diabetes and impaired glucose tolerance) (Leibovitz, 1991), is simply as it sounds – the inability of the body to cope with the amount of sugar ingested. Nurses on general wards will meet patients with this condition frequently. However, during times of physical or emotional upset these patients can become seriously ill, requiring a high level of medical and nursing intervention.

The classification of diabetes has always been somewhat confusing, and unfortunately it still is.

Traditionally diabetic patients are classified into two types:

Insulin dependent diabetes (type 1)

These are patients requiring exogenous insulin. Typically these are young patients needing insulin injections to sustain life.

The second group are known as:

Non-insulin dependent diabetes (type 2)

This type is confined mainly to older adults who are not dependent on insulin to maintain life.

However these categories do occasionally become confused, for instance some non-insulin dependent diabetics may be treated with insulin to improve control, although they are not dependent on insulin to sustain life. For this reason it is generally agreed that the patient is given a category that best describes the onset of his or her condition, rather than the therapy to be used.

This chapter's focus will be upon *type 1* diabetic patients. It is extremely rare for type 2 sufferers to be admitted to the acute high dependency unit. It is important, however, to understand the difference between the two types so that the differential treatment and assessment means can be understood by the nurse.

The action of insulin

Under normal circumstances insulin is produced in the pancreas in small endocrine glands called the islets of Langerhans (of which there are about a million). There are at least four types of cells in the islets of Langerhans; of these the alpha (or A) cells secrete glucagon with the beta (or B) cells secreting insulin. Normal adults secrete approximately 40–50 units of insulin per day. The rise in insulin begins about 8–10 minutes after the ingestion of food (known as stimulated insulin secretion); this peak is primarily in response to plasma glucose levels. When the glucose concentration in the system is increased suddenly, an initial short lived burst of insulin is released – the early phase. If the glucose stays at this level, the insulin production falls and then begins to rise again this time at a more steady rate – the late phase.

It is possible however, to secrete small amounts of insulin without glucose stimulation, and this is referred to as basal insulin secretion.

Insulin facilitates the movement of glucose across cell walls, where, after entering the cell it is utilized to create heat and energy. However, because the glucose only stimulates the B and the D cells in the islets – whereas the amino acids

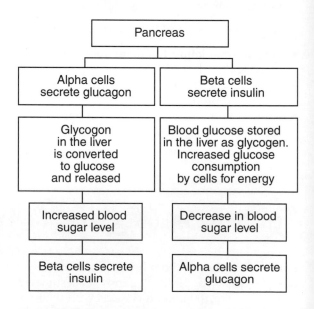

Figure 5.2 Regulation of the secretion of glucagon and insulin

stimulate the A cells for glycogen as well as B cells for insulin – the amount of insulin produced will depend on the ratio of protein to carbohydrate in the meal. The higher the carbohydrate content of the meal the less glycogen will be released by any amino acids absorbed (Fig. 5.2).

The main function of insulin is to promote storage of ingested nutrients, although insulin affects just about every tissue in the body (the reason some experts prefer to call diabetes a state rather than a condition). The main tissues affected when considering diabetes are those used for energy storage. The liver, the muscles and adipose tissues are the most important sites associated with energy storage.

The liver

The liver is the major organ affected by insulin; it is the first organ that insulin reaches via the blood stream. When insulin reaches the liver it promotes glycogen synthesis and storage, and at the same time it inhibits glycogen breakdown. Insulin also acts to reverse the catabolic events, i.e. the breaking down of glucose to release energy

The muscle

The muscle expends its usual glycogen stores with muscle activity. Insulin promotes amino acid transportation and ultimately glycogen synthesis to replace stores lost by muscle activity. The muscle has the capacity to store large amounts of glycogen which cannot be used as plasma glucose, except by indirectly supplying the liver with lactate for conversion to glucose.

Adipose tissue

Adipose tissue is essentially fat in the form of triglycerides. Adipose tissue is the most efficient tissue at storing energy. Insulin acts to promote the storage of triglycerides in adipose tissue

Summary

Insulin:

1 facilitates the movement of glucose across cell walls to be used for energy
2 promotes conversion of glucose to glycogen when glucose is in excess of immediate requirements
3 promotes the storage of fat
4 promotes the synthesis of protein

Type 1 diabetes

Type 1 diabetes (or insulin dependent diabetes – IDDM) is a severe form of diabetes generally diagnosed in children and young adults or less commonly in non-obese adults. About 20 per cent of diabetics in North America and Europe are type 1. It is a catabolic malfunction (the inability to breakdown complex compounds into simple compounds) in which circulating insulin is virtually absent. Due to the absence of insulin the plasma glucose is raised, still the pancreatic B cells fail to respond to insulin secreting stimulus.

It is still not clearly understood what causes type 1 diabetes. Some experts believe that type 1 diabetes might occur post-infection or from an environmental influence upon the pancreatic B cells; whilst the immune cells of the pancreas struggle to overcome this assault, they inadvertently destroy the pancreatic B cells. The viruses that have been associated with altered pancreatic function are rubella, mumps and coxsackie virus.

PATHOPHYSIOLOGY

As a result of the rapid decline or total deficiency of insulin, glucose is unable to transfer effectively into the cells for storage, and ultimately the utilization of glucose for the needs of the cells and its conversion to glycogen in the liver, and storage in the adipose tissue are depressed. Glucose accumulates in the blood and causes hyperglycaemia (a high serum blood glucose).

As insulin levels continue to fall the body uses compensatory factors, energy stores are drawn from the muscle and adipose tissue and broken down to provide a source of energy. Amino acids from the muscle are transported to the liver for conversion to glucose and fatty acids for oxidization and thus conversion to ketones (acetoacetic acid, β-hydroxybutyric acid and acetone). Only a limited amount of ketones can be utilized by the cells; if ketones are produced at a rate exceeding the consumption by the cells ketone acids accumulate in the blood. The effect of the low insulin:glucagon ratio on the liver encourages the further production of ketones leading to ketoacidosis.

In the absence of insulin the insulin antagonist hormones (those hormones which usually work in opposition to insulin) such as corticosteroids, catecholamines and glucagon are consistently raised. Peripheral utilization of ketones and glucose is reduced, and with increased production and decreased utilization, the levels of ketones and glucose in the blood continue to rise.

The hyperglycaemia (high circulating serum glucose) causes osmotic diuresis (as the body attempts to excrete the glucose) and loss of volume from the vascular system. With reduced blood flow, the kidneys' ability to excrete glucose is reduced. Hyperosmolality (a larger than normal concentration of molecules) of the blood worsens, severe hyperosmolality correlates with depression of the nervous system, leading eventually to confusion, stupor, coma and death.

SIGNS AND SYMPTOMS

Signs

When insulin deficiency occurs relatively slowly, the patient may drink enough fluid to maintain normal levels of hydration and normal excretion of glucose from the kidneys may be maintained. In this instance the patient may keep mentally alert and the physical signs be few. If the patient starts to vomit, as a response to raised ketones, dehydration will occur and when compensatory mechanisms can no longer cope, stupor or coma will occur. A patient who is stuporous with rapid breathing and a fruity (pear drops) smelling breath (evidence of acetone) is a classical presentation for a patient who is suffering from the early effects of diabetic ketoacidosis (Cahill, 1976). Due

to the depleted plasma volume postural hypotension may occur. Hypotension when the patient is recumbent is an extremely serious sign, and if present medical assistance should be sought straight away.

Symptoms

Increased urinary production is present in response to sustained hyperglycaemia and the onset of osmotic diuresis. Most type 1 diabetics will suffer polyuria (passing large amounts of urine) and nocturia (getting up at night to pass urine); nocturnal enuresis (bed wetting) may occur in children.

Due to the hyperosmolar state the patient may complain of severe thirst; they may also experience double vision as the lens and retinas are exposed to hyperosmolar fluids. Lowered plasma volume leads to dizziness and weakness due to the postural hypotension mentioned earlier. General weakness and malaise is common and is caused by the general potassium loss and the conversion to energy of muscle protein.

Generally there is no loss of appetite, but weight loss still occurs, initially due to the loss of water, and then of fat stores. Further weight loss will occur as the muscle content of the body is reduced when released for conversion to energy (amino acids to glucose and ketones).

Neurotoxicity (poisoning of the nervous system) occurs from the elevated blood sugars. Paraesthesia (pins and needles or a numbness) may be an indication that the nerves are affected; this is usually temporary, and subsides with insulin treatment. As the patient becomes ketoacidotic, nausea and vomiting may occur; anorexia is induced and dehydration worsens. This further increases hyperosmolarity, and the patient begins to lose consciousness. With increased acidosis, Kussmaul respiration occurs (rapid deep respiration) in an attempt to expel carbonic acid. If the cardiovascular system is overburdened for too long it will be unable to maintain necessary vasoconstriction. Shock will occur and complete circulatory collapse may follow.

At this point the patient will immediately require high level medical and nursing input.

Summary of clinical features of type 1 diabetes at diagnosis

1 Thirst
2 Polyuria and nocturia
3 Weight loss
4 Blurred vision
5 Pruritis
6 Fatigue
7 Peripheral neuropathy

Type 2 diabetes

As mentioned earlier, type 2 diabetes is very rarely seen in the high dependency situation except perhaps as part of a pre-existing condition. It will be discussed briefly here to assist the nurse to differentiate between the two types. Type 2 diabetes comprises of a heterogeneous (several smaller subgroups that may not necessarily have exactly the same features) group of the milder forms of diabetes. This type of diabetes nearly always occurs in adult life. Experts often define type 2 diabetes by the complications that do *not* occur, for instance it may be referred to as non-ketotic, not associated with autoantibodies of the islet cells, and is not dependent on exogenous (injected) insulin (hence the term non-insulin dependent diabetes mellitus or NIDDM) (Fig. 5.3).

No one theory explains the manifestation of diabetes; most suggest that there is an element of insulin insensitivity by the tissues in those suffering type 2 diabetes.

Type 2 diabetes may be classified further into two smaller components: obese NIDDM and non-obese NIDDM.

The patient with type 2 diabetes mellitus has a relative insulin insufficiency; this does not necessarily mean that the islet of Langerhans cells are not functioning properly, in fact insulin production and secretion may be entirely normal or in some cases excessive. The state of hyperglycaemia occurs because the insulin is ineffective. The impaired action of the insulin produces hyperglycaemia and in turn hyperinsulinaemia (the excessive production of insulin by the islets of Langerhans). If the hyperinsulinaemia is enough to cope with the circulating glucose all is well;

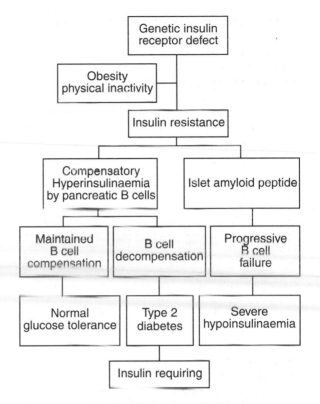

Figure 5.3 Pathophysiology of type 2 diabetes

however if there is still insufficient insulin, type 2 diabetes will manifest (McGee, 1993).

SIGNS AND SYMPTOMS

Summary of clinical features of type 2 diabetes at diagnosis

1 Mild to moderate thirst
2 Increased urine output
3 Tiredness
4 Blurred vision (or diabetic complications spotted at opticians)
5 Often asymptomatic

Diabetes mellitus: the whole picture

INVESTIGATIONS

Tests for diabetes must always be used as part of a clinical examination for diagnosis.

Urinalysis

Glycosuria

Glucose detected in the urine is a measurement which reflects the amount of glucose in the blood at the time the urine was made. This will not prove to be accurate enough for control of some patients with severe uncontrolled diabetes. Indeed in type 1 diabetes blood glucose monitoring has largely replaced urine testing

Ketonuria

In diabetes ketone bodies are excreted into the urine. These can be detected easily on a dipstick test (although these strips have a rather short shelf-life so it is important to ensure they are still accurate). Also it is important to remember other conditions can also cause ketones in the urine, e.g lack of food, fever, high-fat diets and alcoholic ketoacidosis

Proteinuria

A similar dipstick test is available to detect protein in the urine. Protein detected in a diabetic patient is often the first sign of renal complications. If protein is detected in the urine a 24-hour urine sample should be collected to measure the rate of creatinine excretion. Serum creatinine levels must also be monitored to determine creatinine clearance. Often as renal impairment increases, proteinuria develops

Venous blood glucose

Venous blood collected for glucose analysis needs to be collected in a tube containing sodium fluoride to prevent further glycolysis which when measured would make the blood sugar appear artificially low

Capillary blood glucose

This test is available in a paper strip option and most strips marketed at present have portable reflectance meters. These give a digital readout, the latest of which reduce chances of human error by providing a quantitation regardless of the blood volume on the strip, and have an automatic timing function

Glycosylated haemoglobin assays (HbA1c)

The major form of glycosylated haemoglobin is haemoglobin A1c which is approximately 4–6 per cent of the total haemoglobin, and is produced by a reaction between glucose and the amino terminal amino acid of the beta chains of the haemoglobin. The glycosylation of the haemoglobin is dependent on the concentration of the blood glucose. This reaction is not reversible which means that the half-life of the glycosylated haemoglobin is directly related to the life-span of the red blood cells. Red blood cells usually circulate for about 120 days; therefore an HbA1c will reflect the state of glycaemia for the preceding 8–12 weeks

Lipoproteins

Lipoprotein levels are also affected by the action of insulin and dependent upon normal levels. In type 1 diabetes there is often a slight rise in cholesterol and once the hyperglycaemia returns to normal the lipid profile is often generally normal

Table 5.1 Diagnosis of diabetes and impaired glucose tolerance

		Glucose concentration mmol\L (normal ranges)	
		Lab estimation (venous blood)	Finger prick (capillary)
Random/fasting tests for whole blood			
Diabetes	Random	>10.0	>11.1
	Fasting	>6.7	>6.7
Uncertain	Random	6.7–9.9	7.8–11
	Fasting	5.0–6.6	5.0–6.6
Glucose tolerance test			
Diabetes	Fasting	>6.7	>6.7
	2 h level	>10.0	>11.1
Impaired glucose tolerance			
	Fasting	<6.7	<6.7
	2 h level	6.7–10.0	7.0–11.1

Remember the results in Table 5.1 are for whole blood (taken as a venous sample or capillary blood taken as a bedside measurement). If tests are conducted on plasma results may be slightly higher.

Treatment of diabetes mellitus

DIET

The mainstay of treatment for type 1 or type 2 diabetes is diet. For type 1 diabetes, total calories should be calculated to maintain an ideal body weight. Meals are taken at times designed to best complement insulin treatment; most type 1 diabetic patients usually administer insulin twice a day. For type 2 diabetes the emphasis is on weight reduction. If a significant weight loss is achieved, a fall in fasting blood glucose may follow.

INSULIN THERAPY

Insulin therapy is used for all type 1 diabetics and for type 2 diabetics who are unable to adequately control their hyperglycaemia with a combination of diet and oral hypoglycaemic drug therapy. Insulin therapy is usually given by subcutaneous injection, although during the patient's time in the high dependency area a continuous infusion pump will be necessary to control the amount of blood glucose exactly.

Insulin types

Most diabetics in the UK are now treated with human insulin prepared by recombinant DNA technology (a sequence of DNA is artificially added to a DNA chain) with synthetic insulin; very few remain on insulin derived from pork or beef pancreas. The rate of insulin absorption can be prolonged by increasing the particle size, or by combining the insulin with zinc or protamine.

Traditionally insulin has been classified into short, intermediate and long-acting insulin (Table 5.2). In reality long-acting insulin is no longer used, because of the dangers of insulin accumulation and hypoglycaemia. Short-acting insulin is a simple soluble insulin whose action onsets after approximately 30 minutes and peaks at around 1 to 3 hours. Its duration lasts for about seven hours. It is usually administered by subcutaneous injection, but can be given intravenously in a hyperglycaemic emergency.

Intermediate action (or medium action) insulin has a duration of about 14 to 22 hours. Many of these are zinc preparations which prolong the action of the insulin. Isophane insulin is a complex of protamine and insulin; after injection prote-olytic enzymes degrade the protamine and the insulin is absorbed.

Biphasic mixtures are a combination of soluble and isophane insulin in various proportions (for example 30 per cent soluble and 70 per cent iso-phane). The soluble insulin gives the rapid onset, and the isophane insulin prolongs the action.

ORAL HYPOGLYCAEMIC DRUGS (ANTIDIABETIC DRUGS)

Again the use of these types of insulin controlling drugs will not usually be seen in the high depen-dency unit, but will be discussed briefly to enhance understanding.

Traditionally hypoglycaemic drugs have been divided into two categories, that of the biguanides and the sulphonureas.

Biguanides act by an unknown mechanism peripherally to increase glucose uptake. As met-formin (the only biguanide used at present) does not increase insulin release, hypoglycaemia is rarely an issue. The obvious advantage of met-formin is that functioning pancreatic B cells are not a requirement for use. Used as an adjunct to diet, it is particularly suitable for obese patients as it improves both fasting and postprandial hyperglycaemia without apparent weight gain. Adverse reactions are usually gastrointestinal, nausea, diarrhoea, vomiting – which may occur in 20 per cent of patients but is often dose-related and transient. A very rare side effect is lacto-acidosis (see section on lactoacidosis, p. 119) and for this reason metformin is contraindicated in patients with impaired renal, hepatic or cardio-respiratory function.

> **Sulphonureas have a dual action:**
> 1 To enhance the release of insulin from the pancreatic B cells
> 2 To potentiate the action of insulin on its target cells

Diabetic coma

NURSING CARE AND TREATMENT OF COMA

A cause for diabetic coma needs to be established immediately if the correct therapy is to be initi-ated. However coma is a medical emergency and may be due to other conditions such as CVA (cere-bral vascular accident) etc. All comatose patients need initial emergency treatment:

> 1 Establish an airway
> 2 Establish intravenous access
> 3 Positioning of an unconscious patient
> 4 Careful and close blood glucose measurement

Once initial emergency measures are instituted any comatose diabetic patient should have admin-istered 50 mL of 50 per cent dextrose intra-venously, unless bedside monitoring of blood glucose indicates hyperglycaemia.

Table 5.2 Table of insulin therapy

Type of preparation	Onset (h)	Peak (h)	Duration (h)
Short acting: (Soluble or regular) i.e. neutral	1	2–4	6–12
Intermediate acting: Isophane (suspension of insulin/protamine or insulin zinc suspension) (semilente)	1	4–6	14
Insulin zinc suspension (lente)	2	8–12	24
Long acting: Insulin zinc suspension (ultralente)	3	8–12	60–75
Protamine zinc insulin	3	8–12	28–35

CLASSIFICATION OF DIABETIC COMA

Hyperglycaemic coma incorporates:

1 Diabetic ketoacidosis – severe insulin deficiency.
2 Hyperosmolar, non-ketotic – mild to moderate insulin deficiency.

Hypoglycaemic coma is completely different, and results from overdose of insulin or antidiabetic drugs.

Lactic acidosis coma results from severe tissue anoxia, sepsis or cardiovascular collapse.

DIABETIC KETOACIDOSIS

ACTIVITY 5.1 Patient scenario

Callum is an 18-year-old currently studying for A level examinations. He has complained of headaches which he has put down to revision, and complains of feeling tired. He has been burning the candle at both ends and is not unduly surprised when he falls asleep in lesson time. After a heavy lunchtime drinking session, Callum leaves the bar and collapses on the pavement outside. A lollipop lady sees this happen, places him in the recovery position and calls a ambulance.

What would lead you to suspect diabetes? What type of diabetes would be most likely? What would be the immediate treatment and nursing care?

Callum is suffering from hyperglycaemia with ketoacidosis.

Ketoacidosis is an acute complication which usually affects type 1 diabetics, but in rare circumstances may affect type 2 diabetics when under extreme stress: infection, trauma or surgery, for example. Ketoacidosis may be the first manifestation of type 1 diabetes, or may also be the result of severe infection, trauma, surgery or myocardial infarction when insulin requirements are high. It is a life-threatening emergency and should always be treated as such. Elderly patients have a much poorer prognosis than their younger counterparts. Unfortunately, most cases of ketoacidosis are due to poor compliance or poor patient understanding.

Clinical features of diabetic ketoacidosis

1 Usually preceded by polydipsia and polyuria
2 Fatigue
3 Nausea and vomiting
4 Mental stupor
5 Mild hypothermia
6 Coma

Laboratory findings

1 Urine
2 Extreme glycosuria (four plusses or 2 per cent)
3 Large amount of ketones (apart from a fasting patient, ketonuria would indicate a problem)

Blood

1 Hyperglycaemia (usually above 17 mmol)
2 Ketonaemia (any presence of ketones in the blood)
3 Low arterial blood pH (normal = 7.34–7.45)
4 Low plasma bicarbonate (normal = 22–26 mmol/L)
5 Normal or slightly elevated potassium (normal = 3.5–5.3 mmol/L – a shift of potassium occurs from intracellular to extracellular spaces)
6 Serum phosphate may be elevated (whereas total body phosphate may be depleted – normal = 0.70–1.40 mmol/L)
7 Serum sodium is generally reduced (as severe hyperglycaemia draws cellulose water into the interstitial compartment, normal = 135–145 mmol/L)
8 Urea is elevated (dehydration – normal = 1.0–6.5 mmol/L)
9 Nitrogen is elevated (dehydration)
10 Serum creatinine is elevated (normal = 55–120 mmol/L)

Medical management of ketoacidosis

1 Replacement of fluid and electrolytes with intravenous saline and dextrose solutions
2 A constant intravenous infusion of soluble insulin at a rate of 6–8 units per hour
3 Replacement of potassium intravenously

4 In severe cases of profound acidosis (pH < 7.0) replacement of bicarbonate may be necessary in controlled amounts of 50–100 mmol/h

5 A prophylactic regime of heparin may be administered if osmolality is high, or the patient is at risk of thrombosis (i.e. elderly or unconscious)

6 Treat underlying cause, i.e. infection – throat swabs, blood cultures, mid-stream specimen of urine, and broad-spectrum antibiotics whilst awaiting results

Nursing care of the patient

All unconscious patients will need full nursing care. The patient will be nursed in the recovery position. A nasogastric tube may be necessary, and if deeply unconscious the patient may need endotracheal intubation to prevent vomiting and asphyxiation. If no urine is passed within the first four hours of treatment a urinary catheter may be necessary, if still anuric, diuretic treatment should be considered by the physician.

Nursing care requirements

1 Blood sugar should be monitored 1–2 hourly

2 The administration of insulin as prescribed should be monitored and maintained

3 Intravenous infusion of fluids should be given as prescribed

4 Fluids input and output should be recorded

5 Consciousness level should be monitored using Glasgow Coma Scale

6 Patient's vital signs should be monitored hourly

Complications of treatment

1 Hypokalaemia (low serum potassium) should be avoidable by careful monitoring of blood results. Two-hour laboratory measurements may be necessary until sliding scale insulin regime is effective and lower doses of insulin are administered

2 Adult (acute) respiratory distress syndrome is associated with the use of hypotonic fluids in young people in particular. A cautious fluid regime will help prevent this

3 Cerebral oedema is seen mainly in children and again is associated with hypotonic fluids. Also less likely to occur if the blood glucose does not fall <10 mmol/L during the acute phase

Further nursing considerations

Abdominal pain is common in diabetic keto-acidosis; it should be treated conservatively and observed closely until the patient's metabolic disturbance is corrected. Simple analgesia should be given for pain relief. During all stages of the patient's treatment he or she and their family will need constant reassurance and support, as well as physical assistance with all of the activities of daily living.

HYPOGLYCAEMIA

ACTIVITY 5.2 Patient scenario

Freda McIntyre is a 72-year-old woman who has had diabetes for 10 years. Until recently Freda has been fit and well, living and coping on her own. She has never taken medication for her diabetes, but adhered strictly to a diabetic diet. Recently Freda developed a leg ulcer which refused to heal. On investigation by her GP, Freda's diabetes appeared to be poorly controlled, the leg ulcer appeared infected and she was admitted and commenced on sulphonurea medication. This morning Freda complained of hunger pains and sweating; she has now been found in the toilet by the cleaner, unconscious. She has been admitted to your unit from accident and emergency.

Why might Freda be unconscious and what are the likely causes?

Freda has suffered a severe hypoglycaemic attack.

Hypoglycaemia can affect either type 1 or type 2 diabetics. It may be the result of a missed meal, unusual physical activity without sufficient calorie supplementation or an increase in insulin dose. Hypoglycaemia affecting type 2 diabetics occurs more frequently when the patient is taking long-acting sulphonureas, especially in those with impaired liver or renal function. In older patients or those with frequent hypoglycaemic attacks, autonomic responses may be blunted. Signs and symptoms may vary from patient to patient, as may time of onset; however one particular patient may tend to follow a similar pattern to previous hypoglycaemic attacks.

For type 1 diabetics, the normal ability to counter-regulate hypoglycaemia by releasing a surge of glucagon is lost a few years after developing diabetes; for many type 1 diabetics hypoglycaemia is the most frequent complication. From the time of losing the ability to secrete glucagon, the type 1 diabetic patient is solely reliant on autonomic adrenal responses to counteract a hypoglycaemic crisis, and to alert him or her of impending crisis. However, as individuals age the responses to this crisis become blunted and a potentially life-threatening scenario emerges of neuroglycopaenic convulsions or coma.

Clinical features

There are two important issues to be considered when looking for signs and symptoms of hypoglycaemia: those resulting from neuroglycopaenia (which is insufficient glucose for normal central nervous system functioning); and those resulting from stimulation of the autonomic nervous system.

Neuroglycopaenia/autonomic hyperactivity

Adrenergic effects
- Mental confusion
- Impaired thought process
- Bizarre behaviour
- Stupor
- Coma

Autonomic hyperactivity
- Tachycardia
- Palpitations
- Sweating
- Tremulousness

Parasympathetic effects
- Nausea
- Hunger

Treatment of Hypoglycaemia

First and foremost the treatment for hypoglycaemia is *glucose administration*. Patients who remain conscious and able to eat and drink, either by the paramedic on the scene or by staff in the A&E Department, should be given any beverage or food (except pure fructose which does not cross the blood–brain barrier) that contains a high level of sugar, such as orange juice, high sugar drinks, sweet chocolate bar or glucose tablets. As the patient is already depleted of glucose this sugar may be utilized instantly; therefore it is important to follow this with some amount of carbohydrate (even a couple of biscuits) to prevent hypoglycaemia reoccurring.

For the unconscious or stuporous patient, oral feeding is obviously not an option. The more usual treatment is 50 mL of 50 per cent glucose given intravenously over 3 to 5 minutes. If no glucagon is available, small amounts of honey or syrup can be rubbed into the mucosa under the tongue until more appropriate measures can be taken.

Nursing care is that of the patient above *excepting the administration of insulin*.

Prevention of Hypoglycaemia and Patient Education

Management of hypoglycaemia unawareness is paramount. It is pointless educating the patient regarding treatment of hypoglycaemia if he or she is unaware when it is occurring. If the patient is suffering nocturnal hypoglycaemia he or she may be unaware. Monitoring of the blood sugar around 2 or 3 am for at least a week will verify this. If a patient suffers nocturnal hypoglycaemia, the night time insulin dose should be adjusted accordingly. Sometimes the patient will complain of waking with a headache, which may lead you to suspect night-time hypoglycaemic attacks (often referred to as hypos). If the patient is unaware of having hypoglycaemic effects whilst he or she is awake, then regular monitoring of blood sugars should be encouraged to attempt to detect the risk periods. In cases where tight glycaemic control has been sought, it may have to be relaxed a little to prevent such episodes.

Patient education is essential to help prevent hypoglycaemia. The recognition of precursors and more importantly the ability to alter calorie or insulin dose to suit daily lifestyles is imperative.

Patients on discharge from the unit or ward should be encouraged to carry sugar in an easily taken form, i.e. glucose tablets and for some glucagon may be necessary – with the education of patient and family that ultimately corresponds with this. All patients taking antidiabetic drugs or insulin should be encouraged to carry identification stating which type of diabetes they have and what medication they currently take. A talisman necklace or bracelet containing such information helps others and the emergency services to give appropriate treatment.

HYPERGLYCAEMIC, HYPEROSMOLAR, NON-KETOTIC STATE

Although referred to as a state, this condition may present as a coma and may be seen in the high dependency area of the hospital. It is restricted to middle-aged or elderly patients who suffer type 2 diabetes (non-insulin dependent) which is often only mild. Often these patients may have some degree of congestive heart failure or renal failure, and unfortunately the prognosis is worse if this is found to be the case. There may be an event or trauma such as CVA or burns that precipitate the event. Drugs implicated in the development of a hyperglycaemic, hyperosmolar, non-ketotic state (a state that may vary from drowsiness and confusion to complete coma) are thiazide diuretics, phenytoin, glucocorticoids and some others.

Pathogenesis

This type of coma tends to occur in middle-aged or elderly patients, especially those on sulphonureas. The coma is characterized by severe hyperglycaemia, which leads to glycosuria and osmotic diuresis which leads to water loss. It is believed to be the presence of small amounts of insulin which prevents the formation of ketones by inhibiting lipolysis in the adipose stores. As the plasma volume is depleted, renal insufficiency develops which in turn limits glucose excretion and leads to a high serum glucose, and osmolality. Water is depleted from the cerebral neurons, the patient becomes confused, and coma may ensue.

Signs and symptoms

1 Insidious onset
2 Weakness
3 Polyuria
4 Polydipsia
5 Often a history of reduced fluid intake
6 Dehydration
7 Patient may be hypotensive
8 Tachycardia
9 Possible shock!
10 Lethargy, confusion or coma

Laboratory findings

1 Severe hyperglycaemia
2 Increased serum sodium
3 Increased serum osmolarity
4 Serum ketones absent

Treatment

Fluid replacement is paramount. As much as 6 litres of fluid may be necessary in the first 8 hours; if there is no circulatory collapse then a hypotonic fluid should be used. In all cases careful monitoring of the blood pressure and pulse is essential. During fluid replacement, measurement of intake and output is essential, and if necessary a central venous catheter should be used in order to measure the central venous pressure when replacing the fluid.

In some cases replacing the fluid may be enough to aid recovery, but often insulin therapy is necessary and this should be given intravenously or intramuscularly until the patient is stabilized. If the patient is severely ill, it may be necessary to use continuous intravenous infusion of insulin. Insulin would be administered following a sliding scale outline.

Electrolyte replacement should be ensured when fluids are replaced, although the potassium depletion is not severe. Once insulin therapy is commenced, potassium and glucose will be allowed to enter the cells and serum potassium will become depleted.

Once the patient is stabilized, the physician must concentrate on finding the precipitating factors; often this may be obvious such as a severe infection. However, it may necessitate extensive investigations. The nurse must reassure the patient and help provide coping skills, together with a full explanation of any new treatment.

Reassurance is necessary for the patient to return to as normal existence as possible.

LACTOACIDOSIS

In the absence of high levels ketones in the plasma, but when a profound acidosis is present lactoacidosis should be suspected. Lactoacidosis is only usually a complication for an otherwise severely ill diabetic. It is not uncommon in patients suffering from cardiac, hepatic or renal failure. Very rarely, lactoacidosis is found in patients on biguanide therapy (metformin) and it is necessary to consider this.

Pathogenesis

When glucose is metabolized anaerobically, lactic acid is the end-product. It is usually the erythrocytes which lack the enzymes for aerobic oxidization that produce this acid. Usually it is the liver and to some extent the kidneys which remove lactic acid by converting it to pyruvate and then back to glucose, a process which requires oxygen.

Lactic acid which accumulates in the blood either due to overproduction (tissue hypoxia) or under-removal (liver failure) or both (circulatory collapse) causes lactoacidosis.

Signs and symptoms

1 Hyperventilation
2 Mental confusion
3 Stupor/coma

Laboratory findings

1 Plasma glucose is usually raised but can be normal
2 Plasma bicarbonate is low as is arterial pH
3 Ketones are usually absent from the plasma
4 Plasma lactate concentration > 6 mmol/L

The presentation of lactoacidosis is variable as it often incorporates signs and symptoms of the prevailing illness. In the unusual occurrence of the lactoacidosis being spontaneous, the onset is rapid but the cardiopulmonary system is unaffected.

Treatment

Aggressive treatment of the precipitating illness is necessary. An airway should be established and good oxygenation ensured. If the cause is not immediately obvious, swabs and blood cultures should be taken and broad-spectrum antibiotics commenced. If the patient is hypotensive, adequate fluids and pressor drugs if necessary should be given to increase blood pressure and allow proper perfusion. Treatment with bicarbonate remains controversial as there is no evidence to suggest that morbidity or mortality is affected by the administration of bicarbonate.

UNIT MANAGEMENT ISSUES

Each clinical area dealing with unstable diabetic patients needs absolute protocols to enable nurses to instigate immediate resuscitation and emergency measures and treatment. Clear documentation is vital and records for diabetic episodes should be kept prominently on a flowchart to avoid confusion and to aid decision-making.

Diabetes insipidus

Diabetes insipidus and diabetes mellitus are not to be confused; these are two completely different conditions, with only one common characteristic – the production of large amounts of urine. In diabetes insipidus copious amounts of dilute urine are produced.

ACTIVITY 5.3 Patient scenario

Thomas is a 3-year-old boy who has had no serious illness; however his mother complains that he is very thin and she feels he is not thriving as he should. Recently she has tried to toilet train Thomas and says it is hopeless. She claims that although Thomas does not drink any more than her last two children he passes much larger quantities of urine; he has never been dry day or night. On careful history it would appear that in fact Thomas is drinking large amounts of fluid and that his urine is quite dilute; he has had previous tests for diabetes mellitus, all of which have been negative. His GP decides to refer Thomas to a paediatrician. He is then admitted to your unit for treatment.

What might be wrong with Thomas? What would be the reason for referral, and what investigations might Thomas need?

Thomas has diabetes insipidus.

There are two main classifications of diabetes insipidus:
1 Central diabetes insipidus
2 Nephrogenic diabetes insipidus

Central diabetes insipidus is caused by failure of the pituitary gland to secrete adequate quantities of antidiuretic hormone. The purpose of antidiuretic hormone is to increase the water permeability of the luminal duct in the kidney, to encourage reabsorption of water. Without sufficient amounts of antidiuretic hormone, large amounts of dilute urine (free water) are passed. The loss of large amounts of water causes cellular and intracellular dehydration; this is turn stimulates thirst and causes polydipsia.

Nephrogenic diabetes insipidus is usually caused by the kidneys' inability to respond to the actions of ADH. In this instance the ADH levels are normal or elevated. The causes range from chronic renal disease, sickle cell disease, protein starvation and drugs, to congenital defect and familial causes.

Causes of central diabetes insipidus

Causes of central diabetes insipidus may be idiopathic or familial. Familial diabetes insipidus is a rare condition, but may be inherited by either a recessive or a dominant gene and is usually diagnosed early in infancy. Idiopathic diabetes insipidus is usually diagnosed later in life and is associated with a decline in the number of ADH containing fibres in the pituitary gland (Hague, 1987). Other causes include tumours and cysts, granulomas and infections, an interruption of the blood supply, autoimmune causes and occasionally surgery to remove suprasellar tumours.

Primary pituitary adenomas are rarely the cause; however central nervous system lesions and hypothalamic tumours may predispose to diabetes insipidus. Lesions may cause diabetes insipidus when they infiltrate the pituitary stalk as this interferes with the hypothalamic neurohypophysial nerve canals.

Diabetes insipidus caused by trauma is often as a result of surgery for hypothalamic or pituitary tumours. Head trauma may result in diabetes insipidus; the extent of the damage will determine the severity of the diabetes. All of these causes of diabetes insipidus will be due to an underlying ADH deficiency, although the reason for the ADH deficiency will differ.

Diagnosis of diabetes insipidus

A careful history should be taken, involving family history and a detailed account of drinking and urinary habits. Plasma and urine osmolality must be measured. The osmolality of the urine in diabetes insipidus is very low when compared to that of the plasma. These levels are not always conclusive and water deprivation tests may be necessitated. Vasopressin (antidiuretic hormone) trials are also of great value in determining whether the disease is central or nephrogenic. Radioimmunoassays are available that allow us to measure plasma levels of ADH.

If other endocrine disease is present such as anterior pituitary disease, the diagnosis of diabetes insipidus is often difficult to make.

Treatment of diabetes insipidus

A nasal spray containing synthetic vasopressin which is an antidiuretic hormone (such as desmopressin) is administered. This is to replace the absent antidiuretic hormone, which will allow the urine to become more concentrate. The frequency of administration varies with severity of disease, but will hopefully achieve one mild diuresis every 24 hours instead of a constant diuresis. The result is usually good with excellent control of polyuria and polydipsia. Sodium and serum osmolality are measured at frequent intervals, usually initially weekly then monthly etc. Desmopressin can be given subcutaneously if necessary, although the nasal route is usually preferable for most people.

Acute pancreatitis

Acute pancreatitis is a serious condition that is characterized by inflammation of the pancreas.

Pathophysiology

Acute pancreatitis is caused by self-digestion of this organ by the very enzymes that it produces to aid digestion. The pancreas as mentioned earlier is an organ that has more than one function. Its endocrine function of insulin production was discussed earlier on. It is its exocrine function that needs to be understood in this condition. The enzyme it produces principally is called trypsin. The pancreas produces between 1 and 4 litres per day of this substance; pancreatitis occurs usually when there is a blockage of the biliary system causing a backflow of the digestive juices into the organ itself. Other causes include chronic alcoholism, trauma and ischaemic vascular disease.

Signs and symptoms

Severe abdominal pain is the most striking feature of the serious condition. It may occur following a heavy meal or alcohol session. There will be abdominal distension with rigidity. Nausea and vomiting may be present as may fever, jaundice and hypotension. The patient will be acutely ill and may become shocked, tachycardic and show signs of dyspnoea.

Laboratory tests

BLOOD

Serum amylase and lipase will be elevated, peaking at 24 hours, falling rapidly to normal levels within 48 to 72 hours. White cell count will be elevated and hypocalcaemia may correlate with the severity of the condition.

X-RAY

X-Rays of chest and abdomen will be performed to differentiate pancreatitis from other abdominal disorders.

Treatment

Treatment is aimed primarily at prevention or treatment of complications.

- Oral intake is prevented to reduce pancreatic stimulation.
- Intravenous infusion is commenced.
- A nasogastric tube may be passed to remove fluid from the stomach and thus ease distension and nausea.
- Antacids may used after the initial acute episode has passed.

Nursing care of the patient

Nursing care is aimed at supporting the comfort of the patient. Following a careful assessment the following aspects must be considered (Simpson, 1998).

1 *Close observation of vital signs* is essential to prevent worsening of this condition. 1–2 hourly blood pressure, pulse and respiration. In particular respiratory function assessment is vital as respiratory insufficiency may ensue.
2 *Pain relief.* The nurse must provide analgesia as prescribed for this extremely painful condition.
3 *Fluid balance.* All input and output must be carefully monitored. Mouth care and hygiene needs must be met.
4 *Psychological support* of the patient and family is essential.

Disorders of the thyroid gland

The thyroid gland is responsible for regulating homeostatic function (which is responsible for enabling a state of equilibrium in the body) such as the production of heat and energy and metabolism (Behi, 1988). Thyroid disease is perhaps one of the most poorly diagnosed diseases; this may be due to the fact that most of the signs and symptoms can be attributed to minor illness or other diseases. For the most part thyroid disease does not present as a medical emergency, but for those affected it is no less distressing and frustrating. To understand the severity of thyroid disorder it is necessary for the nurse to fully understand the function of the thyroid gland.

The thyroid gland is situated in the neck at the level of the fifth, sixth and seventh cervical vertebrae (Fig. 5.4). It is a bilobular gland and is extremely vascular. To enable the thyroid gland to synthesize the necessary hormones for bodily functions it relies on iodine. Iodine enters the body through food or water as iodide or iodite ion (Hinchliff and Montague, 1994). The thyroid

gland, by means of a thyrotrophin-dependent pump, concentrates and traps iodide in the follicular cells, and stores it in thyroglobulin. Two things happen in the follicular cells: the iodide is

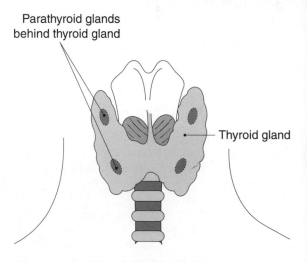

Figure 5.4   Position of the thyroid gland

rapidly oxidized by a peroxidase catalysed reaction, and iodine reacts with tyrosine deposits in the thyroglobulin (by organification) to form tri-iodothyronine (T3) and thyroxine (T4), which are iodinated hormones. The thyroglobulin containing these iodinated hormones is then secreted into the follicles and stored as colloid.

Regulation of thyroid hormones

The release of the T3 and T4 hormones is controlled by a negative feedback system, which is in turn controlled by circulating levels of T3 and T4. When circulating levels of T3 and T4 fall, the hypothalamus gland is stimulated into producing thyrotrophin-releasing hormone (TRH) which in turn travels to the anterior pituitary gland to stimulate the release of thyroid-stimulating hormone (TSH). TSH is the primary factor controlling thyroid growth and hormone production and secretion. TSH rapidly induces the production of pseudopods at the cell colloid border which accelerate the absorption of thyroglobulin. Colloid droplets are formed which fuse with lysosomes, and protease enzymes degrade the thyroglobulin and release it into the circulation. These hormones then go on to influence a range of functions. Just as a low circulating concentration of T3 and T4 will stimulate the hypothalamus to produce TRH, so high circulating levels of T3 and T4 will inhibit this process (Fig. 5.5).

Effects of the thyroid hormones

T3 and T4 circulate in the serum bound to protein carriers, although there is still some available free hormone. It is the free hormones that cross the cell membrane, either through diffusion or by specific transport system (depending on availability) through the cell cytoplasm to bind with the specific receptor in the cell nucleus. Inside the cell T4 is converted into T3 which appears to be the active hormone.

The effects of T3 are felt almost immediately in

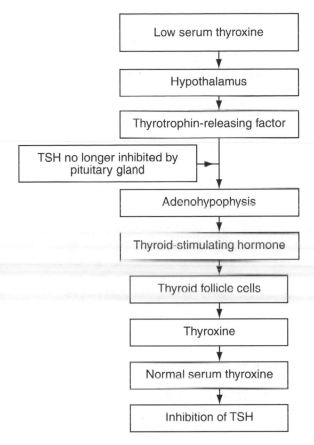

Figure 5.5 Regulation of thyroxin secretion

our early life and continue to affect us (Clancy and McVicar, 1995).

1 *Fetal development.* Before about 11 weeks the fetus is dependant on small amounts of maternal T3 which manage to cross the placental barrier, however after 11 weeks gestation the fetus can depend on its own anterior pituitary TSH system for normal growth and development.
2 *Heat production.* T3 increases the consumption of oxygen and the production of heat and by doing so increases the basal metabolic rate.
3 *Skeletal effects.* T3 stimulates increased bone reabsorption and to some extent bone formation. Therefore untreated hyperthyroidism may result in depletion of calcium from the bone (osteopaenia).
4 *Gastrointestinal effects.* Gut motility is stimulated by the thyroid hormones.
5 *Neuromuscular effect.* Thyroid hormones are

essential for normal growth and development, also for the function of the central nervous system. In hyperthyroidism muscle reflexes become overly brisk (known clinically as hyperreflexia). In hyperthyroidism protein turnover is increased and loss of muscle tissue (or myopathy) results if untreated.

6 *Cardiovascular effects.* The thyroid hormones increase the number of beta adrenergic receptors in the heart, improving contractility of the heart.

7 *Pulmonary effects.* The normal response of the respiratory centre is maintained by thyroid hormones. In severe cases of hypothyroidism patients may need artificial ventilation due to hypoventilation.

Laboratory investigations

Thyroid function tests are most commonly used to determine whether too much or too little hormone is being produced. Sensitive assay tests are now available to aid with accurate diagnosis of underactive and overactive thyroid glands, and also thyroid disease.

These same assays are also used to determine whether treatment used for thyroid disorder is being successful. TSH analysis is probably the best assay when testing for thyroid abnormality, and if abnormal levels of TSH are found (elevated in hypothyroidism and suppressed in hyperthyroidism) then further estimates of T3 and T4 and free thyroxin should be investigated.

Thyroglobulin can be measured in serum by double antibody radioimmunoassay, but depending on the method may give spuriously high and low values. For patients with hyperthyroidism a radioactive iodine uptake test and scan may be of some use.

Normal ranges for serum thyroid hormones	
Total thyroxine (T4)	60–150 nmol/L
Triiodothyronine (T3)	0.8–2.4 nmol/L
Free T4	8.8–23.2 pmol/L
Free T3	0–8.6 pmol/L
T4/TBG ratio	6–12
TSH	0.13–3.54

Hypothyroidism

Hypothyroidism can be either congenital or acquired.

CONGENITAL

1 Congenital absence.
2 Inborn errors of thyroxin metabolism.

ACQUIRED

1 Iodine deficiency.
2 Autoimmune thyroiditis (Hashimoto's disease).
3 Post-radiotherapy for hyperthyroidism.
4 Post-surgical thyroidectomy.
5 Anti-thyroid drugs (i.e. carbimazole).
6 Pituitary tumours and granulomas.

Almost 95 per cent of new patients have primary dysfunction of the thyroid gland itself.

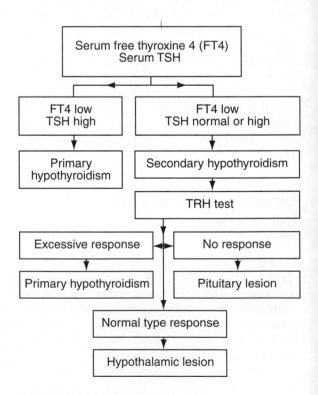

Figure 5.6   Diagnosis of hypothyroidism

PATHOGENESIS

Hypothyroidism may be classified as a clinical syndrome. It affects every system of the body. A lack of thyroid hormones results in hypothyroidism and in turn results in a general slowing down of the body's systems. In an infant this has serious consequences, and results in marked slowing of growth and development both physically and mentally (cretinism). In adults the systems generally slow down and there is depositing of glycoaminoglycans in the intracellular spaces producing the typical picture of hypothyroidism or myxoedema.

The manifestation of myxoedema may vary with the degree and duration of the disease, but corresponds to the lack of thyroid hormone.

There is an abnormal reduction in cellular activity, and lack of thyroxin causes the body to retain water, resulting in the puffy-faced myxoedemic look. The retention of water also brings about an increase in the blood volume; this may lead to hypertension. A slow pulse rate is common with hypothyroidism and rarely low output heart failure may occur. Slow metabolism means low body temperature and the risks of hypothermia, especially for the elderly. Many myxoedemic patients develop a preference for warm climates.

The adult brain has reached maturity and therefore there is no retardation; however in moderately severe cases nerve responses may be dulled and the patient may complain of lack of mental awareness. The skin may become thick and dry and the tongue and lips appear overlarge. The patient's voice may be noticeably hoarse.

SIGNS AND SYMPTOMS

1 Constipation.
2 Weight gain.
3 Hair loss.
4 Angina pectoris.
5 Hoarse voice.
6 Dry flaky skin.
7 Balding and loss of eyebrows.
8 Bradycardia.
9 Xanthelasmas (hyperlipidaemia).
10 Goitre (especially with iodine deficiency).
11 Delayed relaxation phase of tendon reflexes.
12 Effusions (pericardial/pleural).
13 Carpal tunnel syndrome.
14 Menstrual interference – amenorrhoea/menorrhagia.
15 Bizarre psychiatric features classified as myxoedema madness.

TREATMENT OF HYPOTHYROIDISM

Replacement of the deficient hormone is the basis of treatment. In the case of neonatal hypothyroidism, prompt treatment is necessary to prevent abnormal development. This is most satisfactorily achieved by taking thyroxine sodium (Eltroxin) orally, although it can be administered intravenously in the case of myxoedemic coma. Liothyronine sodium has a similar action to thyroxine, but is more rapidly metabolized. Liothyronine sodium may be used in severe hypothyroid states where a rapid response is required. The response of thyroxine may be measured both clinically and biochemically.

For an adult the initial dose should not exceed 100 µg daily, preferably before breakfast. The dose should be increased every 2–4 weeks until normal metabolism is steadily maintained.

NURSING CARE

Nursing care of the patient with hypothyroidism is based upon the symptoms of the condition. It consists of:

1 Ensuring that medication is administered and understood by the patient.
2 Providing support and reassurance for the patient and family.
3 Ensuring the patient is comfortable, warm and assisting with daily living.
4 Close monitoring of the condition and awareness of worsening state. Preventing the onset of myxoedemic coma.

Myxoedemic coma

Myxoedemic coma is a severe medical emergency and should be treated as such. This is the most extreme form of myxoedema and if treated incorrectly may be fatal. In the absence of sufficient

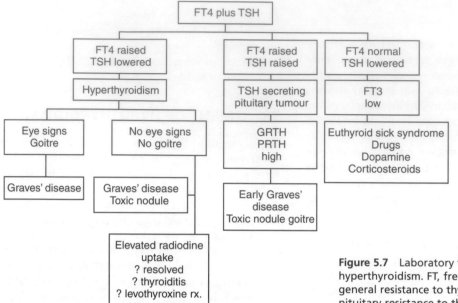

Figure 5.7 Laboratory tests in the diagnosis of hyperthyroidism. FT, free thyroxine; GRTH, general resistance to thyroid hormones; PRTH, pituitary resistance to thyroid hormones

thyroid hormones the body's systems have slowed down to the extent the patient becomes comatose and hypoventilation ensues. These patients often need intubation and mechanical ventilation, and blood gases should be measured regularly. Other complications such as heart disease or infection should be suspected and treated.

Intravenous therapy is commenced with caution; remember these patients are already retaining fluid. Drug absorption is poor, and replacement of thyroid hormone is given intravenously as levothyroxine because of this. These patients have free thyroxine binding sites, with a depletion of serum thyroxine, so intravenous thyroid hormones should have good effect. An echocardiograph (ECG) is often helpful when commencing therapy to assess the risk of angina or cardiac arrhythmias.

The clinical signs of recovery are a return of cerebral and respiratory function, and the return to normal of the body temperature. During the time of unconsciousness the patient will need full supportive nursing care, and careful handling to maintain body temperature.

If the patient was known to have a normal adrenal function before the coma, it is not necessary to investigate for adrenal problems. If however no history is available adrenal insufficiency due to adrenal or pituitary disease should be discounted by measuring the plasma cortisol level.

The prognosis for myxoedemic coma is good provided the need for intubation and mechanical respiration is noted. The patient also has a better chance of survival if underlying diseases or problems are recognized and treated promptly.

Hyperthyroidism

The clinical syndrome opposite to hypothyroidism is that of hyperthyroidism, or thyrotoxicosis (Fig. 5.7). This condition is the result of tissues being exposed to high levels of circulating thyroid hormones. The most common cause of thyrotoxicosis is an overactive thyroid. Less common causes include:

1 Over-ingestion of thyroxine therapy
2 Excessive secretion of thyroid hormones from ectopic sites

Conditions associated with thyrotoxicosis

1 Diffuse goitre (Graves' disease)
2 Toxic adenoma (Plummer's disease)
3 Carcinoma of the thyroid
4 Teratoma of the ovary
5 Hydatidiform mole

GRAVES' DISEASE

This is the most common form of thyrotoxicosis and occurs much more in women than in men. There is a strong familial tendency, with about 15 per cent of new cases having a close relative with the same condition. It is commonly viewed as an autoimmune disease and about 50 per cent of these patients' relatives will have autoimmune antibodies circulating. Graves' disease is a syndrome which consists of one or more symptoms, for example:

1 Thyrotoxicosis.
2 Exophthalmos.
3 Goitre.
4 Dermopathy (pretibial myxoedema).

Pathogenesis

In Graves' disease, T lymphocytes become sensitized to antigens within the thyroid gland and this stimulates B lymphocytes to produce antibodies to these antigens. One of these antibodies is directed at the TSH receptor site, and has the capacity to stimulate it, ultimately stimulating thyroid hormones, and growth and development of the thyroid gland. Although there is an underlying genetic predisposition it is not entirely clear what triggers the disease. The circulating level of antibody correlates directly to its severity.

Signs and symptoms of Graves' disease

Signs

1 Diffuse goitre
2 Conjunctival oedema
3 Lower leg oedema
4 Finger clubbing
5 Oncholysis (Plummer's nails)
6 Lid retraction and lag
7 Ophthalmoplegia
8 Exophthalmos.

Symptoms

1 Heat intolerance
2 Weight loss
3 Nervousness or fidgeting
4 Bounding peripheral pulses
5 Lid retraction and lag
6 Sweating
7 Fine peripheral tremor
8 Brisk tendon reflexes
9 Tachycardia
10 Atrial fibrillation

Treatment of Graves' disease

Although Graves' disease is an autoimmune disease, the treatment for it concentrates on controlling the hyperthyroidism. The three alternate treatments are:

- Surgery.
- Antithyroid drug therapy.
- Radioactive iodine therapy.

Nursing care

These patients need a high level of nursing care, careful monitoring of vital signs, drugs administered and response to therapy. Patient reassurance is essential, as some instances of thyrotoxic crisis are precipitated by emotional crisis.

1 Great effort should be made to keep the patient calm and reassured
2 Adequate dietary and fluid input is required to prevent malnutrition
3 Care should be taken to keep the patient's skin clean and dry
4 Eye care is required to prevent injury to the eyes which will be prominent

Surgical treatment

Because the thyroid gland is a very vascular gland, surgery can be difficult. To help avoid complications, patients are usually given potassium iodide drops daily for about 2 weeks to help reduce the vascularity. The patient will be given antithyroid drugs prior to treatment to stabilize the general condition; this usually takes about 6–8 weeks. Surgery is often an option for those patients who have very enlarged glands, or perhaps marked multinodular goitres.

There is some conflict regarding the amount of thyroid tissue that should be taken; however almost always a subtotal thyroidectomy is all that is necessary (usually leaving a couple of grams of tissue either side of the neck). However, if the patient has particularly progressive complications, rarely a total thyroidectomy may be performed. It is not possible to remove exact quantities and often patients require thyroxine supplements post-surgically. The alternative is to risk too much thyroid tissue remaining and for the disease to relapse.

Antithyroid drug treatment

Most patients with small glands and mild disease can be treated with antithyroid drugs. The drugs (such as carbimazole) are administered until the disease undergoes remission. Thionamides prevent the synthesis of thyroid hormones by inhibiting the peroxidase catalysed reaction necessary for iodine organification. All antithyroid drugs are administered orally, and all accumulate in the thyroid gland. These drugs do not begin to take effect until the thyroid hormones that are already formed are depleted, usually about 4 weeks. This process of treatment needs careful monitoring and has a high relapse rate, as much as 60–80 per cent. Once the patient is deemed to be euthyroid, the dose is reduced to a maintenance dose.

Radioactive iodine therapy

Following the administration of radioactive iodine the thyroid gland will shrink; over a period of 6–12 weeks the patient will usually become euthyroid. Prior to the treatment the patient will be given antithyroid drugs to aim for a euthyroid state; a week before the treatment drugs are stopped. Radioactive uptake and scan are done, and the dosage of radioactive iodine is calculated on the thyroid estimated weight. Again this treatment is not an exact science, and one of the biggest problems is that the patient becomes hypothyroid; however this often happens with any treatment for hyperthyroidism and is at least a reassurance that hyperthyroidism will not reoccur. As with all patients treated for thyroid disorder, a life-time follow-up is essential to ensure the euthyroid state.

During the acute stages of thyrotoxicosis, beta adrenergic drugs (such as propanolol) are often used; these are for treatment of symptoms such as palpitations, tachycardia and atrial fibrillation. They do not help with treatment of the overactive thyroid gland.

THYROTOXIC CRISIS

Otherwise known as a thyroid storm, this condition requires rigorous management. Thyroid storm is rarely seen since the introduction of radioactive iodine and antithyroid drugs. Often it is the result of an underlying illness or infection, and rarely as the result of thyroid therapy or surgery.

Pathogenesis

Thyrotoxic crisis results from a sudden and rapid production and synthesis of thyroid hormones. The metabolic rate rises rapidly and as a result the patient has a multitude of signs and symptoms, all representing the severe form of hyperthyroidism. For example tachycardia, atrial fibrillation, acute restlessness, diarrhoea and vomiting and eventually heart failure and collapse.

Treatment of thyrotoxic crisis

1 Beta adrenergic drugs administered orally/i.v. for control of arrhythmias
2 Antithyroid drugs administered orally, or if necessary as suppository. Control of the hormone synthesis is imperative.
3 Sodium iodide i.v. over 24 hours. Retards hormone release.
4 Antipyretics. To control fever.
5 Intravenous fluids. For nutrition and electrolyte imbalance.
6 Sedatives.
7 Oxygen, digitalis and diuretics for heart failure.
8 Treatment of underlying disease, such as antibiotics/antiallergy drugs etc.

Specific nursing care

The nurse caring for the patient with a hyperthyroid condition under treatment must monitor his or her physical and psychological state at all times. Treatment effectiveness must be watched closely. As with all conditions, reaasurance and supprt is needed both for the patient and their family as this condition can be frightening. If the patient's condition should worsen it is vital that the surgeon or physician is informed immediately.

Hypocalcaemia

Hypocalcaemia usually results from a failure in the normal responses of the parathyroid hormone (PTH) or vitamin D, to maintain a normal serum calcium level. In other words hypocalcaemia may result from a lack of PTH secreted by the parathyroid gland, a failure of the normal responses in recognizing the PTH, or it may result from a lack of vitamin D or a failure of the normal responses to vitamin D. Hypocalcaemia causes neuromuscular excitability and most of the manifestations are as a result of this.

Signs and symptoms

1 Seizures
2 Paraesthesia (pins and needles)
3 Tetany (intermittent tonic muscle contraction)
4 Cataract
5 Organic brain syndrome
6 Calcification of the basal ganglia

NURSING CONSIDERATIONS

Many patients may complain of tingling in their fingers, lips and tongue. The classic sign of tetany is muscle spasm and most commonly recognized is the carpopedal spasm. The thumb is adducted and the metocarpophalangeal joints flexed. The interphalangeal joints are extended and the wrists flexed. Collectively this is known as the 'main d'accoucheur' posture. The hands are typically the most affected area, but potentially any muscle group may be affected. If this involuntary spasm affects the laryngeal muscles the condition becomes life-threatening.

Hypocalcaemia also has dermatological effects; patients often complain of dry and flaky skin and may be predisposed to other dermatological conditions. There are also cardiac implications, with a delay in repolarization (an extended QT interval) and patients with underlying heart problems may suffer heart failure. Cataracts are common and the severity of the cataract will depend on the severity and duration of the hypocalcaemia.

Causes of hypocalcaemia

1 Hypoparathyroidism (a condition caused by a lack of secretion by the parathyroids)
2 Pseudohypoparathyroidism
3 Other disorders, i.e. rhabdomyolysis

Hypoparathyroidism

Hypoparathyroidism may be an autoimmune, familial, idiopathic or most commonly a surgical problem. Surgery to the neck which involves removal or destruction of the parathyroid glands (which are situated to the sides of the thyroid gland) will increase the risk of hypoparathyroidism.

Surgery most often associated with this problem is thyroidectomy, parathyroidectomy or surgery for tumours. If acute tetany occurs it will be approximately 2 days post-operatively and although initially many cases seem dramatic, often many of these patients will recover well enough not to necessitate calcium replacement (seemingly some part of the gland has recovered a blood supply). However for approximately 50 per cent of all these patients some form of replacement therapy will be necessary, although it may not be for a couple of years after surgery.

TREATMENT FOR ACUTE HYPOCALCAEMIA

The mainstay of the treatment is intravenous calcium given as calcium chloride or calcium gluconate. Calcium should be given over a few minutes (200 mg to begin with). Oral calcium and vitamin D should be commenced, but further i.v. calcium may be necessary in bolus doses until this takes effect. Treatment is titrated against serum calcium values. As well as pharmacotherapy, these patients need intensive nursing care as often they are unable to manage even simple tasks when the muscle spasms are present. If the patient has suf-

fered laryngeal spasm, a tracheotomy may have to be performed, which subsequently adds to the patient's requirements.

NURSING CONSIDERATIONS

- The nurse must monitor the patient's vital signs constantly during the acute phase. Blood pressure, pulse, temperature and respiratory function must be regularly checked.
- Treatment as prescribed must be given and carefully recorded. Its effects should be monitored and recorded.
- Constant reassurance is required both for patient and family.
- If the patient's condition should deteriorate, then immediate medical assistance must be sought.

Further reading

Avery, R. 1992 *Principles and practice of clinical pharmacology and therapy*. London: Pharmaceutical Press.

Behi, R. 1988 Treatment and care of thyroid problems. *Nursing* **3**(41) 4.

Brunner, L.S. and Suddarth, D.S. 1992 *The textbook of adult nursing*. London: Chapman and Hall.

Cahill, G.F. 1976 Insulin and glucagon. In: Parsons, J.A. (ed.) *Peptides, hormones*. London: Macmillan.

Clancy, J. and McVicar, A. 1995 *Physiology and anatomy. A homeostatic approach*. London: Arnold.

Craven, R.E. and Hirnle, C.J. 1992 *Fundamentals of nursing, human health and function*. Philadelphia: J B Lippencott.

Epstein, O., Perkins, G.D. *et al.* 1992 *Clinical examination*. London: Gower Medical Publishing.

Goodinson, S. 1996 Assessment of nutritional status. *Nursing* **7**, 252–8.

Hataas, J.L. 1995 Weight reducing effects of the

plasma protein encoded by the obese gene. *Science* 269–343.

Hague, W. 1987 Treatment of endocrine diseases. *British Medical Journal* **294**, 297.

Hinchliff, S. and Montague, S. 1994 *Physiology for nursing practice*. London: Baillière Tindall.

Hinchliff, S., Norman, S. and Schober, J. 1994 *Nursing practice and health care*. London: Arnold.

Leibovitz, H.E. 1991 (ed.) *Therapy for diabetes mellitus and other related disorders*. New York: American Diabetes Association.

McGee, M. 1993 *A guide to laboratory investigations*, 2nd edn. Oxford: Radcliffe Medical Press.

Martindale 1993. *The extra pharmacopoeia*, 13th edn. London: The Pharmaceutical Press.

Neal, M.J. 1992 *Medical pharmacology at a glance*, 2nd edn. London: Blackwell Science.

Simpson, P. 1998 *Introduction to surgical nursing*. London: Arnold.

Young, E. 1988 Goitre. *Surgery* **63**, 1499.

Caring for the neurological system

Jenny Muxlow

Introduction

The aim of this chapter is to explore the issues surrounding the treatment and care of the neurologically ill patient in the high dependency setting. Many patients suffering from head injury, or other neurological assaults, be it due to disease or accident, will require the depth and intensity of care offered by a high dependency unit. Accurate observation, detection and the prompt reporting of changes in neurological status can be life saving. This chapter will focus upon the injuries and acute illnesses most commonly seen in the high dependency unit.

Anatomy and physiology of the nervous system

The nervous system consists of two main parts, the autonomic or automatic part whose function is associated with the control of blood pressure and other vital functions and the central nervous system. The central nervous system comprises the brain and spinal cord. This is often described as being rather like a large telephone network, both transmitting and receiving messages via a complex system of neurones and chemical transmitters.

Overview of the central nervous system

Functional anatomy of the brain

The brain is divided anatomically into three main structures: the forebrain, the midbrain and the hindbrain. Medical science is gaining knowledge relating to the function of the brain. However, there is still much that we do not know about the complex function of the brain and its structures.

THE FOREBRAIN

The forebrain consists of the cerebrum, which is divided into two hemispheres connected by a large bundle of myelinated axons (nerve cells) allowing communication between the two hemispheres. Each hemisphere consists of an outer cortical section and the inner subcortical structure which, it is thought, connects with the midbrain and hindbrain. The cortex is made up of 'grey matter' and is the main information processing area. The surfaces or lobes of the cortex are named after the bones in the skull, namely, the frontal, temporal, parietal and occipital lobes (Fig. 6.1).

The frontal lobes are responsible for the planning, execution and evaluation of actions. The parietal lobes are mostly responsible for sensory reception and perception and make sense of sensations such as touch and pain. They are also thought to be used in the creation of memory. The occipital lobes receive most of the input from the eyes and contain the visual cortex. The temporal

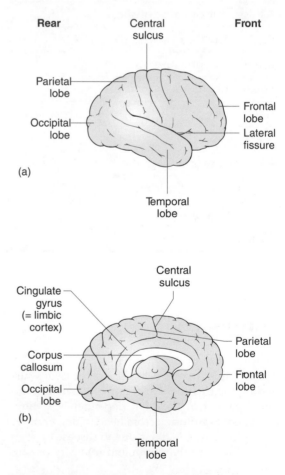

Figure 6.1 Cerebral hemispheres of the forebrain. (a) External features: lateral view. (b) The inner surface of the left hemisphere, with the right hemisphere removed

lobes are also part of the memory system and receive sensory input from the ears.

THE CEREBRAL NUCLEI

Beneath the cortex lies the white matter. This consists of myelinated axons which convey impulses between different parts of the brain. There are also areas of grey matter which comprise processing areas called the basal ganglia and the limbic system. The basal ganglia are involved with the control of movement and interact with the motor cortex. The limbic system consists of the hippocampus and the amygdala. This system has a role in memory, behaviour and the control of emotion. Deep within the forebrain lies the diencephalon; this section of the brain consists of the thalamus and hypothalamus. The thalamus acts as a relay centre for sensory input to the cortex. The hypothalamus lies at the base of the brain. This structure controls the autonomic nervous system and via the pituitary gland release of several of the main hormones.

THE MIDBRAIN

The midbrain lies deep within the brain and consists of the tectum and the tegtectum. The tectum forms the posterior part of the midbrain. The tectum

receives input from the eyes, via the thalamus and helps control eye movement. In addition to this it receives sound input from the ears. The tegtectum helps control movement, relays sensory information and has a role in the control of sleep cycle.

THE HINDBRAIN

The hindbrain is composed of the cerebellum, pons varolii and the medulla oblongata. The cerebellum is a large structure at the back of the brain. This part of the brain receives input from the eyes and ears. The cerebellum controls the fine tuning of movement, and is essential to walking or standing. The pons varolii is part of the relay system transferring information to the cerebellum. The medulla oblongata links the brain with the spinal cord. The medulla controls respiration, cardiovascular acceleration and depression and also transmits impulses from the body via the spinal cord.

THE CRANIAL NERVES

The cranial nerves are part of the peripheral nervous system and connect directly to the brain rather than the spinal pathways (Fig. 6.2). There are twelve pairs of cranial nerves. Ten pairs connect with the

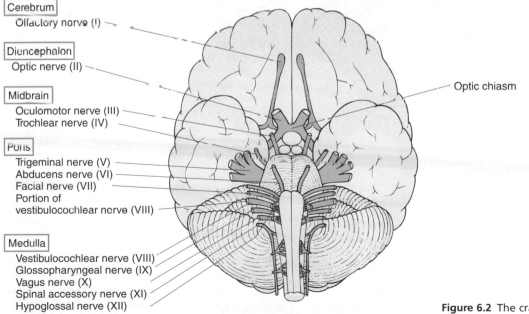

Cerebrum
Olfactory nerve (I)

Diencephalon
Optic nerve (II)

Midbrain
Oculomotor nerve (III)
Trochlear nerve (IV)

Pons
Trigeminal nerve (V)
Abducens nerve (VI)
Facial nerve (VII)
Portion of
vestibulocochlear nerve (VIII)

Medulla
Vestibulocochlear nerve (VIII)
Glossopharyngeal nerve (IX)
Vagus nerve (X)
Spinal accessory nerve (XI)
Hypoglossal nerve (XII)

Optic chiasm

Figure 6.2 The cranial nerves

Table 6.1 Functions of the cranial nerves

Cranial nerve	Branch	Homeostatic Function	Tissues innervated
Olfactory (I)	–	Sensory	From olfactory epithelium of the nose
Optic (II)	–	Sensory	From retinal cells of the eye
Oculomotor (III)	–	Motor	To the rectus muscles (inferior, superior, medial) and inferior oblique muscle that move the eyes. Also to the upper lip area
Trochlear (IV)	–	Motor	To the superior oblique muscle of the eye
Trigeminal (V)	Opthalmic	Sensory	From areas around the orbits of the eyes, the nasal cavity, the forehead, upper eyelids, and eyebrows
	Maxillary	Sensory	From the lower eyelids, upper lip, upper gums and teeth, the mucous lining of the palate, and the skin of the face
	Mandibular	Mixed	*Sensory* from the skin of the jaw, the lower gums and teeth, and the lower lip. *Motor* to the muscles of mastication, and to the floor of the mouth.
Abducens (VI)	–	Motor	To the rectus muscles (lateral that move the eyes
Facial (VII)	–	Mixed	*Sensory* from taste receptors (anterior two-thirds of tongue). *Motor* to muscles of facial expression. Includes visceral efferents (autonomic nervous system) to the submandibular and sublingual salivary glands, and tear glands
Vestibulocochlear (VIII)	Vestibular	Sensory	From the vestibular apparatus (balance organs) of inner ear
	Cochlear	Sensory	From hearing receptors of the cochlea of inner ear
Glossopharyngeal (IX)	–	Mixed	*Sensory* from the pharynx, tonsils, and posterior third of tongue. Includes visceral afferents (autonomic nervous system) from carotid arteries and aortic arch. *Motor* to pharynx (i.e. swallowing movements). Also visceral efferents (autonomic nervous system) to parotid salivary glands
Vagus (X)	–	Mixed	Sensory from the pharynx, larynx, and oesophagus. Also visceral afferents (autonomic nervous system) from the thorax and abdomen. *Motor* to the larynx, pharynx, and soft palate (swallowing movements). Also visceral efferents (autonomic nervous system) to viscera of the thorax and abdomen
Accessory (XI)	Cranial	Motor	To the pharynx, larynx, and soft palate (swallowing movements)
	Spinal	Motor	To the sternocleidomastoid and trapezius muscles of the neck
Hypoglassal (XII)	–	Motor	To the musculature of the tongue

brainstem, two pairs, the olfactory and optic nerves, connect with the forebrain. It is important that the nurse is aware of these nerves as injury may disrupt their functions and alert the nurse to a change in the patient's condition (Table 6.1).

BLOOD SUPPLY

The brain is supplied by four arteries. Two originate from the common carotid arteries, each of which divides into an internal and external branch. The external carotid arteries supply the

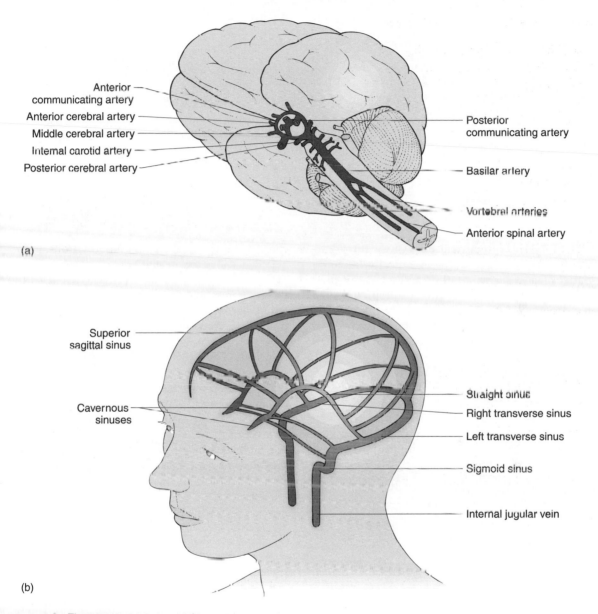

Anterior communicating artery

Anterior cerebral artery

Middle cerebral artery

Internal carotid artery

Posterior cerebral artery

Posterior communicating artery

Basilar artery

Vertebral arteries

Anterior spinal artery

(a)

Superior sagittal sinus

Cavernous sinuses

Straight sinus

Right transverse sinus

Left transverse sinus

Sigmoid sinus

Internal jugular vein

(b)

Figure 6.3 The blood supply to the brain (a) Cerebral arteries. The anterior and posterior communicating arteries join the three pairs of cerebral arteries to form the circle of Willis around the base of the brain (b) Venous drainage

pharynx, larynx and the face. The internal carotid arteries supply the brain. The other two arteries supplying brain are called the vertebral arteries.

In order to maintain normal activity, the adult brain requires 750 mL of oxygenated blood per minute. From the total amount of circulating oxygen, 20 per cent is consumed by the brain. Under normal conditions the cessation of blood flow to

the brain for as short a period as 5–10 seconds is sufficient to cause temporary changes in neural activity. Interruption of blood flow to the brain for 5–10 minutes will result in irreversible brain damage. The major blood vessel structure associated with the flow of blood to the brain tissue is the Circle of Willis (Fig. 6.3).

ACTIVITY 6.1

Make a list of the patients that you have seen who have suffered from brain injuries in the past. Can you associate some of their signs and symptoms with damage to the structures of the brain outlined above?

Assessment of consciousness

One of the most important roles of the nurse caring for the seriously ill, neurologically impaired patient lies with the accurate assessment of their neurological status, and correct interpretation of the observed data. The most widely used tool in the assessment of neurological status is the Glasgow Coma Scale which was developed by Jennett and Teasdale (1974).

Full consciousness is dependent upon the cerebral hemispheres being intact and interacting with the ascending reticular activating system (RAS) (Fig. 6.4). This system runs through the brainstem, the hypothalamus and thalamus; therefore any lesion which affects this communication process will result in impairment of consciousness. Chipps *et al.* (1992) describe a person's state of consciousness as their degree of arousal and awareness. They describe arousal as the measure of being awake, whereas awareness involves the person being able to interpret incoming, sensory data and making sense of it by responding appropriately. A comatose patient is not aware of the incoming stimuli, and therefore there is no response. A patient who is described as being in a persistent vegetative state (PVS) has no awareness, but demonstrates arousal; however, this is not in response to sensory stimuli.

'Locked in' syndrome is where the patient can be aroused and is aware, but because of damage to the motor pathways in the brainstem, they are unable to respond either verbally or through purposeful movement (Viney, 1996).

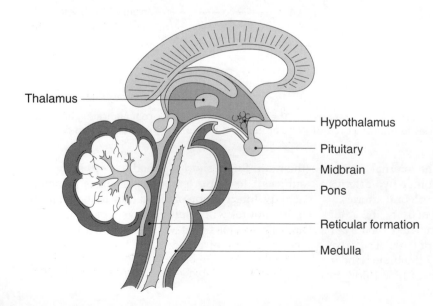

Thalamus

Hypothalamus

Pituitary

Midbrain

Pons

Reticular formation

Medulla

Figure 6.4 Lateral view of the brain identifying the reticular formation system

Neurological assessment

When carrying out neurological assessment, the nurse must observe for the best level of response. The score ratings on the Glasgow Coma Scale (Fig. 6.5) are used to measure consciousness; the patient who scores 8 or less on the scale is considered to be in a coma. On the other hand, the patient who scores 8 or more on the scale and is able to obey commands, thus receiving sensory input and responding appropriately would be considered to be conscious. Most importantly, wherever possible the same nurse should carry out the neurological assessment of a patient for the shift, thus increasing the accuracy of the recordings. When handing over to another nurse, both should undertake the patient's neurological assessment. The chart is intended that the observations of the 'best' response are recorded without any reference to the previous score. However in reality this often is not seen to be the case; therefore an opportunity to hand over should increase the nurse's confidence in the accuracy of their interpretation of the data.

When carrying out neurological assessment, the areas which are assessed are the eyes, verbal response, and motor activity.

EYES

Just because a patient's eyes are open, this does not mean that they are aware, or aroused. Many papers indicate that the majority of head-injured patients, despite the severity of their cerebral injuries, will eventually open their eyes, but not be aware of their surroundings. Usually patients with head injury demonstrate spontaneous blinking and their eyes will move around; again it is essential that this is not interpreted as the patient being aware.

Pupil reaction provides vital information about central nervous function. The use of correct equipment is essential (a pen torch). The pupils should be round and equal in shape and size (2–5 mm), when checking the reaction to light note the speed of constriction.

An expanding mass such as a blood clot may cause pressure to be exerted upon the 3rd cranial nerve (the oculomotor) resulting in lack of response to light. A fixed and dilated pupil may be the result of a herniation of the medial temporal lobe. Remember that the lesion is on the same side as the fixed dilated pupil.

VERBAL RESPONSE

This is performed to assess two parts of the function of the cerebral cortex. It firstly examines the transmission and understanding of verbal and also physical stimuli, it also measures the ability to respond to questions or noise. The outcomes of this may indicate whether the language area of the brain is involved, which is situated in the dominant hemisphere of the brain.

Orientation

The patient will know who they are, where they are, and the time or the day. However other conversation may not be clear.

Confused

The patient is considered to be confused if one or more of the questions cannot be answered correctly.

Inappropriate words

Here speech is used in a jumbled manner, and conversation is rarely possible. Some of the words may however be understood, but they are not appropriate to the question.

Incomprehensible

This is when the only response the nurse can elicit from the patient is noises without any understandable words.

No response

Finally, this is where no verbal response at all can be obtained from the patient.

MOTOR ACTIVITY

Within this catagory of the Glasgow Coma Assessment, the nurse is looking for the best motor response from the patient.

Obeys commands

This involves asking such questions as 'put out your tongue' or 'squeeze my fingers'. It is essential

GLASGOW OBSERVATION CHART

DATE						
TIME						
C O M A S C A L E	Eyes open	Spontaneously				Eyes closed by swelling = C
		To speech				
		To pain				
		None				
	Best verbal response	Orientated				Endotracheal tube or tracheostomy = T
		Confused				
		Inappropriate words				
		Incomprehensible sounds				
		None				
	Best motor response	Obey commands				Usual record the best arm response
		Localizes pain				
		Flexion to pain				
		Flexion abnormal				
		Extension to pain				
		No response				

Blood pressure and pulse rate / Respiration scale: 200, 190, 180, 170, 160, 150, 140, 130, 120, 110, 100, 90, 80, 70, 60, 50, 40, 30, 20, 15, 10, 5

Pupil scale (mm):
- 1 — 40, 39, 38
- 2 — 37, 36
- 3 — 35, 34
- 4 — 33, 32
- 5 — 31, 30
- 6
- 7
- 8

PUPILS	right	Size				+ reacts
		Reaction				− no reaction
	left	Size				c. eye closed
		Reaction				
LIMB MOVEMENT	ARMS	Normal power				Record right (R) and left (L) separately if there is a difference between the two sides
		Mild weakness				
		Severe weakness				
		Spastic flexion				
		Extension				
		No response				
	LEGS	Normal power				
		Mild weakness				
		Severe weakness				
		Extension				
		No response				

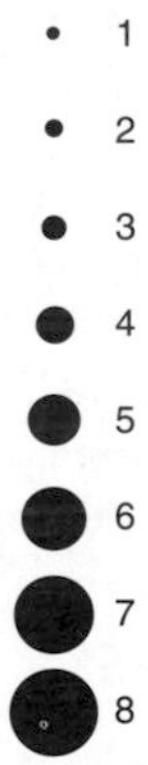

Figure 6.5 Glasgow coma chart

to establish that the response is not a reflex movement; therefore it is important to get the patient to carry out two different commands.

Localizes to pain

This is where a physical stimulus is applied to the patient in order to try to get the patient to move in a meaningful manner in an attempt to locate/remove the source of discomfort. No stimulus should be applied for more than 30 seconds, as this could result in soft tissue damage to the area to which pressure is being applied.

Flexion to pain

The upper limbs will flex rather than try to localize to the site of stimulation. To ensure that this response is accurate, try two different sites of physical stimulus. If on neither occasion does the patient try to move towards the pain, but rather flexes the upper limbs, then this should be recorded.

Extension of limbs

This occurs when the elbow will straighten with internal rotation, indicating subcortical brain damage.

No response

If no response can be obtained it is an indication that the brainstem function is so depressed it is not allowing any sensory input or motor output.

Finally ensure that sufficient painful stimuli has been exerted and that spinal injury and paralysis has been eliminated from the diagnosis (see 'Methods of applying physical stimulus').

Methods of applying physical stimulus

Three commonly used sites for applying a physical stimulus are as follows:

1 *Trapezius pinch.* This involves pinching the muscle on the shoulder, pressure should be increased in order to achieve the best response
2 *Supraorbital ridge pressure.* This method involves resting the hand on the patient's head, with the flat of the thumb or finger placed upon the supraorbital ridge or eyebrow, and the pressure increased. Do not use this method if there is any suspicion of facial damage/fractures
3 *Jaw margin.* Apply pressure with the flat of the thumb or finger into the angle of the jaw, of just behind the ear lobe; again any suspected fractures in this area are a contraindication for its use

Other common sites for applying physical stimuli have been sternal rubbing, applying pressure to the bed of the thumb nails and pinching the ear lobes, these have however been indicated as causing excessive bruising and are generally not recommended.

Care of the unconscious patient

There are several serious considerations to be aware of when caring for the unconscious patient. The first and most important thing to remember is that the nurse is totally responsible for every aspect of the patient's life. As such every aspect of the patient's comfort must be taken care of. The specific nursing care of the unconscious patient is as follows:

• The patient's airway must be protected at all times. The patient must be nursed in the recovery position. An artificial airway may be used to prevent the patient's tongue from blocking the airway.

• Neurological observations must be carried out frequently and recorded on the patient's chart.
• The patient will be immobile and care must be taken to prevent pressure sore formation from occurring.
• The patient will require artificial feeding and this should be commenced early on in their treatment. The nurse must include the dietician in assessing the nutritional and hydrational needs.
• All hygiene requirements must be met by the nursing team. This will include skin, mouth, eye and nasal care.

Summary

- Full consciousness is dependent upon the cerebral hemispheres being intact and interacting with the ascending reticular activating system (RAS)
- Arousal is the measure of being awake
- Awareness involves the person being able to interpret incoming sensory data and making sense of it by responding appropriately
- A comatosed patient is not aware of the incoming stimuli, and therefore there is no response
- When carrying out neurological assessment,

the nurse must observe for the best level of response
- The patient who scores eight or less on the Glasgow Coma Scale is considered to be in a coma
- The majority of head-injured patients, despite the severity of their cerebral injuries, will eventually open their eyes, but not be aware. Usually patients with head injury demonstrate spontaneous blinking and their eyes will rove around; this must not be misinterpreted as the patient being aware

Intracranial pressure

Intracranial pressure (ICP) is the pressure exerted within the skull and meninges by the contents (brain, cerebral spinal fluid (CSF) and the amount of cerebral blood flow).

The skull, along with the meninges, forms a rigid shell; this shell is filled to capacity, and is therefore unyielding to raised volume. The ICP is the pressure exerted by the normal brain components within this closed structure. If any one of the components increase in volume, a decrease in the volume of one or both of the other two components must occur to maintain normal intercranial pressure; this is referred to as the *compensation mechanism*.

Basic components of the brain within the skull

- Brain matter (80% of the total volume)
- Cerebral spinal fluid (10% of the total volume)
- Blood (10% of the total volume)
- Intracranial pressure (Normal range 0–15 mmHg)

McNair (1996)

Raised intracranial pressure

This is defined as occurring when one or more of the components within the rigid structure of the skull increases in volume and displaces the contents, i.e. the brain tissue, blood or cerebral spinal fluid.

This is usually a symptom which occurs as a result of either the drainage system being impeded by a clot, debris, or in congenital malformation of the system as in paediatric hydrocephalus. It also occurs when the brain is swollen following trauma, or as a result of a growing tumour.

THE COMPENSATION MECHANISM

Firstly, a displacement of cerebral spinal fluid (CSF) occurs from the cranial subarachnoid space and basilar cisterns to the spinal subarachnoid space or the lumbar cisterns. As the ICP continues to rise, the CSF produced in the choroid plexus will reduce, and the absorption of CSF into the arachnoid villi will increase. If the pressure continues to rise there will be a reduction in the volume of cerebral blood flow. The venous blood will be shunted away from the affected area into the distal venous sinuses. The decreased cerebral blood flow will lead to further brain tissue ischaemia, due to decreased cerebral perfusion. When the compensation mechanism reaches its maximum capacity, intracranial hypertension occurs, and displacement of brain tissue will occur, resulting in 'coning' or herniation occurring, which is when the brain tissue is displaced from a compartment of high pressure to one of lower pressure (Viney, 1996). When this involves high sustained pressure upon the medulla and pons, cardiac arrest and death will result. Frequent neurological assessment is essential to determine signs of raised ICP.

ACTIVITY 6.2

What are the signs of rising intracranial pressure?

SYMPTOMS

Symptoms include: decrease in consciousness level; decrease in pulse rate; widened pulse pressure; decrease in respiration rate; and a rise in blood pressure (Lee, 1989). These signs are due to increasing pressure upon the medulla oblongata in the brain.

Early detection of raised ICP may be life saving, and may also reduce the likelihood of increasing the brain damage. Following even a minor head injury there is a risk of raised ICP occurring as a result of damage to the dura or cerebral tissue.

Some neurosurgeons advocate the use of intracranial measurement tools; however, this is an invasive procedure and many consider the risk of infection outweighs the benefits. This is carried out only in specialist units and will not be seen in the high dependency unit. However, as previously mentioned early identification of rising ICP may necessitate transfer to a neurosurgical unit.

NURSING CARE

Patients with raised ICP must be nursed with great sensitivity in an attempt not to increase the pressure further. Intracranial pressure rises when patients undergo nursing activities essential to their wellbeing, without a break in between procedures. Oral pharyngeal suction also increases ICP. Communication with the patient, however,

has been shown to reduce the ICP of patients with head injury along with therapeutic touch (Viney, 1996).

Plan the patient's care, ensuring a break of at least 10 minutes between procedures. This will involve working closely with other healthcare professionals, e.g. physiotherapists, to ensure this can be achieved.

Nurse the patient with the head slightly elevated, no more than 30 degrees of tilt, to assist the venous drainage via the jugular and vertebral veins. Drainage can be inhibited by flexing or extending the neck. Therefore particular attention must be paid to ensure that the patient maintains a neutral alignment at all times. This must include log rolling the patient when changing position, and using a small pillow to keep the head in a good position when the patient is on their side. Hip flexion must also be avoided as this has been shown to increase intrathoracic pressure (Brunner and Suddarth, 1995).

Other simple activities may also increase ICP and thus decrease cerebral venous drainage. This includes straining upon a defaecation; thus great consideration must be given to ensure the patient does not become constipated. Any activity which might involve the patient holding their breath, e.g. helping to move their own position, increases the risk of increasing ICP.

ACTIVITY 6.3: Case study

John Smith is a 26-year-old man who has been admitted to the high dependency unit following a fall whilst out climbing. He has reportedly been unconscious for 30 minutes. When he is admitted to the unit he is aware of his surroundings but drowsy. His Glasgow Coma Score is recorded as 12. His blood pressure is 110/70, pulse rate 80 beats per minute and respirations 15 per minute. During the evening he becomes increasingly drowsy. His blood pressure has risen to 140/90, and pulse rate decreased to 60 beats per minute. His respirations are now 10 per minute.

What might be happening to John?

These signs indicate that John's ICP is increasing. The alteration in consciousness indicates a reduction in cerebral blood flow, which could result in tissue ischaemia, which is part of the brain's compensation mechanism in response to a rise in intracranial pressure.

The indications in John's case are that this is as a result of his fall, and may be due to an intracranial bleed, either a dural tear or a subdural haemorrhage.

Nursing action

Immediate intervention is essential to try and prevent displacement of brain tissue and brain damage occurring. John is immediately taken to theatre where a large blood clot is removed.

Summary

- Intracranial pressure is the pressure exerted by the normal brain components within the rigid structure of the skull
- Raised ICP occurs when one of the components of the skull increases in volume thus displacing either brain tissue, blood or CSF
- When the compensation mechanism reaches maximum capacity, intracranial hypertension occurs, resulting in displacement of brain tissue
- Essential signs of raised ICP are: decrease in conscious level; decrease in pulse rate; increase in blood pressure; and a reduced respiration rate
- Frequent neurological observations are essential in patients, even those admitted following a minor head injury

Subarachnoid haemorrhage

This is a common neurological condition which affects 150 people per million each year. This condition can be described as bleeding from vessels within this space or from an associated aneurysm (Marsden and Fowler, 1988).

Classic symptoms

The classic symptom is severe headache, which has a sudden onset, described by some patients as feeling as if they have been 'hit over the head with something very heavy'. The headache tends to be in the occipital or frontal area.

Vomiting is almost always a feature, and occurs as a result of increased pressure upon the brain tissue caused by the bleed.

Blurred vision and papilloedema may occur. Although these symptoms often develop, they may be of a later onset, again caused by raised ICP. Changes in conscious level or seizures may occur. The severity of the symptoms depends upon the extent of the bleed. Because blood is a very irritant substance, meningeal irritation is common, resulting in symptoms the same as those indicated in meningitis.

Other symptoms

- Neck stiffness, this may vary from mild to complete rigidity
- Photophobia, again the degree of which will vary according to the severity of the menigeal irritation
- Kernig's sign, which is a resistance to straight leg raising, again an indication of meningeal irritability

Diagnostic procedures

It is important to note here that patients who suffer from a subarachnoid haemorrhage will not die from the blood loss itself, rather they will succumb to the damage to the cerebral tissue caused by increased ICP and lack of oxygenation to cerebral tissue. Early and correct diagnosis is therefore imperative.

Initial diagnostic procedures will include history taking. The above classic symptoms will usually be present.

A computed tomography (CT) scan will follow, which will identify the location of the bleed, and indicate the extent of the bleed. This procedure will also show that there is no mass present, which may confuse the diagnosis. If the hospital has access to a magnetic resonance imaging (MRI) scanner then this will also be carried out. Following this procedure a lumbar puncture will be performed to confirm the diagnosis, and to collect CSF for cell count, culture and protein and sugar levels. Three samples are taken; uniformly blood-stained samples confirm the diagnosis. Red blood cells are usually found circulating in the spinal CSF about 30 minutes following a bleed and are usually present for several days.

Nursing care

Neurological assessment of the patient should be made using the Glasgow Coma Chart; any changes in conscious level, or other neurological changes should be reported immediately. The frequency of the observations will depend upon the patient's condition, but in the early stages following admission it is usually advisable to carry these out at least hourly, as further bleeding is most likely during the first 24 hours following admission.

Frequent strong analgesia must be prescribed in order to try and minimize the patient's level of pain. This will also help to reduce their anxiety levels and restlessness, both of which are essential to minimize the risk of a rebleed (Andrus, 1991). A high level of fluid intake may be prescribed. The reasons for this are an attempt to minimize vasospasm of the cerebral blood vessels. Increased vasospasm which occurs as a direct response to the bleed will result in increased cerebral ischaemia, through a reduction in perfusion of the brain tissue. This will result in brain damage. Fluids of up to 3 litres in 24 hours may be prescribed. If the patient is unable to tolerate this level of fluids orally, then they should be administered intravenously. A strict intake and output record must be kept in order to monitor the patient's hydration

levels. Where intravenous fluids are prescribed, signs of fluid overload should be looked out for. This would be indicated by the patient becoming increasingly breathless, a sign of pulmonary oedema, distension of the jugular vein and peripheral oedema (Lee, 1989).

Prevention of nausea may be indicated through the administration of prescribed antiemetics. This is because meningeal irritation, usually present in patients who have suffered from a subarachnoid bleed, is often accompanied by nausea and vomiting. It may well be advisable to administer antiemetics at the same time as giving analgesia. Preventing the patient from retching will help to minimize the risk of raising ICP (Brunner and Suddarth, 1995).

Altering the position of the patient is important in order to reduce the risk of their developing red pressure areas. Interventions such as this must be carried out with minimum disturbance to the patient. Nursing care should be planned to allow the patient time to rest between care, to reduce the risk of increasing ICP. Remember to ensure that the patient's head remains slightly elevated (30 degrees max) to increase cerebral venous drainage.

Maintain body temperature, as warmth increases cerebral perfusion. The patient will develop a pyrexia within the first 24 hours following a bleed, as an immune response reaction. The patient must be nursed with consideration keeping him or her comfortable and quiet (Millar and Burnard, 1994).

The environment is an important consideration; therefore where possible the patient should be nursed in a side room where the lighting can be reduced, because the patient may well be photophobic. Attempts to minimize noise should also be made.

Communication with the patient should be subdued, and ward visitors should be restricted to ensure maximum rest. It is important to keep the patient and the surrounding environment as stress-free as possible.

Elimination and the prevention of constipation is essential; the patient should not be allowed to strain as this could lead to a rebleed. Constipation is a common complication not only for the patient on bedrest, but particularly in this group of patients who are usually given analgesia with a codeine base, well-known for its constipating side effects. If the patient is sufficiently conscious, assistance to use the commode is often considered to be preferable to using a bedpan as it is probably less stressful.

Management of the patient post-bleed is con-troversial. Most neurosurgeons prefer to wait for 10–12 days post-bleed before surgically removing, clipping or bandaging the aneurysm. However there remains much debate about the best time for the optimum patient outcome.

Summary

- Frequent neurological assessment is essential to observe for any deterioration in the patient's condition
- Strong analgesia should be prescribed to try to minimize pain and anxiety levels
- Antiemetics should be given to reduce nausea and vomiting
- Minimum disturbance of the patient is important to encourage rest and to reduce the risk of raising intracranial pressure
- The patient's head should be elevated to encourage cerebral venous drainage
- Maintaining body temperature will promote cerebral perfusion
- The patient should be nursed in a quiet environment without strong light
- Constipation should be avoided

Head injury

Patients may be admitted to the high dependency unit following head injury, where the patient may have suspected brain damage and an alteration in conscious levels. Close monitoring of their condition is essential, as changes in condition can be very rapid. Close observation of oxygen saturation levels must be made as there may be a need to transfer the patient to an intensive care unit for ventilation if oxygen saturation levels drop. Oxygen levels may fall due to the nature of the injury, raised ICP or facial injuries (Lee, 1989). Frequent assessment of the neurological status of the patient using the Glasgow Coma Scale is essential in order to detect any signs of deterioration in the patient's condition.

The types of head injury which may be admitted to the high dependency unit are:

Open head injury

This is where skull fractures penetrate the skin, or wounds are caused by penetrating injuries.

Basilar fracture

These fractures most commonly damage the internal carotid artery, and cranial nerves I, II, IV and VIII; these fractures span the paranasal sinuses which include the frontal, maxillary and ethmoid bones. These bones are relatively fragile and account for this being a frequent fracture. The dura is also easily damaged and leakage of CSF through a dural tear should be looked for. Brain contusions result from the brain tissue being bruised and small haemorrhages occur on the brain surface. Lacerations are the actual tearing of the cortical surface. Injuries of this nature result in microscopic haemorrhages around the blood vessels, reducing the oxygen supply and thus increasing the damage to brain tissue.

ACTIVITY 6.4

Plan the care for a patient with a closed fracture of the skull in the first 12 hours following admission

Nursing care

Patients with a head injury should be nursed in a quiet environment, and in a position where they can be easily observed. They may well be restless and precautions must be taken to ensure that they do not injure themselves. The head of the bed should be elevated to promote venous drainage of CSF, and thus reduce the risk of raised ICP.

Neurological assessment and nursing care should follow the principles of care outlined for the patient suffering from a subarachnoid haemorrhage. Urinary output should be closely monitored, as it is possible that the patient may develop urinary retention and may require catheterization. The head injury may affect the function of the pituitary gland either causing high or low urinary output. Some neurosurgeons restrict fluid initially following head injury.

Calorific requirements are dramatically increased following major trauma, and where the patient is unable to eat due to altered levels of consciousness, other means of feeding should be commenced as a matter of urgency (Millar and Burnard, 1994). Relatives will be very anxious, especially if their loved one is either unconscious or confused. It is very important that the nurse ensures that they are fully informed regarding the diagnosis and medical and nursing intervention. Wherever possible the same nurse should communicate with the patient to ensure continuity.

Documentation of the information the relatives have received is very useful, as they may well require reinforcement of information given earlier. Documenting what has already been told to them helps to avoid confusion and reduces the risk of conflicting information being given. A useful method of ensuring this is to put the information onto a different coloured sheet within the nursing notes. This may be accessed by anybody giving the relatives information, and kept updated and signed by the person providing the information (Watson *et al.*, 1992).

Summary

- Close monitoring of all head injuries is essential in order to quickly identify any change in their condition
- Oxygen saturation levels may drop due to a rise in the intracranial pressure or the nature of the injury, and may necessitate transfer to an intensive care unit for artificial ventilation
- Frequent neurological assessment must be undertaken using the Glasgow Coma Scale
- Patients should be nursed in a quiet environment
- The head of the bed should be elevated to aid venous drainage of CSF (30° max)
- Precautions must be taken to avoid the restless patient from further injuring themselves
- Calorific needs are high following injury
- Monitor urinary output, and report diminished or vastly increased output

Meningitis

Meningitis is inflammation of the meninges which cover the brain and spinal cord. There are several causes of meningitis. It may develop as a result of bacteria viruses, fungi or other toxins. However the most common and alarming is that caused through bacteria, and requires urgent medical intervention as it is a life-threatening condition. Bacteria can enter the CNS through trauma, where the CSF is in direct contact with the external environment. It can also be transmitted to the meninges through the blood vessels, or indirectly through the nose and mouth.

The most common types of meningitis are:

1 *Meningococcal*: caused by the meningitis bacteria. This infection is transmitted through respiratory droplets
2 *Haemophilus*: caused by the *Haemophilus influenzae* organism; again this bacterium is transmitted via direct contact with respiratory secretions
3 *Pneumococcal*: caused by the *Streptococcus pneumoniae* bacteria. This is also transmitted through secretions of the respiratory tract, and this may be either direct or indirect contact
4 *Viral*: this is not transmitted from person to person and can be caused through most viral infections

Meningococcal meningitis is the most virulent type of meningitis, and is particularly common in children and teenagers. One of the most valuable signs in diagnosis is the now well-publicized rash which does not blanche when compressed by a drinking glass. This form of meningitis is accompanied by blood coagulation problems and may result in circulatory collapse. However the actual neurological complications are not common, and recovery is usually complete within 2 weeks without the other complications.

Patient symptoms

- General discomfort including headache which will be severe and photophobia. Limb pain, back ache and fever
- Neck stiffness, from a general stiffness up to flexion and total rigidity
- Nausea due to cerebral/meningeal irritation
- Deterioration in conscious level, disorientation, drowsy
- Meningeal irritability may lead to seizures
- There is a potential risk of raised intracranial pressure due to intracranial inflammatory processes, which may result in the impediment of CSF flow due to blockages in the choroid plexus
- Non-blanching widespread rash

Diagnosis

This is confirmed through the performance of a lumbar puncture, blood cultures and nose and throat swabs. If the cause of meningitis is not clear, occasionally computed tomograph (CT scan) or magnetic resonance imaging (MRI) may show the original site of the infection.

Complications include the development of seizures caused by cerebral irritability, and blocking of the arachnoid villi with debris of white cells, which will result in the prevention of CSF flow, resulting in the development of hydrocephalus. This will be indicated by the patient becoming increasingly drowsy, the blood pressure rising, the pulse and respirations decreasing (raised ICP).

Nursing assessment and care

Baseline observations must be made which include temperature, respiration and pulse rate. The Glasgow Coma Scale should be used to ascertain the level of consciousness. These observations should be repeated frequently to observe for any signs of neurological deterioration, including motor and sensory function.

If meningitis is suspected, then the patient must be nursed in a side room, and barrier nursing principles strictly adhered to until the diagnosis is confirmed, or there is no longer a risk of infection to others. This is dependent upon the infective organism, and may be for several days (Brunner and Suddarth, 1995).

An acute ward is usually a busy environment and therefore fairly noisy. If the patient is ill enough to be admitted to your unit then careful attention needs to be given towards providing an environment which is both quiet and shielded from bright lights (Millar and Burnard, 1994). Noise will only increase the patient's irritability. The patient will be complaining of severe headache and neck stiffness which indicate meningeal irritation. Analgesia and antiemetics must be prescribed as soon as possible to reduce the patient's discomfort.

The patient will be suffering from an elevated

temperature, and may well be hot and uncomfortable. A fan could be used to cool the patient down; however caution needs to be taken to make sure that it cannot be knocked over by a restless patient. Pressure area care is important, although the patient may be restless and changing their own position frequently, friction may soon cause red areas to develop, especially if the patient's skin is moist through sweating.

Nausea and vomiting are common in patients who have meningeal irritation, and therefore the patient is likely to be dehydrated. Fluid replacements, either oral or intravenous, are essential to correct this. If the patient is unable to tolerate oral fluid then intravenous fluid replacements should be considered. Close monitoring of fluid intake and output must be made and recorded on a fluid balance chart (Brunner and Suddarth, 1995).

Elevate the head slightly to promote venous drainage and to reduce the risk of cerebral oedema. Safety measures should be taken to avoid the patient injuring themselves if they are restless. The patient is also at risk from seizures resulting from cerebral irritation; therefore again it is advisable to place cot sides *in situ* to prevent them falling out of bed if they do suffer from a seizure. If the patient does start to have seizures, it is essential that the nurse documents the time, duration and the patient's body movements. Any pattern to the seizures should also be documented, i.e. factors which may trigger the event.

Treatment of bacterial meningitis is through antibiotics. High levels of antibiotics in the CSF are essential in the successful treatment of patients; however there are limited drugs which can cross the blood–brain barrier. Treatment with parenteral antibiotics is a current popular course of medical intervention. Dexamethazone may also be prescribed with the aid of reducing cerebral oedema. This has been indicated as a successful mode of action in the treatment of some cases of bacterial meningitis.

Summary

- There are several types of meningitis
- Barrier nursing is indicated until the diagnosis is confirmed including the type of infection
- Frequent neurological observations are essential to monitor for changes in conscious level
- The patient will be sensitive to noise and light, therefore should be nursed in a quiet environment without bright lights
- Fluid intake and output should be recorded and the patient who is nauseated may require intravenous fluid replacements
- Severe headache should be treated with analgesia
- Venous return should be encouraged by elevating the patient's head
- Safety precautions should be taken where the patient is drowsy, and where seizures are likely in order to minimize the risk of the patient injuring themselves

Epilepsy/status epilepticus

Epilepsy can be described as paroxysmal episodes involving sudden, violent, involuntary contractions of a group of skeletal muscles and disturbances in consciousness, behaviour, sensation and autonomic functioning (Chipps *et al.*, 1992).

Epilepsy is very common, with the incidence of chronic epilepsy being about 4–10 per 1000 (Hart and Shovan, 1990).

Types of seizures

TONIC–CLONIC (GRAND MAL)

The most common type of seizure suffered by the patient admitted to hospital is tonic–clonic (grand mal) fit. The patient may or may not prior to the seizure have a feeling of warning that an attack is coming. The patient will go through a tonic phase when they will fall to the floor, often uttering a cry. The body goes rigid and the patient becomes cyanosed, due to spasm of the respiratory muscles. This stage usually lasts up to two minutes. The next stage is the clonic phase when the muscles relax and there are rapid uncontrolled movements of the limbs. This is often accompanied by incontinence of urine. This stage lasts for several minutes, followed by a period of relaxation/unconsciousness. This stage may last for a varying period of time, and it is important that the patient is placed in the recovery position to prevent them from obstructing or aspirating. The patient may then become confused and remain drowsy before falling into a deep sleep. Upon awakening they usually have no recollection of the preceding events.

PARTIAL (FOCAL)

These seizures involve a specific usually small part of the cerebrum. The most common areas to be affected are the frontal lobes and the temporal lobes. The characteristics exhibited determine the area of the brain involved. This type of seizure is divided into the simple partial seizure (when the patient does not lose consciousness) and the complex partial seizure (where the patient does lose consciousness). It is this second type of seizure which usually arises from the temporal lobe of the brain, and is often associated with bizarre behaviour and memory disturbances including déjà vu.

ABSENT (PETIT MAL)

These seizures are particularly common in children. The person experiences a sudden interference in consciousness, becoming blank, remaining unresponsive and still for several seconds, and then continuing unaware that anything untoward has occurred.

Patients who are admitted to hospital suffering from epilepsy are admitted due to poor control of seizures, and require stabilization on medication, or for observation of their seizure pattern in order to attempt to clarify the diagnosis. Some people who suffer from poorly controlled epilepsy (because of the nature of the condition) are sometimes incorrectly admitted to hospital following a seizure and require discharging home as soon as they feel safe to leave the ward. It is important to note that there may be other medical reasons, other than neurological for seizures to occur, e.g. hypoglycaemia.

STATUS EPILEPTICUS

Status epilepticus is described as serial seizures without recovering full consciousness between the fits. It is classed as a medical emergency, and death is still high from these episodes with a mortality of about 30 per cent (Cascino, 1996). The main cause of status epilepticus is the abrupt withdrawal of treatment; compliance is well-documented as being a problem with sufferers of epilepsy. Other fairly common causes are alcohol withdrawal, brain tumours or as the result of previous brain assault. However the diagnosis of the present state is essential and investigations should be commenced at the same time as drug treatment to stop the seizures (Marsden and Fowler, 1998).

People suffering from status epilepticus will require the attentions of a high dependency unit where their epilepsy is uncontrolled, when seizures do not resolve and require major patient supervision and medical intervention in an attempt to reverse the crisis and avoid brain damage.

Principles of nursing care

The patient will require nursing in a safe environment, with suction and oxygen at hand. An airway may also be necessary for when the patient has stopped convulsing in order to maintain a clear airway. Cot sides must be *in situ* at all times and pillows strategically placed to try to prevent the patient from injuring themselves whilst they are in the clonic phase of the seizure.

Intravenous therapy to endeavour to stop reverse the seizure must be commenced as soon as possible to reduce the risk of brain damage or death. The nurse must therefore remain with the patient to ensure that the intravenous infusion is not displaced. Neurological assessment is also essential but not practical whilst the patient is in a clonic phase. Observations of the duration and any special focal signs should however be recorded as this may assist with diagnosis.

Summary

1 Status epilepticus is life-threatening and requires prompt intervention
2 Patient safety is paramount
3 It is important to record patterns of all seizures
4 Patient education regarding medication compliance is essential
5 Referral to an epilepsy specialist nurse is recommended

Guillain–Barré syndrome

This acute illness develops through the widespread inflammation of ascending or descending nerves in the peripheral nervous system. It is also known as acute inflammatory polyneuritis.

This disease is classed as fairly rare, with an incidence of 1.7 per 100 000 people (Marsden and Fowler, 1988).

The aetiology is not fully understood; however it is considered to be an autoimmune response to a viral infection. This explanation has been derived from the history of patients, over 50% of whom remember having experienced a non-specific infection 10–14 days prior to their current symptoms. It is considered that the lymphocytes may attack the myelin sheath of the neurones causing demyelination.

Ascending Guillain–Barré

- Most common
- Weakness and numbness starts in the lower extremities and progresses upwards to the trunk and arms and then affects the cranial nerves
- Patients may present with either paresis or in extreme cases quadriplegia. These motor deficits are symmetrical
- Sensory symptoms include a mild numbness which is worse in the toes
- Reflexes may be deficient or absent
- Respiratory function is often insufficient in half of the patients

Descending Guillain–Barré

- Initial cranial nerve involvement affecting cranial nerves VII, IX, X, XI, XII; weakness develops in a downwards progression
- Sensory deficits include numbness, most often in the hands and feet
- Reflexes diminished or absent
- Rapid respiratory involvement

Neurological assessment

The patient's cognition and conscious levels are not affected, nor are the pupils. Assessment of the involvement of the cranial nerves should be made frequently.

ACTIVITY 6.5

What are likely to be the most frightening features of the condition, and how will you help overcome them?

Nursing care

It must be recognized that as the patient's condition may deteriorate rapidly, the patient and their family will be very anxious. The patient may well require artificial ventilation should their respiratory effort become inadequate. Therefore close monitoring of their condition is essential.

Complete flaccid paralysis can develop, which includes respiratory failure within 48 hours of initial symptoms developing. In some cases paralysis develops more slowly over several weeks. With this condition there is no change in the patient's level of consciousness, and understandably the experience is one of great fear. Therefore psychological nursing support is of paramount importance for the welfare of the patient and their relatives.

Once the diagnosis has been confirmed, the patient and relatives must be prepared for the possibility of the patient requiring ventilation. The patient also needs to know that the symptoms may well continue to develop even after hospital admission (Chipps *et al.*, 1992).

Summary

- Considered to be an autoimmune response to a viral infection causing demyelination of the neurones
- Ascending Guillain–Barré is the most common
- Weakness may progress rapidly even after admission to hospital
- Mechanical ventilation becomes necessary in 50 per cent of sufferers
- The patient's level of consciousness is not affected by this illness

Myasthenia gravis

Myasthenia gravis (MG) is a neuromuscular, autoimmune condition. This disease is caused as a result of a deficiency in the transmission of nerve impulses at the synapse between the axon at the lower motor neurone and the muscle at the motor end-plate. Autoantibodies attach to the receptor sites on the post-synaptic membrane, which results in a decrease in the number of acetylcholine receptor sites available for neurotransmission across the synapse.

Signs and symptoms

The most prominent symptom of the patient suffering from MG are excessive muscular fatigue and weakness upon exertion. However there is some recovery after resting. Although the pattern of onset varies, the muscles supplied by the cranial nerves are often the first to be affected.

Patients may often be observed to be holding their head up, or trying to support it with their hand. Muscles of the limbs and trunk may also be affected; however smooth muscle of the heart, gut,

The patient may present with:

- Diplopia
- Difficulty in mastication
- Ptosis
- Difficulty in swallowing
- Voice weakness/neck/face weakness

blood vessels and uterus are not affected by this condition (Marsden and Fowler, 1998).

The severity of the condition varies from intermittent mild ptosis to that of generalized muscular weakness; this may become life-threatening if the respiratory muscles are affected.

Diagnosis

Initial diagnosis is through the conduction of electromyographic conduction studies (EMG). In the patient suffering from MG there is a decreasing response to repetitive nerve stimulation.

Edrophonium chloride (Tensilon) challenge tests are also performed. In the patient with MG

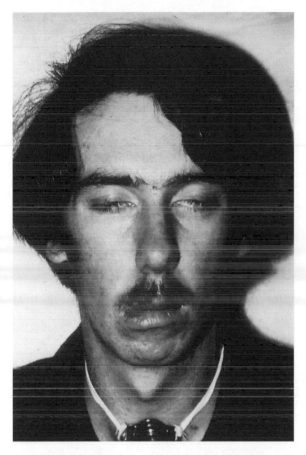

Figure 6.6 Bilateral ptosis and facial weakness in myasthenia gravis

their strength dramatically improves following the injection of intravenous Tensilon, 2–4 mg. (Up to 10 mg can be injected if no initial positive response is evident.) It is essential that before commencing this test full resuscitation equipment is available in case of patient collapse.

A CT scan is undertaken to exclude a tumour of the thymus gland.

Treatment

Surgical removal of the thymus gland is recommended in many patients with a reported high level of success in the reduction of symptoms.

Medication can usually keep the symptoms under control (discussed later in the chapter).

Nursing care on admission

Patients admitted to the high dependency unit are ill and frightened. It is essential that medication is administered on time. They are usually feeling weak and dependent upon the nursing staff for all their activities of living.

Assessment of their needs should be made upon admission, as the patient will usually be able to tell the nurse when the times are when they feel least fatigued, and therefore these times are best used for activities requiring most exertion, e.g. eating, washing.

Medication

Anticholinesterase drugs are used in the treatment of MG; their function is to increase neuromuscular transmission at the synaptic junctions.

Pyridostigmine bromide is the oral maintenance drug of choice. Dosages vary between 60 and 90 mg every 3–4 hours. Side effects include muscle cramps and gut hypermotility. Patients also often suffer from increased production of saliva, excessive perspiration, muscle twitching and cramps. Atropine helps to reduce these side effects (Marsden and Fowler, 1998).

Overdose of the drug causes the potentially fatal cholinergic crisis.

Signs and symptoms of cholinergic crisis
1 Respiratory distress including dyspnoea and wheezing
2 Abdominal cramps including nausea and vomiting
3 Excessive salivation, bronchial secretions and sweating
4 Vertigo
5 Restlessness and apprehension
6 Blurred vision
7 Dysarthria
8 Dysphagia
9 Bradycardia
10 Decreased blood pressure

These symptoms must not be ignored. On the slightest deterioration medical assistance must be sought in order to determine the cause; resuscitation equipment must be accessible; and an anaesthetist should be informed. To determine the nature of the deterioration a Tensilon test will be performed by medical staff. This process involves the administration of intravenous Tensilon which is administered in small doses in order to monitor any changes in the patient's condition. If the symptoms improve within 30 seconds the reason for the deterioration is myasthenic crisis; if the symptoms worsen a diagnosis of cholinergic crisis will be assumed. At this stage the patient may require ventilating. Reassessment of medication will be undertaken as the cause of these crises is too much medication. The patient will be extremely anxious and will require the total care of one nurse in an attempt to reduce the patient's fear. Myasthenic crisis is the result of a lack of acetylcholine; this can be caused by a change in medication, or a lack of medication, stress, either physical or emotional (which includes surgical intervention), or physical illness.

frequently, and may well benefit from the use of a bed indicated for patients at high risk of developing a pressure sore. Frequent pressure area care is essential not only to change the patient's position, but also to aim to keep the skin dry and clean, as the patient is likely to perspire. Fluid intake may be difficult to maintain because of difficulty with swallowing, therefore small frequent sips of fluid should be offered. A fluid balance chart should be recorded in order to monitor fluid intake and output. Dietary intake will also be difficult for the patient and therefore supplement drinks may be prescribed. Food should be selected which requires either no chewing or minimum chewing, dependent upon the patient's condition. Assistance may be required with eating and drinking.

Elimination needs will again depend on the condition of the patient; however they may well prefer to be assisted to use a commode rather than using a bedpan. Normal patterns of bowel movement should be identified (Brunner and Suddarth, 1995).

Signs and symptoms of myasthenic crisis

- Increased blood pressure
- Tachycardia
- Muscle weakness, resulting in dysarthria and dysphagia
- Excessive salivation, bronchial secretions and sweating
- Lack of cough reflex
- Restlessness and apprehension

NURSING CARE

Frequent observations should be undertaken to observe for an increase in weakness. Oxygen saturation levels must be observed as these may well decrease due to weakness of the respiratory muscles.

The patient will require their position changing

Summary

- Myasthenia gravis is caused by an autoimmune condition affecting nerve transmission at the neuromuscular junction of the lower motor neurone and the motor end-plate
- Myasthenia gravis sufferers complain of excessive muscle fatigue
- Weakness can affect the respiratory muscles and is therefore life-threatening
- Medication of anticholinesterase drugs must be administered on time
- When a myasthenia gravis patient is admitted to hospital with an exacerbation of the disease, ITU should be informed in case of mechanical ventilation should be required
- Signs of cholinergic and myasthenic crisis must be observed for
- Patient education is important to try to minimize disease exacerbation

Conclusion

Diseases of the neurological system are often very challenging for the nursing team to deal with. However, with a unified team approach, patients and their families can be cared for in a sensitive and focused way. Patients who are suffering with diseases of the brain and central nervous system are often extremely frightened and upset by their illness. This is also very true for the families as well. This chapter has explored the most commonly seen neurological diseases and provided the reader with the essential information to care for and support the patient and their family through this difficult time.

Further reading

Andrus, C. 1991 Intracranial pressure: dynamics and nursing management. *Journal of Neuroscience Nursing* 23(2), 85–91.

Brunner, L.S. and Suddarth, D.S. 1995 *Textbook of adult nursing*. London: Chapman and Hall.

Cascino, G.D. 1996 Generalised convulsive status epilepticus. *Mayo Clinic Proceedings* 71(8), 787–92.

Chipps, F., Clanin, N. and Campbell, V. 1992 *Neurological disorders*. St. Louis, Baltimore: Mosby's Clinical Nursing Series.

Hart, Y. and Shorvon, S.D. 1990 *Epilepsy*, 2nd edn. London: Reed Business Publishing Group.

Jennett and Teasdale 1974 Assessment of impaired consciousness: A practical scale. *Lancet* 2, 81–4.

Judrez, V.I. and Lyons, M. 1995 Interrater reliability of the Glasgow Coma Scale. *Journal of Neuroscience Nursing* 27(5) 283–6.

Kernich, C.A. and Kaminski, H.J. 1995 Myasthenia gravis: pathophysiology, diagnosis and collaborative care. *Journal of Neuroscience Nursing* 27(4), 207–18.

Lannon, S.L. 1998 Epilepsy in the elderly. *Journal of Neuroscience Nursing* 25(5), 273–81.

Lee, S. 1989 Intracranial pressure changes during positioning of patients with severe head injury. *Heart and Lung* 18, 411–14.

Lisak, R.P. 1983 Myasthenia gravis mechanisms and management. *Hospital Practice* 18(3), 101–109.

Marsden, C.D. and Fowler, T.J. 1988 *Clinical neurology*, 2nd edn. London: Arnold.

Millar, B. and Burnard, J.P. 1994 *Critical care nursing*. London: Baillière Tindall.

McNair, N. 1996 Horizons. Review of coma guidelines. *Journal of Neuroscience Nursing* 28(4), 275.

Viney, C. 1996 *Nursing the critically ill patient*. London: Baillière Tindall.

Watson, M., Horn, S. and Curl, J. 1992 Searching for signs of revival. *Professional Nurse* July, 670–74.

7

Nursing the high dependency patient with spinal cord injury

Paul Harrison

Introduction

This chapter will discuss the planning and delivery of care for individuals who are admitted to the high dependency unit following traumatic spinal cord injury. There is a high chance of the spine-injured patient being admitted to the high dependency unit. This chapter is written to provide the nurse with a good basic level of understanding and knowledge to provide a high level of nursing care for the patient and their family. It presupposes that collaborative communication with a nominated spinal injuries unit was established at the moment of diagnosis and will continue until transfer of the patient to a specialist centre can be effected.

More than 700 people sustain a traumatic spinal cord injury each year in the UK (Masham, 1997). The effects of a traumatic spinal cord lesion are usually permanent and currently there is no cure for this condition. The potential impact of this injury upon an individual and their family increases when one considers that spinal cord injury is most prevalent amongst active males between 15 and 35 years of age.

Twelve centres provide comprehensive acute, rehabilitation and continuing care facilities for all individuals with spinal cord injury in the UK and Eire. Between them they provide a network of regional and supraregional specialist care facilities and services. Since their inception, the survival and quality of life after discharge for these individuals has increased phenomenally.

Historical background

Fifty years ago a diagnosis of spinal cord paralysis was akin to a death sentence. Of those who managed to survive their accident and transportation to hospital, less than half survived the rudimentary and uninformed hospital care and rehabilitation which followed. Within 12 years of their injury, most had succumbed to the mortal effects of chest infections, renal failure, pressure sores and contractures that were prevalent at the time.

Today, as a direct consequence of the knowledge and experience which has accumulated between these specialist centres, the life expectancy of these individuals is at least equal to that of their fellow citizens. Undertaking the acute rehabilitation and continuing care of people with spinal cord injury within dedicated specialist centres of excellence has reduced the incidence of both acute and chronic complications amongst their population to a minimum (Spinal Injuries Association, 1997).

Spinal cord injuries and high dependency care

At present there is an expectation upon UK acute healthcare providers to transfer any patient with an actual or potential spinal cord injury to a specialist spinal injuries unit. The Spinal Injuries Association (a consumer body) and the British Association of Spinal Cord Injury (a body of consultants) recommend that this transfer should be made as soon as possible after the diagnosis of spinal cord injury is made (Spinal Injuries Association, 1997). However, the current prevalence of casualties presenting with ever increasing levels of accompanying multitrauma can create a situation whereby transfer of an individual with a diagnosed or suspected spinal cord injury to a specialist centre may have to be delayed.

Multitrauma can be present in up to 30 per cent of new admissions to a spinal injuries unit (Aung and El-Masry, 1997).

> The most common blunt or penetrating injuries, which may accompany spinal cord injury, are:
>
> • Chest injuries – haemothorax / pneumothorax
> • Complex limb or pelvic fractures
> • Abdominal injuries
> • Head injury

Associated trauma

For this reason, most spinal injuries units now possess dedicated intensive care or high dependency areas within their infrastructure to enable them to continue receiving patients as soon as possible after referral. Despite this and recent improvements in the rapid evacuation and transport of spinal cord injury patients, the admission of a spinal cord injury patient to a local high dependency unit (HDU) is still a possibility.

There are three main scenarios within which a patient with actual or potential spinal cord trauma may be admitted to the high dependency unit of a local district general hospital.

> **Scenario 1**
>
> Multiple-trauma patient with actual or potential spinal column trauma but without evidence of spinal cord trauma

Where doubt exists over the presence of spinal column or spinal cord trauma, experience has proved time and again that it is better to err on the side of caution. In the presence of a traumatic head injury, spinal cord injury should continue to be suspected until consciousness returns.

> **Scenario 2:**
>
> Multitrauma patient with or without spinal column trauma but with evidence of spinal cord paralysis

The presence of spinal cord paralysis in the absence of bony trauma is not uncommon, especially where the cervical spine is involved. Where spinal cord trauma is present, it must be considered in context within all care and therapeutic interventions in order to prevent any deterioration in the patient's neurological or physiological status.

> **Scenario 3**
>
> Patient with evident spinal column and spinal cord trauma without accompanying multitrauma

The patient here presents only with a discrete spinal column trauma with accompanying spinal cord paralysis. The reduction of traumatic forces through the presence of safety equipment, or modifications to personal risk taking behaviour, means that soft tissue trauma resulting in the disruption of spinal ligaments and musculature makes injuries such as these more common.

Admission to the high dependency area in this instance is usually in appreciation of the potential, at this time, for such patients to deteriorate neurologically post-admission with subsequent respiratory or cardiovascular complications.

Potential consequences of the non-specialist environment

The first 2 weeks following spinal cord injury are the most important for the person who has sustained spinal cord injury. It is during this time that the vast majority of immediate and secondary complications can occur. There may be complications if initial management is undertaken in a non-specialist environment. It is also the time when the injured individual and their family will be seeking an accurate and informed opinion of their full potential for recovery, rehabilitation and future quality of life. Failure to appropriately address the full needs of this individual and their family at this time cannot only affect their immediate physiological and psychological status, but also have detrimental effects upon their potential for recovery of function, rehabilitation achievements and quality of life after discharge.

Delay in transfer to a specialist care facility has been established as the key cause of increases in the incidence of post-injury complications, failure to achieve rehabilitation outcomes, extended length of stay and increased care costs (Tator *et al.*, 1995).

In addition, the increasingly litigious society which prevails today means an increasing number of professionals are facing accusations of actual or potential mismanagement, or even negligence, in their delivery of care. The evidence which underpinned care practices at the time of the alleged incident is often called into question in these cases. Close and regular liaison with colleagues in specialist units during pre-transfer care is recommended for ensuring an informed evidence basis for care in such instances.

Clarke *et al.* (1996) suggest that increasing the current level of knowledge and awareness of spinal cord injury amongst acute sector professionals could reduce the incidence of 'preventable complications resulting from critical events' by at least 8 per cent and increase the 'implementation of appropriate nursing interventions' by at least 30 per cent when compared to existing care provision.

The spinal column

The spinal or vertebral column supports the upright posture of the body, and acts as a protective shell or cover for the spinal cord. It is of course flexible and can move fairly freely within certain limits. The flexibility is provided by the individual bones (vertebrae) that make up the column. The column is made up from 33 bones: seven cervical, 12 thoracic, five lumbar, five sacral and four coccygeal (Fig. 7.1). Each vertebra articulates with its neighbour; it has bony processes that provide muscular attachment. The main body provides considerable strength and also acts as a shock absorber. A central cavity exists; this cavity is where the spinal cord runs. Spaces between the adjacent bones allow access for blood vessels and spinal nerves. The first two vertebrae, C1 and C2 are modified and produce a flexion–rotation joint with the base of the skull. Between the vertebrae there is an intervertebral disc made of fibrocartilage with a semi-solid core. The function of this is to provide shock absorption, and to aid movement. Should the tough outer layer of this disk rupture pressure is exerted on the spinal nerves causing severe pain. This is known as a 'slipped' or prolapsed disc.

ACTIVITY 7.1

What do you think are the most likely causes of spinal cord injury?

(a)

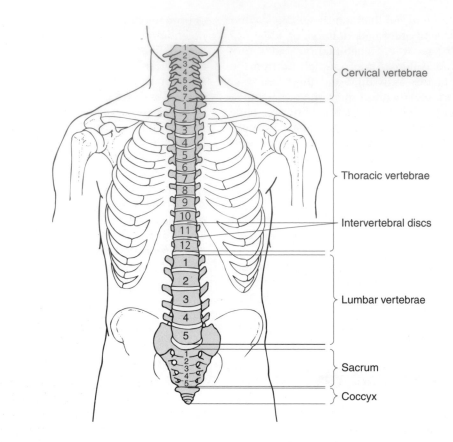

(b)

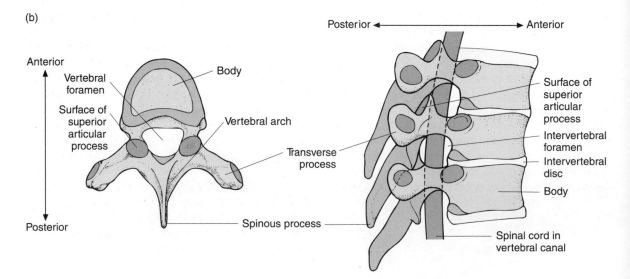

Figure 7.1 The vertebral column. (a) General structure. (b) General structure of a vertebral bone.

Causes of spinal cord injury

The most common mechanism of injury within the UK population is a sudden, unexpected impact or deceleration collision. Velocity is not relative to injury, but may influence the extent of cord trauma within each individual case. The potential for spinal cord injury is the same following a fall at home as following a motorway collision.

Causes of spinal cord injury

- Moving vehicle accident (vehicular occupant)
- Moving vehicle accident (motorcyclist)
- Moving vehicle accident (pedestrian/cyclist)
- Falling or jumping from a height
- Diving or jumping into shallow water
- Sporting accidents
- Industrial accidents
- Blunt assault
- Penetrating trauma
- Surgical accident

Pathophysiology

There is a common misconception about the nature and presentation of spinal cord lesions. The use of the words 'transection', 'cutting' and 'severing' in much of the literature suggests to the reader that the spinal cord is physically divided at the moment of injury. Whilst possible in the event of penetrative trauma or gross traction forces, physical disruption of the spinal cord following blunt trauma is a rare occurrence. In truth, the process of lesion formation is that of ischaemic necrosis.

Displacement of one or more vertebral bodies results in compression of the underlying spinal cord. Alternatively, the cord may be stretched or 'concussed' without any visible disruption of the spinal column. The resulting oedema and vascular damage begins a complex series of physiological and biochemical reactions within the spinal cord. There is little room for swelling within the structural confines of the vertebral canal and the oedematous spinal cord is quickly compressed against the surrounding bone. Circulation of blood and oxygen within the spinal cord is disrupted and ischaemic tissue necrosis quickly follows. There is an almost immediate cessation of conductivity within the spinal cord neurones. This is termed 'spinal shock'. Neurologically, at this time, the patient presents with the loss of all voluntary movements and sensation below the level of their injury. There is also a progressive loss of sympathetic and parasympathetic activity throughout the same area. At this stage it is difficult to be certain of the extent or permanence of functional loss within the spinal cord neurones. The presence of paralysis or paraesthesia does not imply any finality to the process. In some instances, spinal cord oedema and spinal shock can resolve over time with a subsequent improvement in neurological function.

Spinal shock usually persists for between 2 and 6 weeks, dependent upon the age of the casualty and the extent of accompanying trauma. During this time it is impossible for the clinician to provide an accurate diagnosis of the extent of permanent loss of function.

Main presentations of neurological deficiency

Quadriplegia/quadriparesis (also called tetraplegia/tetraparesis)

The complete or partial loss of all movements and/or sensation from the neck downwards affecting all four extremities and the trunk

Paraplegia/paraparesis

The complete or partial loss of all movements and / or sensation from the chest downwards and affecting only the lower limbs

The term *complete spinal cord lesion* is used to define the diagnosis of transverse (complete) ischaemic necrosis which has resulted in the permanent loss of all voluntary movements and sensation below the level of lesion. However, the process by which spinal cord oedema occurs and progresses towards ischaemia is unique in each case. There always exists the potential at this stage that the oedema will resolve with the subsequent return of some neurological function due to the survivability of some nerve fibres. Where this occurs, a diagnosis of *incomplete spinal cord lesion* is given.

Central cord syndrome

This peculiar presentation of incomplete spinal cord lesion usually occurs in elderly or spondylotic patients following minor trauma to the neck. The patient presents with significant loss of function in their upper extremities with partial preservation of function in their lower extremities.

Being able to move their lower limbs whilst being unable to move their upper limbs may result in the inappropriate diagnosis of hysterical paralysis or malingering in these patients.

Initial management

Reduction of spinal cord compression is a priority in these cases. Early reduction of an existing vertebral displacement and stabilization of the fracture site is usually undertaken in the casualty department or emergency room before transfer to the HDU.

Initial orthopaedic management is usually conservative in nature, utilizing in-line traction and closed manipulation under continuous radiological monitoring. There are strict criteria governing surgical intervention at this early stage as inappropriate surgical procedures at this time could cause further (surgical) oedema at the lesion site with a resulting extension of ischaemic effects.

Recent research studies have found that high-dose steroid therapy (methylprednisolone) has a role to play in reducing the effects of spinal cord oedema post-trauma (Bracken *et al.*, 1990).

However, they also identified a window of clinical effectiveness, which limits the commencement of this therapy to within the first 8 hours of injury. Influencing the extent and impact of post-traumatic cord oedema in this way could mean a significant increase in neurone survival. Whilst far from being the magical 'cure', preservation of these additional fibres may have a significant impact upon rehabilitation outcomes and quality of life post-injury.

Example of a local protocol for the administration of methylprednisolone

1 Methylprednisolone administration must commence within 8 hours of the injury/event which is known or suspected to have resulted in spinal cord injury – the earlier, the better.
2 A bolus dose of 30 mg/kg should be given intravenously in 100 mL of 5 per cent dextrose over 30 minutes (3.3 mL/h) followed by:
3 An intravenous infusion of 5.4 mg per kg/h in 230 mL of 5 per cent dextrose over 23 hours (10 ml/h)
4 Local spinal injuries unit can advise further

When utilizing manual transfer techniques, it takes at least five experienced staff to maintain spinal alignment throughout the procedure. In addition they must have supreme confidence in their ability to work as a team.

A wide range of equipment is now available to facilitate the movement and transfer of a patient with an acute spinal cord injury, increasing both staff and patient safety in these situations. Unfortunately, not all of these devices meet the standards of expert practitioners. Before investing in any equipment of this nature it is recommended that staff in general areas consult with their specialist peers for advice.

Moving patients

Careful handling, positioning and turning on every occasion can prevent secondary cord trauma during patient transfers and movements.

ACTIVITY 7.2

Make a list of the effects that spinal cord injury will have on the patient admitted to the high dependency unit

Systemic effects of spinal cord injury

The loss of all voluntary movement and sensation below the level of lesion following spinal cord injury is probably familiar to most professionals in non-specialist areas. Less common however, is an awareness and appreciation of the effects of spinal shock upon the internal systems of the body, especially its effects upon autonomic and reflex functions. The effect of spinal shock upon each individual system is described below.

Orthopaedic

Conservative fracture management is the preferred primary method for all UK spinal injuries units. About 90 per cent of all spinal fractures heal spontaneously after conservative reduction and the maintenance of adequate alignment throughout a period of bed-rest. Throughout this period there exists the potential for secondary injury to

the spinal cord due to inappropriate handling and turning of the patient.

If cervical skull traction has been applied, a careful check must be made of the security of pins, cord, knots and weights before any further movement is attempted. If traction is not going to be utilized for an individual then a properly sized and fitted hard cervical collar must remain *in situ* until all investigations to determine spinal column stability have been completed.

Following the initial reduction and stabilization of the injury site, spinal alignment must be maintained at all times to prevent secondary trauma to the spinal cord. In addition to the cervical traction in place, a neck roll made from gamgee roll, and pillowcases should support the cervical curve. For thoracolumbar injuries, a lumbar pillow of appropriate thickness should support the lumbar curve.

A hard collar should also be applied before a spinal cord injury patient is transferred between

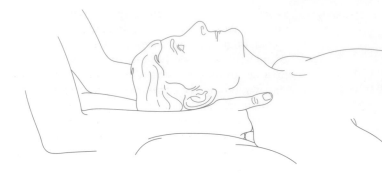

Figure 7.2 Cervical hold procedure for patients with spinal injury.

surfaces or transported from one area to another. Manual support of the head and neck should be applied as illustrated in Figure 7.2 during transfers as an additional safeguard. Hands support the cervical curve from the occiput to C7. The head is supported between forearms. Alignment of the body from head to toe is visible from this position.

During spinal shock, paralysed limbs are com-pletely flaccid and care should be taken to prevent the limbs falling from the surfaces of trolleys or beds or becoming trapped in bed rails. A patient whose flaccid arm falls from a trolley can suffer disruption of his rotator cuff and shoulder joint, resulting in a second disabling condition. A leg allowed to fall under the same circumstances could pull a paralysed patient from a trolley and onto the floor.

Nursing considerations

ACTIVITY 7.3

Spend some time thinking about the whole condition of the patient. Make a list of the important aspects of care. Then devise a care plan that will meet the patient's needs.

Complications of bed-rest

Visitors to any UK spinal injuries unit will discover that the incidence of complications amongst this patient group reduces significantly after early transfer. Bed-rest complications usually associated with spinal cord injury are mostly preventable through collaboration with spinal injuries units.

Prevention of pressure sores

People with spinal cord injury are at the greatest risk of developing pressure sores when hospitalized outside spinal injuries units (Gunnewicht, 1997). Part of the explanation for this is the low priority which skin care is afforded in the pre-admission area, due to the critical status of the patient on arrival in the A&E department. This situation should not be allowed to continue into the high dependency area.

The patient's skin condition should be checked for the effects of pressure on arrival and documented. A note should be made of the estimated time which a patient has spent in a particular position and upon what kind of surface, e.g. supine upon a spine board. If the patient has spent time in the operating theatre, consider their position upon the theatre table and in recovery. Particular attention should be paid to weight-bearing surfaces and bony prominences.

There are three simple but effective instructions for the prevention of pressure sores in people with acute spinal cord injury at this time:

1 Turn the patient regularly, avoiding friction and shearing
2 Avoid turning the patient onto a discoloured area of skin wherever possible
3 Minimize the incidence of the other contributory factors of pressure sore formation

There is still considerable anxiety and uncertainty within general care areas in respect of the manual turning of people with acute spinal cord injury. Clinical experience gained over many years has demonstrated that routine 2 hourly turning for pressure relief is the optimal practice for this period. Two turning techniques are recom-

mended – logrolling for patients with thoraco-lumbar injuries and pelvic twisting for patients with cervical injuries. These manoeuvres are illustrated and described in Figures 7.3–7.8.

As the pelvic twist does not allow for the full visualization of the upper back and occipital area, it is essential to logroll tetraplegic patients once a day for a complete skin check. This manoeuvre requires five or six members of staff and should be planned accordingly to incorporate a daily back wash and sheet change.

It is both inappropriate and unprofessional to implement a practice learned solely from a text-book such as this. A request to your local spinal injuries unit will usually enable you to organize a practical moving and handling workshop with an experienced facilitator. Most units are also able to provide opportunities for clinical placements as developmental opportunities.

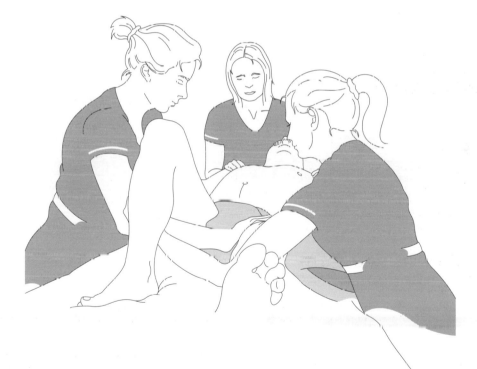

Figure 7.3 Pelvic twisting manoeuvre (stage 1). Utilized for cervical injuries only. Patient's shoulders are 'pinned' by nurse standing at head of bed. Second nurse raises and holds patient's right leg upright in bent position. Third nurse passes her right hand beneath patient's right leg and her left hand beneath patient's lumbar curve – for which the second nurse provides counter traction. Both hands join over the patient's right hip. The twist is accomplished by a sliding upward rotation of the nearside hip.

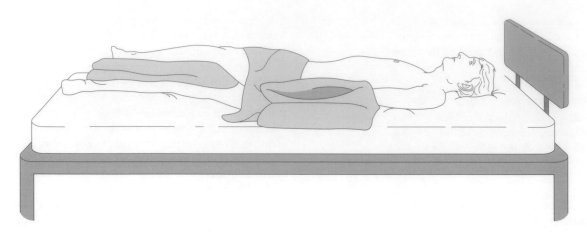

Figure 7.4 Pelvic twisting manoeuvre (stage 2). First two nurses hold their positions whilst the third nurse places a foam wedge or folded pillow *in situ* beneath the patient's buttock – above the sacrum. Sacrum is free from pressure and buttocks are kept apart. Two pillows are placed to support the upper leg. Twist should not be so far as to place weight onto the lower trochanteric pressure area.

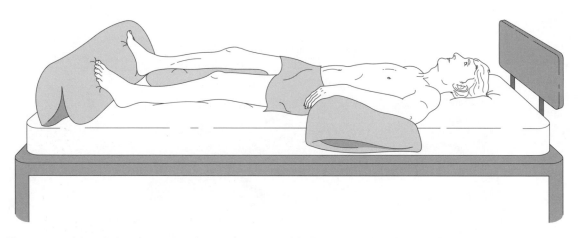

Figure 7.5 Pelvic twisting manoeuvre (stage 3). Feet are 'blocked out' with pillows at the end of the manoeuvre to prevent foot drop. Patient's top leg rests behind his lower leg for stability and comfort. Patient's arms rest on pillows. This procedure can also be utilized for non-spinal injured patients with arthritic or painful shoulders, hemiplegia, fractured or fixated limbs, chest drains or with head/brain injuries. The figure shows the final resting position (although it looks similar to a left-hand turn).

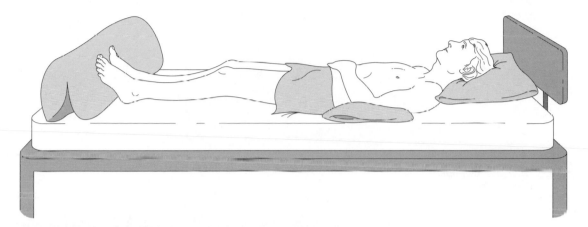

Figure 7.6 Logrolling (stage 1). Supine acute paraplegic patient with all pillows *in situ*. Lumbar pillow assists postural reduction and support of thoracolumbar injury site.

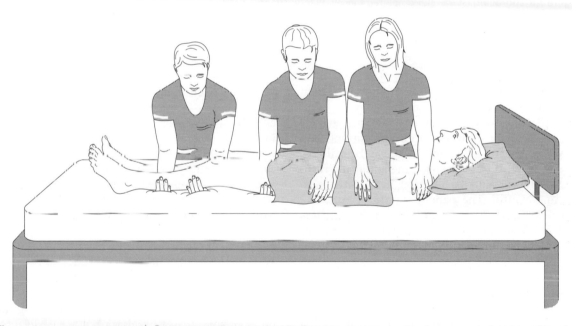

Figure 7.7 Logrolling (stage 2). Preparing to logroll an acute paraplegic patient with three nurses. Lumbar pillow is utilized during the turn to support lumbar curve for patient comfort. Upper leg must be kept in alignment throughout the turn to prevent movement at a thoracolumbar fracture site. An additional person is required to support the cervical spine when logrolling a tetraplegic patient.

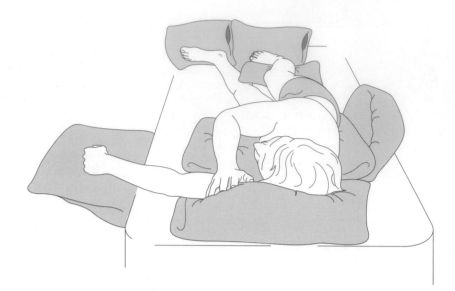

Figure 7.8 Logrolling (stage 3). Completed logroll. Pillows support patient in lateral position. Lateral positioning can vary between 30° and 90° dependent upon skin condition, comfort and clinical need, although a position between 30° and 50° is preferred to prevent pressure on the trochanter. Upper leg is positioned behind the lower one for both pressure relief and spinal alignment.

Where a patient presents with injuries to both their cervical and thoracolumbar spine or with multiple injuries, which make positioning on their side difficult or painful, an electric turning bed (such as Egerton's Paragon 9000) can be utilized. Wherever such beds are used the automatic turning facility should be omitted in preference to manual control. The patient should be turned 2 hourly between 20° to 30° only. This is because it is impossible to guarantee that a paralysed patient will maintain their alignment against gravity if the bed is turned beyond this angle, increasing the risk of secondary cord trauma due to lateral movements of the spine. With care, a patient with complicated chest problems may be supported for short periods during the day at a 40–50° angle for the purposes of active chest physiotherapy.

Before and after each turn the patient's position and alignment should be checked and their skin loading adjusted as required. Particular care must be taken to ensure that the patient's buttocks are not allowed to compress against each other when supine, contributing to the formation of natal cleft sores. Manual separation of each buttock from its neighbour at the end of each turn usually suffices.

Lack of sensation in paralysed limbs means that where limb fractures are being managed in cylinder or backslab casts the patient is at an increased risk of developing plaster sores. All casts should be well-padded. Backslab splints should be removed at least twice each day and the underlying skin inspected for the effects of pressure. Cylinder casts should be bivalved at the earliest opportunity for the same purpose.

Prevention of contractures

Joint contractures can occur rapidly following the onset of spinal cord paralysis but are easily prevented. The departmental physiotherapist should ensure that each acute patient receives a full range of daily passive movements for their paralysed limbs within the limitations of any accompanying injuries. Shoulder abduction should be restricted to 90° following cervical trauma and hip flexion to 50° following thoracolumbar trauma during these exercises. Movements in excess of these ranges can be relayed to the injury site, resulting in pain or even secondary cord trauma.

Additional passive movements can be undertaken by nursing staff before and after turning the patient. Conscious, cooperative patients should be encouraged to exercise non-paralysed limbs through active exercises and involvement in care processes as appropriate to their level of injury. Tetraplegic patients with spinal cord lesions above C7 are at high risk of developing biceps muscle contractions due to their lack of an active opposing triceps muscle. Arm or wrist splints and bandages are not recommended at this stage due to their great potential for skin damage. Instead, both staff and relatives of the patient should passively extend the patient's forearms whenever it is noticed that flexion has occurred. Although time-consuming, perseverance in this endeavour is rewarded during rehabilitation. The potential for an individual with tetraplegia to undertake a range of personal and meaningful tasks such as feeding oneself, brushing teeth etc. could be denied to them by a contracture which developed during their initial period of bed-rest. A rolled crepe bandage placed in the tetraplegic patient's hand is sufficient to prevent finger contractures.

Management of pain

Despite their paralysis, patients with spinal cord injury still experience pain, especially from around and above the site of their spinal injury. As with any other orthopaedic trauma, immobilization of the site of a spinal injury, as described earlier, contributes significantly to the reduction of post-trauma pain. Where severe pain is experienced, due to the presence of complex or multiple injuries, an electric turning bed is beneficial for relieving discomfort experienced during manual turning. Opiates should be avoided in cases of tetraplegia or high paraplegia in case they cause respiratory depression. Diclofenac is the drug of choice for these patients, although dihydrocodeine or buprenorphine can be used for more severe pain.

Tetraplegics are also particularly prone to shoulder pain due to a form of adhesive capsulitis ('frozen shoulder'). This is easily prevented in most cases by regular, passive repositioning of their arms at rest after every turn. Figure 7.9 illustrates an appropriate range of resting arm positions for acute tetraplegic patients.

Some complaints of shoulder pain in spinal cord injury patients may be referred from the abdominal viscera (*see* Acute abdominal complications on p. 171).

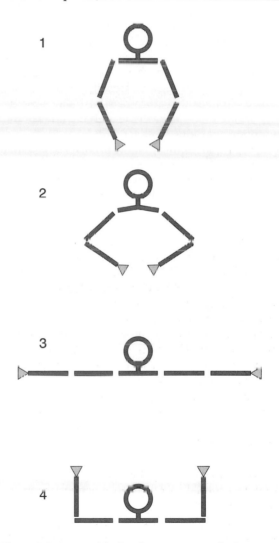

Figure 7.9 Arm positioning for acute tetraplegic patients

Neurological function

To facilitate the reduction of cord oedema, administer methylprednisolone as previously described. Monitor the patient's neurological level every 15 minutes initially, reducing over time where there is no evidence of further neurological deterioration. Sensation should always be assessed against that present in a non-paralysed part of the body – such as the face of a high tetraplegic patient. Motor function should always be assessed against the full range and strength expectations for an individual of a certain age and capability.

The significant feature of spinal shock is the way that it affects the activity and functions of the autonomic nervous system (Zeidlik, 1992).

Sympathetic activity below the level of a spinal cord lesion is suppressed. The effects of this are manifested most in injuries above the sixth thoracic nerve (T6) – the base level of the body's main sympathetic outflow. Parasympathetic activity is not greatly affected by spinal cord injury and therefore dominates all autonomic activity.

On average, the duration of spinal shock is between 48 hours and 14 days post-trauma. In some instances it can persist for up to 6 weeks or more. Notably, these instances are usually when the injury involves a child or where there is significant accompanying trauma requiring major surgical intervention in the immediate post-trauma period. Careful monitoring for the return of reflex activity, sensation or voluntary movement should begin in earnest after 48 hours. Do not confuse reflex spasticity with voluntary movement of limbs. Do not equate the return of sensation to a part of the body with the potential return of voluntary movement to the same.

Respiratory function

All patients with cervical spinal cord lesions suffer the loss of their accessory muscles of respiration. Tetraplegia at or above the level of the third cervical nerve (C3) results in respiratory insufficiency due to diaphragmatic paralysis, necessitating mechanical ventilation.

From the level of C4 down however, the patient should be able to breathe without ventilator assistance, except where pre-existing disease or accompanying trauma require it. Management at this stage is designed to develop the patient's respiratory capacity and ability. Humidified oxygen via face mask or nasal cannulae should be given over the first 24–48 hours to maximize blood oxygen levels at the lesion site in the spinal cord. Half-hourly deep breathing exercises should also be encouraged.

Paralysis of their abdominal and intercostal muscles means that most spinal cord injury patients will be unable to cough effectively to clear any accumulation of secretions in their lungs. The departmental physiotherapist should be asked to instruct nursing staff in delivering ½ hourly assisted coughing where competence is lacking. Figure 7.10 illustrates hand positions for assisted coughing on a supine patient by one or two persons. Force is directed upwards against the diaphragm. Patients with cervical injuries will need an additional person to brace their shoulders against the force of an assisted cough to prevent movement of their neck during the procedure. Regular turning or changes in position, where possible, also contributes to the mobilization of pulmonary secretions.

A mini-tracheostomy may be utilized to facilitate clearing excessive pulmonary secretions. In patients with tracheostomies or mini-tracheostomies *in situ* over stimulation of the vagus nerve can occur during suctioning, leading to cardiac syncope. To reduce this risk, hyperoxygenate the patient before

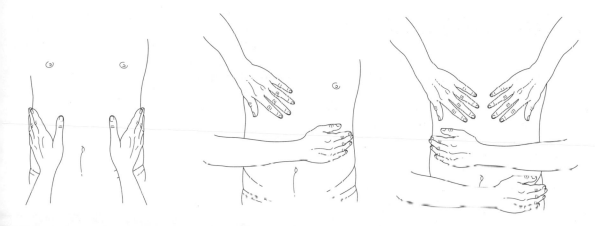

Figure 7.10 Assisting coughing.

suctioning, minimize the time the catheter is in the patient's trachea and monitor their heart rate throughout the procedure. Give prophylactic atropine if this is a persistent problem. An increase in tracheal pressure due to the tracheotomy becoming obstructed due to accumulated secretions can also induce vagal over stimulation.

Associated chest injuries

Rib or sternal fractures, along with haemo/pneumothorax may often accompany spinal cord injury. There is little additional information to add to existing care and management guidelines except to continue monitoring the patient's respi-ratory effort for signs of slowly developing respiratory complications. In the event of respiratory distress, do not attempt to raise or sit the patient up in bed whenever spinal column trauma is suspected.

Pulmonary embolism

Where appropriate prophylactic anticoagulation is undertaken, pulmonary embolism is rare following spinal cord injury. When it does occur it is usually silent in nature and may present initially as an acute disturbance in the patient's normal behaviour.

Cardiovascular function

The loss of vasomotor tone throughout the paralysed areas of the body provides the nurse with the classic diagnostic observations of spinal shock – hypotension, bradycardia and poikilo-thermia. The impact of this effect varies depending upon the level of injury. It is most pronounced in cases of tetraplegia. The loss of tone throughout the majority of the body's antigravity muscles, combined with the passive dilation of its vascular network can result in an average (tetraplegic) blood pressure of 80/50. Unopposed vagal nerve activity results in a (tetraplegic) bradycardia averaging 52 bpm. This effect requires a reinterpretation of anticipated base-line observations whenever a patient with spinal cord injury is admitted to the HDU. Monitor and record observations every 15 minutes initially, reducing over time as appropriate to the patient's progress. Wherever possible, avoid turning the patient onto their left side for prolonged periods (such as during a back wash or sheet change) as this can increase vagal stimulation and may induce cardiac syncope. Turning the patient onto their right side does not have the same effect and this is not usually a problem during routine turning or twisting for pressure relief.

Circulation

Do not confuse spinal shock with hypovolaemia. Massive fluid replacement in the absence of actual blood loss is a common error at this point, resulting in pulmonary overload and subsequent pulmonary oedema. In the presence of actual multitrauma, fractures or abdominal injuries, proceed with caution when replacing lost fluid. Application of TED stockings can replace some of the lost muscle resistance as well as reducing the risk of deep vein thrombosis.

Deep vein thrombosis

Deep vein thrombosis (DVT) is another potential complication following spinal cord injury, but the incidence can be minimized through good prophylactic management. Apply appropriately measured thigh-length TED stockings but ensure that the skin beneath the stockings is checked at least twice a day for the effects of pressure.

Routine anticoagulation with subcutaneous heparin 5000 u three times a day or enoxaparin 20 mg daily should commence on admission and its effectiveness should be monitored. A full range of passive movements to the paralysed lower limbs, as described earlier, will also improve venous return. Detection of an actual DVT in a patient with spinal cord injury is difficult. A swollen lower limb will only be apparent about ten days after the clot has formed. The only reliable diagnostic indi-

cator of early DVT formation is a sudden, unexpected pyrexia (Weingarden *et al.*, 1988).

As this may be masked in the presence of an apparent or detectable infection, every pyrexial episode should be considered as a potential DVT episode as a precaution. Ultrasound scanning has proved significant in detecting thromboses in spinal cord injury patients. The risk potential for deep vein thrombosis increases significantly following spinal surgery.

Thermoregulation

Sweating, shivering and piloerection (goose-flesh) all depend upon spinal nerves for stimulation. In addition, peripheral vasodilation means that the patient's core temperature can soon equal the environmental temperature through circulatory conduction. This is termed *'poikilothermia'*. It is the responsibility of every healthcare professional to ensure that the patient's body temperature is maintained at an appropriate level during all procedures, treatments and investigations. It should be anticipated that the patient's body temperature will drop significantly both during and following the administration of an anaesthetic in theatre.

Immune response

Severe central nervous system trauma has an adverse effect upon the body's immune response mechanism, therefore, all procedures and invasive investigations should be conducted with scrupulous attention towards asepsis. Catheters, drains, central venous pressure lines, parenteral feeding lines, intravenous and arterial lines each have their own potential risk of infection. In combination they put the acute spinal cord injury patient at high risk of developing septicaemia if infection control procedures are neglected.

Gastrointestinal function

Every spinal cord injury patient will present with an initial loss of peristalsis due to spinal shock. Vomiting post-injury is a potential hazard for tetraplegic patients, but the incidence is such that the routine passing of a nasogastric tube is not always essential. A nasogastric tube should only be passed if the patient complains of nausea or has ingested significant amounts of food or fluids pre-injury. There is potential for vagal over-stimulation both during and following the passing of a nasogastric tube.

A spinal cord injury patient should be kept nil-by-mouth for the first 48 hours post-injury without exception – even if bowel sounds are present upon admission. In the absence of actual fluid loss, intravenous fluids prescribed at this time should be for hydration only and should not exceed 2 litres over 24 hours. Observe the patient carefully for signs of abdominal distension during this period as this may impair diaphragmatic breathing. After 48 hours, where crisp, clear bowel sounds are detectable, a graduated oral fluid regime, similar to that followed by patients who have undergone abdominal surgery, can commence. If tolerated, this can be followed by a gradual return to full diet. If the paralytic ileus persists beyond 72 hours then total parenteral nutrition (TPN) should be commenced to offset post-traumatic catabolism. A peripheral line is preferred as it has a lower infection potential for short-term use.

Bowel management

The rectum and anus are also flaccid initially following spinal cord injury. Accumulation of faeces in the rectum can lead to over-distension of stretch receptors in the bowel wall and frustrate the return of reflex anorectal activity. In addition, obstruction of the bowel can weaken the bowel wall and increase the risk of perforation.

A gentle digital check per rectum (PR) to determine the presence of the anal sphincter reflex should be commenced following admission. A gentle digital evacuation of any faeces present at this time should be undertaken with sufficient lubrication. Glycerin suppositories should be utilized to soften the stool if required. Any attempt to stimulate a bowel action using suppositories or enemata at this stage will fail. As digital evacuation of the bowel usually falls outside of the scope of practice for most general nurses, here is another incentive to liaise with a specialist centre – where such procedures are routinely undertaken – to advance local practices.

The anal reflex is the first spinal reflex to return, usually about 48 hours after injury. At this point reflex bowel emptying can be undertaken in line with the patient's oral intake. Alternate day microenemas are utilized in combination with digital stimulation in most cases. This is the beginning of a complex programme of rehabilitation with implications for the patient's future quality of life and such techniques should only be undertaken in collaboration with specialist spinal cord injury practitioners.

Acute abdominal complications

Unopposed vagus nerve activity is thought to be a key factor in the high risk post-injury of stress ulceration. This risk is particularly high for tetraplegics. The administration of a prophylactic antacid (sucralfate) along with an H_2 blocker (ranitidine) from admission has proven successful in reducing this risk.

In the event of an actual visceral ulcer or trauma occurring, the tetraplegic patient may complain of referred visceral discomfort. Visceral ulceration or perforation is usually perceived as a 'burning' or 'persistent' pain in or around the anterior or outer shoulder unrelated to movement. If an ulcer is suspected, the administration of a single dose of an antacid preparation may give relief, confirming the suspected problem exists.

Traumatic abdominal or visceral injuries, sustained at the time of the accident, may be perceived by the patient as a non-specific abdominal discomfort. Any such complaints should be investigated further. Hypergylcaemia due to accompanying pancreatic trauma may manifest itself as acute lethargy in the spinal cord injury patient.

Genitourinary function

The bladder is flaccid throughout the period of spinal shock. Insertion of an indwelling urethral catheter enables continuous bladder drainage and monitoring of urinary output. Experience has demonstrated that reduced bladder activity increases the incidence of sedimentation and catheter blockage. This increases the risk of urinary retention and urinary tract infection following spinal cord injury. An adult urinary catheter gauge of 14–16 ch is therefore recommended. Silicone catheters are also recommended for their durability.

At this stage post-injury, the vast majority of patients with spinal cord injury have the potential to recover reflex bladder function during their rehabilitation at a specialist centre. Over-distension of the bladder during initial management can result in the over-stretching of nerve and muscle fibres within the bladder wall, reducing their potential to recover reflex function. Reflux of stale urine towards the kidney can lead to renal complications. In view of the effect of spinal shock upon diuresis, hourly monitoring of urinary output is essential during the first few days post-injury. The sudden hypotension which accompanies spinal shock stimulates the production of large quantities of antidiuretic hormone (ADH) by the pituitary. Levels of ADH production increase in relation to the level of spinal cord injury. Therefore, in the event of tetraplegia an initial urinary output in the region of 30–50 mL/h should be expected. Indiscriminate increases in fluid infusions and the use of diuretics where there is no clear evidence of renal or cardiac problems are discouraged. ADH secretion increases further following surgery during the post-injury period.

Psychological and emotional support

The initial impact of spinal cord injury upon an individual is sudden and unexpected. The fear and anxiety which follows the realization that one has suffered a serious injury with an apparent and severe loss of movement and sensation throughout a significant proportion of one's body cannot be imagined. Fear and frustration are compounded by the seeming inability of doctors and nurses to give a clear diagnosis due to the presence of spinal shock.

Psychological management and support of the spinal cord injury patient at this time should aim to inform both the patient and their family enough to gain their cooperation. For most patients in the acute stage, awareness of the extent of their injury is distracted by the combined onslaught of examinations, investigations and treatments and dulled by analgesics or anaesthesia. Many patients report post-traumatic amnesia and the young age of many of these individuals means a lack of developed coping mechanisms. Following spinal cord injury each individual strives to 'cope' with their situation appropriate to their individual character.

The following advice is offered for staff supporting the spinal cord injury patient in the high dependency unit:

- Be truthful with all information given to the patient within the limitations of your own knowledge and experience of this condition. Utilize the delay in providing an accurate diagnosis and prognosis to hold out some hope to your patient initially. Ensure that all care-team members give the same advice at this time.
- Care for your patient with both competence and confidence in your abilities so that the patient feels 'safe in your hands'. This is difficult where knowledge and experience is limited and further supports the requirement for early contact with specialist colleagues.
- Make every reasonable effort to reduce the effects of sensory deprivation.
- Involve patients in simple decision making and encourage their active participation in personal care activities where possible.
- Inform your patient and their family of your intention to transfer them to your local spinal injuries unit as soon as possible. Explain why this is necessary.

- Utilize your local spinal injuries unit for additional advice or support as required.

A number of spinal cord injury patients will present with pre-existing psychological or psychiatric conditions, which may have contributed to their accident or injury. They may also complicate both the diagnosis and initial management of spinal cord injury. The contribution of the local mental healthcare team should be sought.

Enabling patients with spinal cord injury to gain early access to specialist staff and environments can reduce the potential for long-term psychological problems post-injury. This is because the confident and familiar approach of specialist practitioners, which has been gained through experience, reflects a positive outlook and approach towards spinal cord injury. Peer support for both patients and their relatives is available from the resident patient population, all of whom share this specialist condition.

Children and elderly adults

Spinal cord injury is not confined to any particular age group. Accurate diagnosis of spinal cord injury within these age groups is often difficult and these patients are more vulnerable than others to its systemic effects.

Children and elderly adults are particularly susceptible to the enhanced effects of spinal shock upon their respiratory and cardiovascular systems

with an increased potential for developing early complications. The effects of spinal shock in these two groups are also more prolonged. The complications of spinal cord injury occur with greater frequency amongst these two age groups, more than any other, whenever there is a delay in transferring them to a spinal injuries unit.

Further activities

ACTIVITY 7.4

What are the acute effects of a traumatic spinal cord injury?

- Spinal cord injury is characterized by the complete loss of all sensation, voluntary and involuntary movements and all reflexes below the level of lesion.

- This is the usual condition of such patients when admitted to the high dependency unit and this condition, known as 'spinal shock', can persist for between 2 and 6 weeks post-injury.
- Rapid transfer to a spinal injuries unit is the best option for such patients.

In some circumstances, stabilization of the patient's condition, sufficient to make the above journey, can delay their transfer initially.

ACTIVITY 7.5 PULLING IT ALL TOGETHER

Before undertaking this activity:
- Can you identify the nominated Spinal Injuries Unit for your hospital?
- Do you know how to contact them for advice or to arrange the transfer of a patient?
- Do you know what criteria they utilize to determine the suitability of a patient for transfer?
- Does your area of practice have an existing collaborative protocol/care plan for patients admitted with spinal cord injuries?

Formulate an evidence-based plan of care for the following patient case study:

John is an 18-year-old student and is admitted to your HDU from Casualty at 06.00 hours after crashing his car into a tree at 23.30 hours last night. John is lying supine, strapped onto a spine board with a cervical collar *in situ*.

His neurological examination suggests that he has sustained a complete lesion of his spinal cord at the level of C6 although there is no fracture visible on X-ray examination.

What might be the significance of the following extracts from John's nursing records and what nursing actions do you feel are required?

---

1 John's observations from A&E are temperature 35.8, pulse 52, respirations 30 and shallow, and blood pressure 80/50.
2 He has an undisplaced closed fracture of his left tibia which has been immobilized in a below-knee plaster cast.
3 He vomited twice in A&E and was given 15 mg of morphine intravenously just before transfer to the HDU.
4 John received 3 litres of intravenous fluid in A&E and has the first of 4 units of blood in progress, each to be transfused over an hour, as the trauma medical team suspect that his persistently low blood pressure is due to internal bleeding.
5 The admitting nurse reports that the skin over John's sacrum and heels is red.
6 She also reports that John is demanding a drink of water and that according to his A&E record he has not voided since admission to A&E.

Answers

1 John's observations from A&E are temperature 35.8, pulse 52, respirations 30 and shallow, and blood pressure 80/50.
Pulse and BP are within expected limits for John's suspected neurological lesion. John's respirations are high and may be diaphragmatic in nature. Temperature suggests hypothermia.
2 He has an undisplaced closed fracture of his left tibia which has been immobilized in a below-knee plaster cast.
Check padding of cast. Bivalve cast as soon as possible. Remove cast to check skin at least twice daily.
3 He vomited twice in A&E and was given 15 mg of morphine intravenously just before transfer to the HDU.
Consider insertion of nasogastric tube to reduce risk of inhalation pneumonia. May need atropine before procedure. May also need prophylactic antiemetic. Monitor John's respirations as may suffer from respiratory depression – have naloxone to hand. Change to non-narcotic analgesia. Check to see if antiemetic was prescribed and given with morphine when administered.
4 John received 3 litres of intravenous fluid in A&E and has the first of 4 units of blood in progress, each to be transfused over an hour, as the trauma medical team suspect that his persistently low blood pressure is due to internal bleeding.
Stop the transfusion and get expert medical opinion immediately. John's persistent hypotension is not indicative of blood loss; neither is it falling continuously. In addition, he is bradycardic and not tachycardic. This suggests spinal shock rather than hypovolaemia. If there is a suspicion of internal

haemorrhage then an ultrasound scan or peritoneal lavage should be ordered. Monitor John's respirations and listen regularly to his chest for signs of pulmonary oedema due to over-infusion.

5   The admitting nurse reports that the skin over John's sacrum and heels is red.
Document condition of John's skin upon arrival. Begin to pelvic twist or turn him, side to side only, as soon as possible after admission to the HDU. Do not place him in a supine position, except to facilitate essential procedures, until all red or pink marks have disappeared.

6   She also reports that John is demanding a drink of water and that according to his A&E record he has not voided since admission to A&E.
Keep John nil by mouth until peristalsis resumes. Explain to John and his family why he is unable to have oral fluids at present. Give John regular mouth care.

Check that John has a urinary catheter in situ and that it is patent. Monitor his urinary output hourly and liaise with specialist medical staff. Oliguria is not uncommon following SCI.

Conclusion

The rapid transfer of people with acute spinal cord injury from a general hospital to a specialist facility is the most effective method of reducing the effect and incidence of complications associated with this condition. The comprehensive lifetime management of these individuals by spinal injuries units has increased their survivability, longevity and quality of existence. In some post-injury scenarios, transfer to a spinal injuries unit may be delayed due to the patient's initial physio-logical status. Admission of these patients to a high dependency unit should be anticipated.

Inappropriate management of these patients during the initial post-trauma period can affect their ability to achieve expected rehabilitation outcomes. Where such a delay occurs, it is essential that nurses and other professionals who work in high dependency care environments are appropriately prepared for the challenge.

Further reading

Alderson J.D. and Frost, E.A.M. (eds) 1996 *Spinal cord injuries: anaesthetic and associated care.* London: Butterworths.

Aung, S. and El-Masry, W.S. 1997 Audit of a British centre for spinal injury. *Spinal Cord* **35**, 147–50.

Bracken, M. *et al.* 1990 A randomised control trial of methylprednisolone and naloxone in the treatment of spinal cord injury. *New England Journal of Medicine* **322**, 1405–11.

Bromley, I. 1991 *Tetraplegia and paraplegia: a guide for physiotherapists.* London: Churchill Livingstone.

Clarke, T., Abbenbroek, B. and Hardy, L. 1996 The impact of a high dependency unit continuing education programme on nursing practice and patient outcomes. *Australian Critical Care* **9**, 138–42.

Crossman, M.W. 1996 Sensory deprivation in spinal cord injury. *Spinal Cord* **34**, 573–7

Clancy, J. and McVicar, A. 1995 *Physiology and anatomy.* London: Arnold

El-Masri, W., Cochrane, P. and Silver J.R. 1983 Gastro-intestinal bleeding in patients with acute spinal cord injuries. *Injury: The British Journal of Accident Surgery* **14**, 162–7.

Grundy, D. and Swain, A. (eds) 1996 *ABC of Spinal Cord Injury*, 3rd edn. London: BMJ.

Gunnewicht, B.R. 1997 Prevention of pressure sores in acute spinal cord injury; outside the specialist unit. *Journal of Tissue Viability* **7**, 124–9.

Hughes, M.C. 1990 Critical care nursing for the patient with a spinal cord injury. *Critical Care Nursing Clinics of North America* **2**, 33–40.

Masham, S. 1997 Specialists only. *Nursing Standard* **12** (6), 17.

McClelland, M.R. 1991 Acute spinal cord injury. *Surgery* **90**, 2158–63.

Ravichandran, G. and Silver J.R. 1982 Missed injuries of the spinal cord. *British Medical Journal* **284**, 953–6.

Silver, J.R., Doggart, J.R. and Burr, R.G. 1995 The reduced urinary output after spinal cord injury: a review. *Paraplegia* **33**, 721–5.

Spinal Injuries Association 1997 *The Spinal Injuries Association recommendations regarding NHS treatment of people confirmed, suspected or potentially experiencing spinal cord injury.* London: Spinal Injuries Association.

Tator, C.H., Duncan, E.G., Edmonds V.E. *et al.* 1995 Andrews DF. Neurological recovery, mortality and length of stay after acute spinal cord injury associated with changes in management. *Paraplegia* **33**, 254–62.

Tehranzadeh, J. and Palmer, S. 1996 Imaging of cervical spine trauma. *Seminars in Ultrasound, CT and MRI* **17**(2), 93–104.

Trieschmann R.B. 1988 *Spinal cord injuries: psychological, social and vocational rehabilitation.* New York: Demos.

Weingarden, S.I., Weingarden, D.S. and Belen, J. 1988 Fever and thromboembolic disease in acute spinal cord injury. *Paraplegia* **26**, 35–42.

Zeidlik, C.P. 1992 *Management of spinal cord Injury* 2nd edn. Boston: Jones and Bartlett.

Caring for the enteral system

Sue Zmarzty

THE ENTERAL SYSTEM

There are few factors more important to the critically ill patient than the provision of adequate nutrition (Garrow and James, 1993). Therefore the aim of this chapter is to help nurses understand the principles of good nutrition, and together with a working knowledge of the anatomy and physiology of the gastrointestinal (GI) tract, be able to effectively manage the nutritional status of a critically ill patient (Zainal, 1994)

Nutrition is an integral part of health, and public interest in and awareness of nutrition, is increasing. Nurses have a major role in promoting and maintaining good nutritional practices in the clinical setting. Knowledge of the physiological processes relevant to nutrition helps provide an understanding of how the body meets its needs. An understanding of what constitutes 'good nutritional status' and 'adequate functioning' of the enteral system are essential for assessing a patient's needs and planning nursing interventions.

In addition to the general recomendations for health (DOH, 1992), it is known that between 30 and 50 per cent of inpatients suffer some degree of malnutrition and as a result, have a higher risk of complications and higher mortality than well-nourished patients. Nurses have a fundamental role in combating and preventing malnutrition yet often lack knowledge and understanding of the problem.

Nutrients are chemical substances in food that provide energy, act as building blocks in forming new body components, or assist in the functioning of various body processes (Berne and Levy, 1990). There are six major classes of nutrients: carbohydrates (CHO), fats (lipids), proteins, minerals, vitamins, and water.

Dietary fibre, both soluble (e.g. gums, mucilages, most pectins) and insoluble (e.g. cellulose, lignin), is an important component of a healthy diet despite the fact that the body is unable to digest it. Insoluble fibre holds water and increases stool bulk, reduces colonic intraluminal pressure and binds metals, e.g. zinc, bile acids and cholesterol. Soluble fibre slows gastric emptying, provides fermentable material to support colonic

bacteria, with the production of gas which aerates the stool and aids defaecation. Both forms of fibre are important in helping to prevent gastrointestinal (GI) disease such as diverticulosis, and aid management serum lipid and glucose levels related to chronic conditions such as heart disease and diabetes mellitus.

Nutrients present in food are made available to the body cells by the enteral (digestive) system (Fig. 8.1).

The transit times for food products vary with the type of macronutrient predominant within the meal (e.g. high fat and to a lesser extent protein rich meals, stay in the stomach for a much longer period of time than high carbohydrate meals). Meals taken late at night also stay in the stomach for a prolonged period. This is due to the lowered metabolic rate during sleep. The general rule relating to metabolic rate is the higher the individual's metabolic rate the faster the transit time of food through the gastrointestinal tract. On average, vegetarians experience a faster transit time than non-vegetarians.

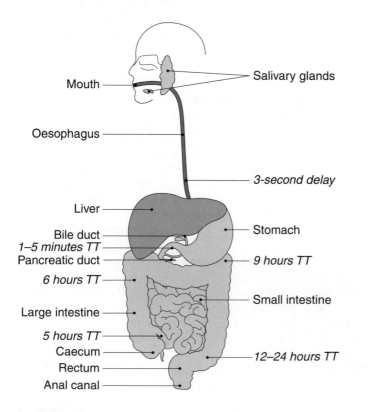

Figure 8.1 Diagram of the enteral system with transit times. TT: transit time.

Table 8.1 Nutrition at a glance

Nutrient	Source
Protein – Nutrient for growth and repair of muscle tissues, bone, enzymes, hormones, blood cells etc.	Found in: milk and dairy products, meats, fish, eggs, nuts, pulse vegetables, cereal products made from wheat, rye or oats
Carbohydrate – for energy	Milk, yogurts (especially sweetened fruit varieties), pulse vegetables, breads, biscuits, breakfast cereals, sago, barley, rice, oatmeal, wheat, pastas, potatoes, fruits, cakes and puddings, cordials and fizzy drinks, sugar
Fat – a concentrated source of energy (calories) important for the fat soluble vitamins A, D, E, K	Butter, margarines, cooking and salad oils, cream and cream cheeses, mayonnaise, oily fish (sardines, tuna, mackerel etc.), fat on/in meats and patés, full- and medium-fat cheeses, egg yolk, chocolates, toffees, rich cakes/pastries, avocado and coconut
Vitamin A – for skin and mucosal integrity, regeneration of the visual pigment rhodopsin, and it can be converted from carotene and stored in the liver	Cooking and salad oils/fats, liver, oily fish, red meats, egg yolk, milk and dairy products and yellow/red fruits and vegetables
Vitamin B complex/Vitamin B1 (thiamin) – involved in the chemical breakdown of carbohydrate foods in the release of energy	Most cereals and foods made with them, yeast and yeast extracts, red meats and offal, pork and bacon, eggs, milk, potatoes, nuts, peas and beans
Vitamin B2 (riboflavin) – involved in cellular aerobic activity, the health of the eyes, the nervous system and during pregnancy	Liver, kidney, milk and yogurt, green vegetables and beer
Nicotinic acid – involved in tissue oxidation and fat metabolism. The amino acid tryptophan can be converted to nicotinic acid	Wholewheat cereals, fish, meat and offals, yeast and yeast extracts, oatmeal, pulse vegetables, dried fruits and cocoa
Vitamin B6 (pyridoxin) – for healthy nervous system and the utilization of iron	Very widely distributed in all foodstuffs of plant and animal origin
Folic acid – involved in oxidation reactions and protein synthesis	Liver, spinach, green vegetables, white fish, wholemeal flours/breads, eggs, ham and pork
Vitamin B12 (cyanocobalamin) – formation of mature red blood cells and nervous system	Widespread in all foods of animal origin but not in plant foods
Vitamin C (ascorbic acid) – for growth and for integrity of connective tissue, wound healing, resisting infections and absorption of iron	Widespread in fresh/frozen fruit and vegetables, and fruit juices
Vitamin D (cholecalciferol) – essential for absorption and deposition of calcium into bone and can be stored in the liver. It is essential for the absorption of calcium	Synthesized in the skin when it is exposed to sunlight, offal meats, egg yolk, fats and dairy products, fish oils and malted drinks
Vitamin E (tocopherol) – antioxidant properties	Vegetable fats/oils, nuts, wheatgerm and eggs
Vitamin K (phytomenadione) – essential for the formation of prothrombin which is involved in blood-clotting	All fresh/frozen dark green leafy vegetables and cauliflower. It is synthesized by intestinal bacteria
Calcium and phosphorus – calcification of bone and teeth	Hard cheeses, milk, yogurts, fish bones, bread and flour products, malted milks, nuts, dried fruits, 'hard' water
Iron – the 'haem' part of haemoglobin, the oxygen-carrying protein in red blood cells	Red meats and offals, egg yolk, oily fish, beef extracts, cocoa and chocolate, dried fruits, flour products, pulse vegetables, 'fortified' breakfast cereals, cider and red wine

Principal physiological processes of digestion

The digestive process comprises five principal physiological processes, all of which may become disrupted during critical illness:

1 *Ingestion (eating)*: the process of taking food into the mouth.
2 *Movement*: the neuromuscular activity of the gut wall (known as peristalsis) necessary to move the food through the GI tract in a unidirectional manner from mouth to anus.
3 *Digestion*: the physical and chemical breakdown of food involving the muscular movements of segmentation and peristalsis, and the action of various enzymes respectively, to render the food into an absorbable form.
4 *Absorption*: the passage of the end products of digestion from the GI tract into the blood stream and the lymphatic vessels which distribute these metabolites to the cells that require them. The liver assimilates and processes these substances in order to keep blood levels optimal for cellular metabolism.
5 *Defaecation (excretion)*: the elimination of indigestible and unabsorbed substances from the body.

The macronutrients in food are broken down by digestive juices into smaller units: proteins into amino acids, fats into fatty acids and glycerol, and carbohydrates (complex sugars and starches – CHO) into simple sugars (glucose and galactose). In these forms nutrients pass from the intestine into the bloodstream. Vitamins and minerals occur in food as micronutrients and pass through the intestinal wall without the aid of digestive juices. Effective digestion requires that all five physiological stages be adequately completed (Todorovik and Micklewright, 1997).

It is important to understand the function of the digestive organs as this knowledge will enable a much better assessment of the patient's nutritional problems (*see* Table 8.2; Fig. 8.2).

The motility of the GI tract is of vital importance to propel food products with adequate time for digestion and absorption (Fig. 8.1). The gut can be thought of as a muscular tube, and from pharynx to rectum it is made up of layers of circular and longitudinal smooth muscle. At various points along its length there are tight bands of muscle (sphincters), which can constrict and dilate according to gut activity. In addition to

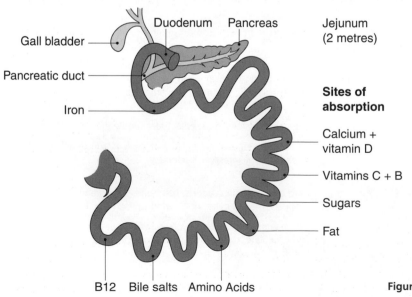

Gall bladder
Duodenum   Pancreas
Pancreatic duct
Iron
Jejunum (2 metres)
Sites of absorption
Calcium + vitamin D
Vitamins C + B
Sugars
Fat
B12   Bile salts   Amino Acids

Figure 8.2 Sites of absorption

Table 8.2   The functions of the organs of digestion

Organ	Exocrine secretions	Functions
Mouth and pharynx, teeth, tongue, facial muscles and salivary glands.	Saliva: Salt, water and mucus **Salivary amylase (ptyalin)**	Chewing, mastication, initiation of swallowing reflex. Moistening and lubricating food. Carbohydrate (CHO) digesting enzyme.
Oesophagus. Smooth and muscular with mucus glands.	Mucus	Moving the lubricated bolus of food to the stomach by peristaltic waves.
Stomach. Thick muscular wall with extra oblique muscle layer, large mucosal folds (rugae), exocrine cells.	Gastric juice: Hydrochloric acid (HCl) **Pepsin** Mucous Intrinsic factor	Storing, mixing and dissolving food. Regulating emptying of liquid food (chyme) into the duodenum. Dissolving food particles, killing microbes, lowering pH. Protein-digesting enzyme. Lubrication and protection of epithelial surface. Necessary for the absorption of vitamin B12 from the diet.
Duodenum. Abundance of villi, vastly increasing luminal surface area, exocrine cells, ducts from gall bladder and pancreas enter here.	Duodenal juice: Bicarbonate **Enterokinase** **Cholecystokinin (CCK),** **Secretin**	Receives chyme from the stomach, muscular contractions (segmentation) mixes food with alkaline juices, neutralizing the strong acid. Activates the protein-splitting enzymes contained in pancreatic juice. Chemical messenger which stimulates contraction of gall bladder and release of bile into the duodenum. Chemical messenger (hormone) which stimulates release of pancreatic juice into the duodenum.
Pancreas. Exocrine and endocrine producing organ.	Pancreatic juice: Bicarbonate **Amylase** **Lipase** **Trypsinogen** and **chymotrypsinogen**	Secretion of enzymes and bicarbonate to digest nutrients and neutralize stomach acid. CHO digestion. Fat digestion. Protein digestion when activated in the presence of enterokinase in duodenum to form **trypsin.**
Gall bladder. Stores bile which is made in the liver.	Bile: Bicarbonate Bile salts Organic waste products	Stored bile is released during a meal and serves to neutralize the acid chyme. Emulsification of fats, facilitating action of pancreatic lipase. Elimination from the body.
Ileum. Villi and microvilli. Exocrine cells, Brunner's glands.	Intestinal juice: **Amylase,** **Trypsin** Salt, water and mucus	Digestion and absorption of most substances, mixing and propulsion of contents. Further digestion of CHO. Further digestion of protein. Lubrication. Action of pancreatic lipase continues.
Colon. Large lumen with no villi.	Mucus (contains bacterial flora)	Storing and concentration of undigested matter by absorption of salt and water. Propulsion of contents. Protection from pathogens. Produces Vitamin K and B complexes.
Rectum		Defaecation reflex initiated by distension.

these there is an extra layer of muscle in the wall of the stomach, the fibres of which are arranged obliquely to facilitate strong contractions of the stomach wall in all directions. The autonomic nervous system (ANS) innervates the whole of the gut and generally the parasympathetic branch stimulates peristalsis, whereas the sympathetic branch inhibits it. Hormones such as catecholamines affect motility once the receptors on the smooth muscle in the wall of the GI tract are stimulated. Spasm of this smooth muscle might occur if the tract is over stimulated by dilation inside the tract, e.g. accumulation of gas or fluid or blockage by foreign body, impacted faeces or tumour. Such dilation can result in painful stimuli known as colic.

Regulation of food intake

Regulation of food intake involves two centres in the hypothalamic region of the brain – the hunger centre and the satiety centre. The hunger centre is constantly active but may be inhibited by the satiety centre. The centres are stimulated by glucose, amino acids, lipids, body temperature, distension of the gut, and cholecystokinin (CCK), and also by psychological influences.

Energy is required by the body to maintain basal metabolic activities and to sustain an increase in those activities when necessary. The amount of energy required by an individual is therefore dependent upon two factors: the basal metabolic rate (BMR) and the physical activity level (PAL) (Todorovik and Micklewright, 1997).

BMR × PAL = estimated average requirement for energy which is expressed in kcalories or/and kjoules (1 kcalorie = 4.2 kjoules)

The caloric value represents the energy incorporated in chemical bonds that is released during metabolism, e.g.

1 g CHO produces 4.1 kcal, 1 g of protein produces approximately the same, and 1 g fat produces 9.2 kcal during metabolism

Metabolism refers to all chemical reactions of the body and has two phases: *catabolism* and *anabolism*.

Anabolism consists of a series of synthesis reactions whereby small molecules are built up into larger ones that form the body's structural and functional components. Anabolic reactions require energy whereas catabolism refers to 'breakdown' reactions that release energy.

Catabolic reactions supply the energy required for anabolic reactions and most metabolic reactions are catalysed by enzymes which are proteins that speed up chemical reactions without themselves being changed.

Metabolic rate varies between individuals and tends to slow with advancing age. PAL values are slightly higher for men than for women, and also tend to decline with advancing age resulting in a reduced energy requirement.

Carbohydrate metabolism

During digestion, polysaccharides and disaccharides are converted to monosaccharides which are transported to the liver. Carbohydrate metabolism is primarily concerned with glucose metabolism.

FATE OF CARBOHYDRATES

- Some glucose is oxidized by cells to provide energy; it moves into cells by facilitated diffusion; insulin stimulates glucose movement into the cells.
- Excess glucose can be stored by the liver and the skeletal muscles as glycogen, or converted to fat.

Glucose catabolism

1 Glucose oxidation is also called cellular respiration.
2 The complete oxidation of glucose to CO_2 and H_2O involves glycolysis, the Krebs cycle and the electron transport chain.

Glycolysis is also called anaerobic respiration, because it occurs without O_2. Glycolysis refers to the breakdown of glucose into two molecules of pyruvic acid. When O_2 is in short supply, pyruvic acid is converted to lactic acid; under aerobic conditions pyruvic acid enters Krebs cycle. Glycolysis yields two molecules of ATP (energy).

Krebs cycle begins when pyruvic acid is converted to acetyl coenzyme A. Then a series of oxidation and reduction reactions take place, and the energy originally in the glucose and then the pyruvic acid is transferred to the reduced coenzymes. The electron transport chain is a series of oxidation–reduction reactions in which the energy in the coenzymes is liberated and transferred to ATP for storage. The complete oxidation of glucose can be represented as follows:

$$Glucose + O_2 \rightarrow 38\ ATP + CO_2 + H_2O$$

N.D. Krebs cycle and the electron transport chain require O_2.

Glucose anabolism

- The conversion of glucose to glycogen for storage in the liver and skeletal muscle is called glycogenesis, and is stimulated by insulin. The body can store 500 g of glycogen, and the conversion of glycogen back to glucose is called glycogenolysis; it occurs between meals and is stimulated by the hormone glucagon.
- Gluconeogenesis is the conversion of fat and protein molecules into glucose.

Lipid metabolism

1 Lipids are second to carbohydrates as a source of energy.
2 During digestion, fats are ultimately broken down into fatty acids and glycerol.

FATE OF LIPIDS

- Some fats may be oxidized to produce ATP.
- Some fats are stored in adipose tissue, mostly in the subcutaneous layer.
- Other lipids are used as structural molecules or to synthesize essential molecules, e.g. phospholipids of cell membranes, lipoproteins that transport cholesterol, thromboplastin for blood clotting, and cholesterol used to synthesize bile salts and steroid hormones.

Lipid catabolism

1 Fat must be split into fatty acids and glycerol (by enzyme action/chemical digestion in the gut), before it can be catabolized. Glycerol can be converted into glucose by conversion into a substrate in the gluconeogenesis pathway or similarly, it can enter the pathway in the direction of glycolysis, and yield ATP anaerobically or in the presence of O_2, enter Krebs cycle and the electron transport chain to maximize energy yield aerobically. Fatty acids are catabolized through beta oxidation, yielding acetyl coenzyme A, which enters the Krebs cycle.
2 The formation of ketone bodies by the liver is a normal phase of fatty acid catabolism, but an excess of ketones in the body is called ketosis, and may cause acidosis.

Lipid anabolism/lipogenesis

The conversion of glucose or amino acids into lipids is called lipogenesis and is stimulated by insulin.

Protein metabolism

- During digestion, proteins are broken down into amino acids.
- Protein anabolism and catabolism must be balanced through daily dietary intake to prevent protein depletion.

FATE OF PROTEINS

1 Amino acids that enter cells are almost immediately synthesized into proteins.
2 Proteins function as enzymes, hormones, structural elements etc. and any excess is stored as fat or glycogen, or used for energy.

Protein catabolism

- Before amino acids can be catabolized, they must be converted to substances that can enter Krebs cycle.
- Amino acids may also be converted into glucose, fatty acids, and ketones.

Protein anabolism

1 Protein synthesis is directed by DNA and RNA and carried out on the ribosomes of cells.
2 Before protein synthesis can occur, all the essential and non-essential amino acids must be present.

Regulation of metabolism

• Absorbed nutrients may be oxidized, stored, or converted, based on the needs of the body.
• The pathway taken by a particular nutrient is controlled by enzymes and regulated by hormones.

MINERALS

1 Minerals are inorganic substances that help to regulate body processes.

2 Minerals known to perform essential functions are calcium, phosphorus, sodium, chlorine, potassium, magnesium, iron, sulphur, iodine, manganese, cobalt, copper, zinc, selenium, and chromium.

VITAMINS

• Vitamins are organic nutrients that maintain growth and normal metabolism, and many function in enzyme systems.
• Fat-soluble vitamins (A, D, E, K) are absorbed with fats.
• Water soluble vitamins (B, C) are absorbed with water.

Severe illness and nutrition

This chapter will now explore the effects that sudden and critical illness has on the nutritional requirements of a patient. It will first consider a fever situation, then explore the effects of critical illness on the body's ability to maintain itself.

Metabolic requirements during a fever

A fever is an abnormally high body temperature; the most frequent cause being infection by bacteria and viruses. Other causes are myocardial infarction, tumours, tissue destruction by X-rays, surgery or trauma, and reactions to vaccines. In response to tissue damage or/and infection, the inflammatory process results in the release of cytokines. One of the cytokine functions is to act as a chemical messenger, attracting phagocytes to the area and triggering the release of prostaglandins.

These reset the hypothalamic thermostat at a higher temperature, and temperature-regulating reflex mechanisms will then act to bring the core temperature up to this new setting. Aspirin, paracetamol etc. reduce fever by inhibiting synthesis of prostaglandins. Up to a certain point, fever has a beneficial effect on the body, as high body temperature is believed to inhibit the growth of some bacteria and viruses. Fever also increases the heart rate so that white blood cells are delivered to sites of infection more rapidly. Also, antibody production and T cell proliferation are increased. Heat speeds up the rate of chemical reactions that may help body cells repair themselves more quickly during a disease. Among the complications of a fever are dehydration, acidosis, and permanent brain damage.

NOT in ?

Nutritional impact of a critical illness

There is a difference between the response of an otherwise healthy individual to starvation and the starvation in the presence of critical illness (stress starvation), which is commonly found in clinical practice. The normal response to starvation is designed to conserve body protein by reducing the rate of depletion and its effect on body weight. Energy requirements are reduced (i.e. basal metabolic rate is reduced) and fat becomes the preferred fuel. Body function is therefore preserved and total starvation can be tolerated for up to 60 days, with compromise of functions such as immune competence around 30 days. The response is regulated by reduced substrate levels, decreased insulin secretion and increased levels of glucagon in the blood. Ketones are the preferred energy fuel at 14–20 days with some degree of glucose intolerance. Introduction of a sufficient level of substrate (nutritional food) restores metabolic normality. In stress starvation, the metabolic response to critical disease overrides the normal response to starvation and conservation of body protein and energy is no longer possible. Weight loss and depletion of body protein is accelerated and significant impairment of body function may appear early in the course of the illness. The catabolic nature of the response is related to the disease processes and is unaffected by nutritional intake.

All diseases associated with an inflammatory response or tissue repair such as trauma or operative surgery, induce a metabolic response. The magnitude of the response is related to the severity of the clinical condition. The issue of greatest importance, clinically, is the catabolic phase seen during acute illness when the rate of tissue loss and protein depletion can be rapid. Just as important to the patient is the anabolic phase which follows, and which is associated with recovery, weight gain and rehabilitation.

Features of the metabolic response to stress illness

PROTEIN

Tissue loss occurs mainly in skeletal muscle and is associated with increased urinary excretion of nitrogen, potassium, magnesium, sulphate, phosphate and creatinine. Protein turnover is increased, and the breakdown (catabolism) of protein is increased to a much greater extent, resulting in a net loss of protein from the body.

In severe critical illness, the requirements for protein may be increased by 50–80 per cent.

CARBOHYDRATE

There is a state of glucose intolerance with hyperglycaemia, hyperinsulinaemia and insulin intolerance. This is associated with an increase in gluconeogenesis by the liver, principally from tissue protein. Uptake of glucose by the body tissues is reduced due to glucose and insulin intolerance, despite the fact that the tissues are desperate for energy for recovery to take place.

FAT

Lipolysis (fat breakdown) is increased with raised blood levels of free fatty acids and glycerol. By contrast with non-stressed starvation, ketones remain low or absent.

ENERGY

Resting energy expenditure may increase by 18–30 per cent in multiple fractures, 30–60 per cent in severe infections, and 50–100 per cent in severe illness.

The mechanisms which bring about this metabolic response to illness are not fully understood, but certainly, stimuli such as pain, anoxia, hypercarbia, hypovolaemia and hypotension all operate where there is tissue damage and physiological stress/injury. These all trigger release of ACTH and growth hormone from the hypothalamus, resulting in increased circulating levels of cortisol, glucagon and insulin. Tissue cytokines, released in response to tissue damage and the inflammatory response, are also thought to be involved.

ACTIVITY 8.2

What does critical illness mean to the severely ill patient in your care?

CLINICAL IMPLICATIONS

- Loss of body weight at an accelerated rate, which reflects the reduction in skeletal muscle mass (i.e. a loss in lean body mass).
- Muscle function is impaired and experienced as weakness. This has direct implications for respiration and all activities of daily living. Immune function is impaired by traumatic stimuli and by malnutrition, and the cause of death in the critically ill is commonly an infection on top of the stress starvation.
- Mental acuity and performance are impaired, resulting in apathy and depression with loss of morale and the will to recover. A general sense of weakness and illness impairs appetite and the ability to eat.
- A severely malnourished person does not have the nutritional reserves to cope with the increased metabolic demands of severe injury, resulting in organ failure and infection. Organs

with rapid cell turnover are the first to fail, e.g. the GI tract epithelium becomes flattened and the ability to absorb nutrients rapidly declines.

The nutritional status of a patient is therefore of paramount importance as malnourishment prolongs recovery, increases the need for high dependency nursing care, increases the risk of serious complications of illness and at worst, leads to death. However, assessing those patients at risk of malnutrition is difficult because of the many factors involved. In the past, nursing assessment has tended to rely on general observation of nutritional status rather than accurate and systematic screening and early referral to a dietician (Reilly, 1996).

ACTIVITY 8.3 Patient scenario

Cathy Slater has been admitted to your unit suffering from a severe respiratory disorder. She is very dyspnoeic and agitated. As part of her overall nursing assessment, you need to assess her nutritional status and needs during her stay with you. How can the patient's nutritional status be effectively assessed by the nurse?

In order to care for your patient's nutritional needs it is essential to be able to assess your patient's nutritional status.

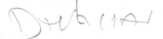

Effective assessment of nutritional status

Effective nursing assessment of nutritional status will involve the following factors.

- Height and weight to calculate body mass index (BMI = weight (kg) divided by height (m) squared. BMI normal range 19–25). (N.B. There is some debate relating to the use of BMI as the calculations are based on healthy young males; however, it is a standard measure and should be used).
- Direct observation of muscle bulk, subcutaneous fat, dehydration and grip strength – if possible carry out anthropometric measure-

ments using skin calipers and tape measure. Assess mobility.
- Biochemical profile to determine urea and electrolytes, albumin and retinol binding protein which give an indication of body protein status, total lymphocytes etc.
- Disease and treatment (drugs, investigations and therapy).
- Dietary history investigating the patient's 'normal diet' (question and answer, 24-hour recall and diet diary), recent changes and weight loss. Include family and friends if possible.
- Fluid balance/food intake charts.

- Include the dietician to consider nutritional assessment tools.

The nurse must be vigilant and observe his or her patient for signs of poor nutrition. Poor nutrition may be pre-existing or as a result of their hospitalization and illness. Poor dietary intake over a period of time can result in the signs and symptoms shown in Table 8.3.

It is important to note too, that there are many diverse conditions likely to result in nutritional

Table 8.3 Nutritional deficiencies and their effects

Deficiency	Effects
Potassium	Confusion, constipation, cardiac arrythmias, muscle weakness
Folate	Anaemia, confusion
Vitamin D/Calcium	Fractures or bone pains associated with osteomalacia
Vitamin C	Haemorrhages, impaired wound healing and immune response
Iron	Anaemia, lethargy, confusion
Protein	Thinness, wasting, low plasma albumin resulting in oedema

Table 8.4 Potential causes of inadequate intake

Quantity

Mechanical feeding problems
Inadequate intake may be caused by mechanical feeding problems due to poor functioning of oral mucous membranes, teeth, tongue or salivary glands, receding gums, ill-fitting dentures or mouth ulcers

Physical disabilities
Physical disabilities may also prevent adequate nutritional input. Dysphagia due to neuromuscular disorders including stroke, head injury, Parkinson's disease, achalasia, multiple sclerosis or scleroderma.

Obstruction
Obstruction may be an issue causing inability to take adequate nutrition. This may result from

goitre, acute tonsillitis, cancer neoplasm, chronic oesophagitis or aortic aneurysm.

Psychological
These causes may include the eating disorders such as bulimia and anorexia nervosa, dementia, clinical depression, general loss of appetite and nausea.

Quality
This category may include simple factors such as poor dietary feeding habits or food allergies. Issues such as lack of adequate dietary knowledge may be apparent or the person may be from an institutionalized setting where nutrition is not correctly balanced

Increased metabolism
Fever, infections or malignancy will cause a metabolic increase as will hyperthyroidism, surgical stress, trauma and burns

Increased dietary loss
The patient may be nauseated causing vomiting, or they may have diarrhoea. Decreased transit time through the gut may be caused by pathogenic organisms (e.g. *Salmonella*), gastrointestinal irritation, drug therapy. The patient may have an ileostomy or suffer from malabsorption syndrome

Defective utilization
This may result from metabolic disease, hepatic insufficiency or renal tubular acidosis

Defective absorption
This may be caused by pancreatic disease, biliary obstruction, coeliac disease, Crohn's disease. Infections could also be to blame, e.g. tuberculosis or *Giardia*. Systematic conditions may reduce absorption, e.g. scleroderma, diabetes. Certain drugs may be responsible, e.g. antibiotics or excess laxatives. Surgical procedures such as short bowel syndrome, fistulae or aggressive gastric surgery could have this effect.

Defective functions of major organ systems
Serious conditions such as severe heart disease, chronic obstructive pulmonary disease, liver disease, renal and brain damage may all have a significant effect on nutritional condition and must be taken into consideration by the nurse in his or her assessment

deficiencies. The nurse needs to be aware of all of these conditions when making the initial assessment, during continual reassessment, and at the evaluation of his or her nursing actions. A systematic assessment of the intake will enable a clearer decision to be made relating to choice of feeding method (Sidenvall and Ek, 1993). The nurse must also be clear about the potential causes of inadequate intake. These causes may be as simple as poorly fitting dentures or sore mouth.

As shown in Table 8.4, two issues arise, the first being related to quantity, the second quality.

Good nutrition is dependent on partnership

While patients at high risk are automatically referred to the dietician, the nurse plays a crucial role in the care of patients at moderate or low risk by monitoring their nutritional status and maximizing their nutritional support. Determining the appropriate action is a very important stage in the patient's treatment.

Providing nutritional support

Artificial nutritional support refers to nutritional support administered via a tube, whether *enteral* – feeding into the stomach or intestine – or *parenteral* – feeding into the circulation.

It is an important aspect of the modern management of high dependency patients to supply additional food as soon as possible (Hinchliffe *et al.*, 1994). Nutritional support does not have therapeutic properties, i.e. it cannot treat primary disease, but rather should be seen in the context of other supporting actions such as pain control, antisepsis, control of circulating blood volume by intravenous infusion, or dialysis in renal failure. In the last 20 years modern management has enabled patients to survive acute episodes of critical disease where impaired nutritional status would have had a serious impact upon survival.

GOALS FOR NUTRITIONAL SUPPORT

1 Achieve nutritional balance, i.e. maintain status quo and prevent further depletion.
2 Restore depleted tissue, i.e. regain the negative protein balance and return to normal function.

OPTIONS FOR ACTION

The options are:

- Hospital/normal diet, with or without the addition of frequent small appetising snacks between meals.
- Sip feeding with a balanced composition similar to a normal diet or/and fortified liquid foods, e.g. Complan, Fortimel, Hical, Fresubin etc., or special liquid feeds composed of amino acids, glucose and lipid which reduce intestinal inflammation in some patients with Crohn's disease.

There are also special preparations for patients with renal failure and other metabolic disorders.

1 *Enteral tube feeding* – administration of specially formulated liquid nutrients through a tube directly into the gut either by nasogastric, nasoduodenal or nasojejunal routes suitable for short term measures, or by percutaneous endoscopic gastrostomy (PEG) and jejunostomy for long-term measures.
2 *Parenteral tube feeding* – introduction of digested nutrients directly into a vein, so bypassing the intestine.

ACTIVITY 8.4

When choosing the most appropriate method of nutritional support for your patient, what is the first fundamental question that you require an answer to?

In order to choose the most appropriate method of nutritional support the answer to this fundamental question is required:

Is the enteral system/gut functional?

If so, then enteral feeding is the optimal course of action in order to promote and maintain a healthy functioning GI tract.

How do we feed our patients?

Enteral feeding is indicated in those patients with increased nutritional needs and whose GI tract is functioning (Finlay, 1997), but who might have compromised oral access to the GI tract, an inability or unwillingness to eat, and where there is a danger of aspiration. Insertion of nasoenteric tubes may be generally carried out by qualified and experienced nurses; however doctors are

Table 8.5 Potential complications of enteral feeding

Complication	Prevention/Treatment
Tube blockage	Flush tube with water when feed is interrupted/stopped, maintain a continuous flow using correct tube/nutrient solutions combinations, and replace tubes regularly
Misplacement/displacement	Insert correct type/length tube with patient in an upright position, check tube position by aspiration and pH/X-ray, and secure firmly.
Aspiration	Elevate head of bed during continuous feeding, check position of tube before each feed, avoid large-bore tubes and use nasojejunal feeding if patient is supine, unconscious or when the cardiac sphincter is incompetent.
Discomfort	Secure tube firmly to avoid mucosal erosion, encourage nose breathing, ensure hydration, oral hygiene, lubricate lips and inspect nares daily
Contamination	Good personal hygiene practices when handling feeds and equipment, avoid non-sterile feeds, change giving sets regularly, aseptic care of PEG tube site and change bags/bottles every 24 hours
Nausea and vomiting	Avoid high lipid or hyperosmolar feeds, use low lactose or lactose-free formulas and dilute when necessary; avoid rapid infusion rates, increase concentration and rate slowly, and use an enteral pump if available
Diarrhoea	Dilute feed or change to lactose-free and isotonic formula if appropriate, monitor antibiotic therapy and hydration and consider i.v. fluids for better absorption. Check feed for contamination
Constipation/overflow	Monitor hydration and use fibre-containing feed
Bowel distension/colic	Dilute feeds at reduced infusion rate and use lactose-free feed

responsible for the insertion of fine bore feeding tubes in patients who have maxillofacial disorders or following surgery, laryngectomy, and any disorder of the oesophagus. Patients who require prolonged enteral nutrition will have a percutaneous endoscopic gastrostomy tube (PEG tube) inserted by medical staff expert in the technique. PEG is a procedure performed under local anaesthetic whereby the tube is placed endoscopically. Some tubes are kept in place by means of a retention balloon while others are sutured in place. Drug therapy in solution can also be administered via the tube. It is essential that the nurse monitors constantly the function and safety of the method of feeding; he or she must be fully aware of the potential complications of enteral feeding as shown in Table 8.5 (Palmer and MacFie, 1997).

Composition of an ideal enteral diet

An average patient will need 8.4–12.6 MJ (2000–3000 kcal) and 10–15 g nitrogen, corresponding to 60–90 g protein in 2–3 litres of fluid.

The proportion of energy provided by fat should be about 30–40 per cent. The mixture should contain essential minerals, trace elements and vitamins.

Total parenteral nutrition

Total parenteral nutrition (TPN) is indicated in those patients with increased nutritional needs and whose GI tract is not functioning, and who may have fistulae, multiple trauma/burns, inflammatory bowel disease with complications, ITU patients, multiple organ failure, pancreatitis, prolonged paralytic ileus, peritoneal sepsis and short bowel syndrome.

HOW IS TPN GIVEN?

Central venous catheters are inserted by experienced medical staff and managed by suitably qualified medical and nursing personnel. The subclavian vein is the preferred site, but for patients with poor venous access or for whom a central line is contraindicated, a peripherally inserted central catheter (PICC) may be used though should ideally be only for a limited period The infusion enters the vein at a point where it will be rapidly diluted by high volume flow past the catheter tip. The potential complications of TPN are listed in Table 8.6.

Nutrients used in parenteral feeding

The feed is tailored to a patient's individual requirements. A stable patient with intestinal failure usually requires about 10.5 MJ (2500 kcal) of energy and 12 g of nitrogen as crystalline amino acids in 2500 mL of fluid. Energy is provided using glucose and lipid emulsion (usually soya bean oil). Lipid usually provides about 30 per cent of the calories infused. Amino acid provision includes all the essential amino acids and a wide range of the non-essential ones. Mixed into the bag with the above are the normal daily requirement of electrolytes, trace elements and vitamins. For patients with sepsis and increased metabolic requirements, the feed needs to be modified with additional amounts of vitamin B complex, trace elements and electrolytes. Nutrients are administered to the patient from a 3 litre bag and all feeds are specially prepared by the pharmacist according to medical prescription and dietetic

Table 8.6 Potential complications of TPN

Complications of:	Prevention/Treatment
Catheterization Air embolism, arterial puncture, chylothorax, haemothorax, pneumothorax, nerve injury, arrhythmias	Correctly insert central line, confirm position and document and firmly secure. Tilt patient into a 20° head-down position prior to venepuncture. Use silicone catheters in preference to plastic in order to minimize damage to the lining of the vein.Withdraw catheter slightly as the catheter tip can be too close to the sinoatrial node (pace-maker). The catheter tip should lie in the superior vena cava.
Indwelling catheter Sepsis, septicaemia	Insert catheter under full sterile conditions, cover entry site with a sterile adhesive dressing and change when necessary in accordance with strict aseptic technique. Ensure infusion solutions are sterile, and change infusions and giving sets only by experienced nurses wearing sterile gloves.Monitor patient for pyrexia, inspect catheter site, swab and culture blood and catheter tip for microorganisms and sensitivity
Catheter blockage Air embolism, blood clot	Maintain adequate infusion rate using a volumetric infusion pump; check clamps, taps and devices and heparinize 12-hourly; change empty fluid containers promptly. Ensure there are Luer locking connections to prevent accidental disconnections
Metabolic disturbances Hyperglycaemia, hypoglycaemia, urea and electrolyte imbalances, hyperosmolar diuresis, nutritional deficiencies, overhydration and circulatory overload	Ensure feed solution meets the specific needs of the patient and control rate of infusion. Disturbances may be due to the nutrient proportions in the feed – too much glucose can cause dehydration, respiratory distress due to CO_2 build-up, and coma. Energy can be provided in the form of more lipid and proportionally less glucose. Feed composition is very important and comprises pre-digested macronutrients: glucose, lipid emulsions, L-amino acids; and micronutrients: electrolytes, trace elements and vitamins and water

Table 8.7 Effects of drugs on nutritional status

Drug	Effect on nutritional status
Aspirin and non-steroidal anti-inflammatory drugs (NSAIDs)	Blood loss and iron deficiency
Digoxin	Lowers appetite
Purgatives	Potassium loss
Cancer chemotherapy	Anorexia
Diuretics	Potassium loss
Phenformin and Metformin	Vitamin B12 malabsorption
Co-trimoxazole	Can antagonize folate

recommendations based on individual patient needs, extent of trauma, pre-operative repletion, post-operative management etc. A regular rate of infusion is ensured by using a constant volume infusion pump, which incorporates alarms to warn of air in the infusion system and changes in flow rate. Dietary interventions/therapeutic diets are considered for: acute renal failure, cancer, cirrhosis of the liver, Crohn's disease, coeliac disease,

ACTIVITY 8.5

My patient is on medication. Will drug therapy affect her nutritional status?

constipation, diabetes mellitus, diverticulitis, gastrectomy, hyperlipidaemia, liver transplantation, malabsorption syndrome and obesity.

As with all aspects of nursing, it is absolutely essential to be aware of side effects of any medication that the patient is taking. Some drugs commonly prescribed can lead to malnutrition (Table 8.7).

General nursing considerations

Foods can also affect the absorption of certain drugs; however it is true to say that most drugs are best taken with, or just after meals. This is because it is the easiest way to remember to take any drug and some are gastric irritants such as aspirin and NSAIDs (non-steroidal anti-inflammatory medications such as Voltarol or Neurofen). Absorption of some drugs is a little delayed, but this is unimportant and a few are better absorbed when taken with meals, e.g. beta blockers. Plenty of water should be taken with diuretics and bulk formers like methyl cellulose, Fybogel. A few drugs should be taken half an hour before meals such as antibiotics which are labile in acid, ampicillin, benzylpenicillin, cloxacillin, erythromycin, tetracycline, rifampicin and isoniazid; also antidiabetic agents such as glibenclamide, and of course, appetite suppressants. Particular drugs can affect the nutritional state. Appetite may be decreased by bulking agents, amphetamines, cardiac glycosides, glucagon, morphine, indomethacin, cyclophosphamide, cytotoxic therapies, salbutamol, levodopa etc. Appetite may be increased by chlorpromazine, androgens, anabolic steroids, corticosteroids, insulin, lithium, amitriptyline, benzodiazepines and metoclopramide. Malabsorption for one or more nutrients may be induced by neomycin, chlortetracycline, cyclophosphamide, methotrexate and methyldopa. Hyperglycaemia (high blood glucose) may be produced by corticosteroids, thiazide diuretics, and phenytoin. Hypoglycaemia can arise with alcohol, propanolol, sulphonylureas and insulin. Plasma lipid levels may be raised by chlorpromazine, phenytoin, cimetidine and propanolol, and lowered by aspirin, colchicine, phenformin and propanolol. A negative protein–nitrogen balance can arise with corticosteroids, vaccines and tetracyclines, and a positive protein–nitrogen balance with insulin and anabolic steroids. Plasma phenylalanine can be raised by trimethoprim and methotrexate. Vitamin and mineral levels are affected by a great variety of medications and it is always worth bearing this in mind when considering the nutritional status of a patient, and how best to offer nutritional support during high dependency care.

Food and your patient's comfort

Consuming food satisfies physical needs and also mental needs as well. People eat for comfort as well as energy. It is highly important that the nurse does not forget this fact. Physiological studies have shown that the ingestion of food causes relaxation, sleepiness and friendliness. Meals high in fat tend to induce these feelings in particular (Wells and Read, 1995). The pleasure of eating a tasty meal is known to induce the release of endorphins (the body's own opioids/pain killers), and it seems that a sweet taste in the mouth enhances this effect (Barr et al., 1994). Furthermore, certain foods seem to have an analgesic effect and reduce pain perception to noxious stimuli such as intense cold and intestinal distension. The analgesic effect is only apparent if food is taken orally, and probably initiated by oral stimulation of endorphin production and amplified by intestinal activity following the meal (Zmarzty et al., 1997, 1999). Patients who are ill have a poor appetite. Stimulation of appetite so that they eat more would avoid the need for artificial nutritional support in some cases, and moreover, allow the very act of eating to stimulate pleasure, comfort and perhaps analgesia too. In so doing, recovery time might well be reduced. Further research is required to explore the effects of nutritional deprivation and replacement on the outcome of illness. Such research would benefit patient care and improve the efficient use of resources.

Nutrition, the nurse and the future

It is unfortunately true that sometimes our patients do not receive adequate nutrition during their hospital stay. This is not acceptable and it is hoped that by reading this chapter, the issues surrounding diet and nutrition will be pushed to the forefront of the nurse's thoughts. There is an urgent need for more post-registration nursing courses in clinical nutrition. Some hospital trusts now employ a nutrition nurse specialist, and offer inservice teaching programmes with a system of 'link nurses'. Here a ward nurse accepts particular responsibility for nutritional care in that clinical setting, and meets the nutritional team for regular teaching, updating and briefing. These measures can go some way towards reducing the current level of malnutrition in our hospitals.

Further reading

Physiology

Berne, R.M. and Levy, M.N. 1990 *Principles of physiology*. London: Mosby.

Clancy, J. and McVicar, A.J. 1995 *Physiology and anatomy: a homeostatic approach*. London: Arnold.

Mackenna, B.R. and Callander, R. 1992 *McNaught Callander illustrated physiology*, 5th edn. London: Churchill Livingstone.

Vander, A.J., Sherman, J.E. and Luciano, D.S. 1990 *Human physiology*, 5th edn. Maidenhead: McGraw-Hill.

General nutrition

Department of Health 1991 *Dietary reference values: a guide*. London: HMSO.

Department of Health 1992 *Health of the Nation: A strategy for health in England*. London: HMSO.

Department of Health 1994 *Eat Well!: an action plan from the nutrition task force to achieve the Health of the Nation targets on diet and nutrition*. London: DOH.

English National Board for Nursing, Midwifery and Health Visiting 1995 *Nutrition for Life: Issues for debate in the development of education programmes*. London: ENB.

Garrow, J.S. and James, W.P.T. (eds) 1993 *Human nutrition and dietetics*, 9th edn. London: Churchill Livingstone.

Hinchliffe, S., Norman, S. and Schober, J. 1994 *Nursing practice and health care*. London: Arnold.

Rodwell Williams, S. 1994 *Essentials of nutrition and diet therapy*, 6th edn. London: Mosby.

Truswell, A.S. 1992 *ABC of nutrition*, 2nd edn. London: BMJ.

Effects of malnutrition

Anderson, M.D., Collins, G., Davis, G. and Bivins, B. 1985 Malnutrition and length of stay – a relationship? *Henry Ford Hospital Medical Journal* **33**(4), 190–3.

Beese, G. 1997 Energy crisis. *Nursing Times* **93**(49), 55–7.

Delmi, M., Rapin, C.H., Bengoa, J.M. *et al.* 1990 Dietary supplementation in elderly patients with fractured neck of femur. *Lancet* **335**, 1013–16.

Dempsey, D.T., Mullen, J.L. and Buzby, G.P. 1988 The link between nutritional status and clinical outcome; can nutritional intervention modify it ? *American Journal of Clinical Nutrition* **47**, 352–6.

Guest, C. and Pearson, S. 1997 Recovery on a plate. *Nursing Times* **93**(46), 55–7.

Haydock, D.A. and Hill, G.L. 1986 Impaired wound healing in surgical patients with varying degrees of malnutrition. *Journal of Parenteral Nutrition* **10**, 550–4.

McWhirter, J.P. and Pennington, C.R. 1994 Incidence and recognition of malnutrition in hospital. *British Medical Journal* **308**(6934), 945–8.

Reilly, J.R., Hull, S.F., Albert, N., Waller, A. and Bringardener, S. 1988 Economic impact of malnutrition: a model system for hospitalised patients. *Journal of Parenteral Nutrition* **12**, 371–6.

Reynolds, J.V., O'Farrelly, C., Feighary, C. et al. 1996 Impaired gut barrier function in malnourished patients. *British Journal of Surgery* **83**(9), 1288–91.

Shaw-Stiffel, T.A., Zarny, L.A., Pleban, W.E., et al. 1993 Effect of nutrition status and other factors on length of hospital stay after major gastrointestinal surgery. *Nutrition* **9**(2), 140–5.

Assessing nutritional status

Allison, S.P. 1995 Malnutrition in hospital patients. *Hospital Update*, February, 55–61.

Campbell, M.K. and Kelsey, K.S. 1994 The PEACH Survey: a nutrition screening tool for use in early intervention programmes. *Journal of the American Dietetic Association* **94**(10), 1156–8.

Cotton, E., Zinober, B. and Jessop, J. 1996 A nutritional assessment tool for older patients. *Professional Nurse* **11**(9), 609–12.

Detsky, A.S., Smalley, P.S. and Chang, J. 1994 Is the patient malnourished? *JAMA* **271**(1), 54–8.

Fulham, C. 1992 Postoperative nutrition. *Surgical Nurse* 22–5.

Lupo, L., Pannarale, O., Altomare, D., Memeo, V. and Rubino, M. 1993 Reliability of clinical judgement in evaluation of the nutritional status of surgical patients. *British Journal of Surgery* **80**, 1553–6.

Reilly, H. 1996. Nutritional assessment. *British Journal of Nursing* **5**(1), 18–24.

Shireff, A. 1990 Pre-operative nutritional assessment. *Nursing Times* **86**(8), 68–72.

Sidenvall, B. and Ek, A.C. 1993 Long term care

patients and their dietary intake related to eating ability and nutritional needs: nursing staff interventions. *Journal of Advanced Nursing* 18, 565–73.

Smith, L.C. and Mullen, J.L. 1991 Nutritional assessment and indications for nutritional support. *Surgical Clinics of North America* 71(3), 449–57.

Thomas, E.A. 1987 Pre-operative fasting – a question of routine? *Nursing Times* 83(49), 46–7.

Torrance, C. 1991 Pre-operative nutrition, fasting and the surgical patient. *Surgical Nurse* 5–7.

Wynn, M. and A. 1993 Catering concerns. *Nursing Times* 89(20), 61–4.

Artificial nutritional support

Archer, S.R., Burnett, R.J. and Fischer, J.F. 1996 Current uses and abuses of total parenteral nutrition. *Advances in Surgery* 29, 165–89.

Briggs, D. 1996 Nasogastric feeding practice in intensive care units. *Nursing Standard* 10(49), 42–5.

Brown, F. and Howe, A. 1996 Preventing malnutrition in patients on CAPD. *Professional Nurse* 11(6), 354–6.

Finlay, T. 1997 Making sense of parenteral nutrition in adult patients. *Nursing Times* 93(2), 35–6.

Holmes, S. 1996 Percutaneous endoscopic gastrostomy; a review. *Nursing Times* 92(17), 34–5.

Lennard-Jones, J.E. 1992 *A positive approach to nutrition as treatment*. London: King's Fund Centre Report.

Palmer, D. and MacFie, J. 1997 Alternative intake. *Nursing Times* 93(49), Suppl.

Payne-James, J., Grimble, G. and Silk, D. (eds). 1995 *Artificial nutrition support in clinical practice*. London: Edward Arnold.

Rollins, H. 1997 A nose for trouble. *Nursing Times* 93(49), Suppl.

Shaw, J.E. 1994 Identifying gaps in knowledge: nurses knowledge of enteral feeding practices. *Professional Nurse* 9(10), 665–8.

Sizer, T. 1996. *Standards and guidelines for nutritional support of patients in hospital*. Maidenhead: BAPEN.

Todorovik, V.E. and Micklewright, A. (eds) 1997 *A pocket guide to clinical nutrition*. London: British Dietetic Association.

Zainal, G. 1994 Nutrition of critically ill people. *Intensive and Critical Care Nursing* 10(3), 165–70.

Ziegler, T.R., Gatzen, C. and Wilmore, D.W. 1994. Strategies for attenuating protein-catabolic responses in the critically ill. *Annual Review of Medicine* **45**, 459–80.

Food and mood

Barr, R.G., Quek, V.S.H., Cousineau, D. *et al.* 1994 Effects of intra-oral sucrose on crying, mouthing and hand-mouth contact in newborn and six-week-old infants. *Developmental Medicine and Child Neurology* **36**, 608–18.

Bell, A.M., Pemberton, J.H., Hanson, R.B. and Zinsmeister, A.R. 1991 Variations in muscle tone of the human rectum: recordings with an electro-mechanical barostat. *American Physiological Society* G17–25.

Oberlander, T.F., Barr, R.G., Young, S.N. and Brian, J.A. 1992 Short-term effects of feed compo-sition on sleeping and crying in newborns. *Pediatrics* **90**, 733–40.

Read, N.W., French, S. and Cunningham, K. 1994 The role of the gut in regulating food intake in man. *Nutrition Reviews* **52**(1), 1–10.

Wells, A.S. and Read, N.W. 1995 The influ-ences of dietary and intraduodenal lipid on alert-ness, mood and sustained concentration. *British Journal of Nutrition* **74**, 115–23.

Zmarzty, S.A., Wells, A.S. and Read, N.W. 1997 The influence of food on pain perception in healthy human volunteers. *Physiology and Behav-iour* **62**(1), 185–91.

Zmarzty, S.A. and Read, N.W. 1999 An exami-nation of the effects of isoenergetic intragastric infusions of pure macronutrients on cold pain per-ception in healthy human volunteers. *Physiology and Behaviour* **65** (4/5), 643–8.

Supporting the patient and their family

Robert McSherry

Introduction

Providing first-class care for high dependency patients is not just a question of understanding the nature of illnesses and their treatment. Just as important is the absolute requirement that the nurse is aware of the role that she/he has to play in supporting both patients and their families throughout the period of care in the high dependency unit. The aim of this chapter is to provide the nurse with a framework to assist in supporting the dependent patient and their family within the high dependency setting. This chapter will:

- provide guidelines that will promote the effective use of communication;
- discuss the barriers to communication;
- provide case studies, reflective questions and activities, along with examples of good practice to illustrate specific situations in supporting the dependent patient and their family.

Need for effective communication

As healthcare processes and organizations become increasingly complex, so the need to communicate with patients clearly about the clinical and non-clinical aspects of their care grows. But provision has not kept up with the growing need, and lack of information and problems in communicating with health professionals usually come at the top of patients' concerns. (Audit Commission, 1993, p. 1.)

The above quotation from the Audit Commission's (1993) Report on 'What Seems to be the Matter: Communication between Hospitals and Patients' could not be more true; experience within the clinical specialties of general medicine, elderly care and acute stroke and rehabilitation nursing would support this statement. This issue seems to have worsened over the past 5 years or so and has prompted the introduction of several significant reforms such as the 'White Paper Working For Patients' (1989); 'The Patients Charter: Raising The Standard' (1992) and most recently 'The Code on Openness in the NHS' (1997). These reforms are aimed at increasing the efficiency and effectiveness of the NHS by making smaller units directly responsible for their own existence, rather than being funded by central organizational bodies such as the old Regional Health Authorities.

The drive for an improved, efficient and effective NHS has also seen the introduction of advanced supporting technology and surgical interventions. (e.g. pressure-relieving equipment, minimal invasive surgery and daycare surgery). This means that an individual patient's average length of stay in hospital for some major operations and medical treatment has reduced markedly. The reforms have led to availability of continuing care/rehabilitation and long-term care beds within many hospital and community trusts being reduced by up to 40 per cent, as the demand for more acute emergency beds increases. This reduction in patients' stay is exacerbated by the fact that patient dependency is rising due to demographic changes within society.

According to the Department of Health (1993) 'Health of the Nation' report: 'between 1981 and 1989, the number of people aged 75–84 has risen by 16 per cent, and those 85 and over by 39 per cent'. This phenomenon is predicted to continue well into the 20th century. The increased life expectancy means that patients who are admitted to acute medical, surgical, orthopaedic and elderly care wards increasingly have multiple pathologies, and often have complex social circumstances, requiring greater support in a shorter period of time from the health professionals around them. This, according to the study of Tierney (1994) accounts for an estimated readmission rate of 27 per cent soon after discharge. It therefore becomes imperative for all health professionals to work in a collaborative way, thereby ensuring that all care available to the patient is focused, which in turn would aid greater patient comfort and satisfaction. As patient empowerment and expectation increases, more questions are being asked about specific care and treatments, all placing a significant amount of pressure on the health professional to deliver an even higher standard and quality of care to the patient. The outlined evidence suggests that in order to become efficient and effective 'supporters' of patients, and of dependent patients in acute services over shorter periods of time, first-rate communication is certainly the way forward.

Communication

According to the UK Central Council for Nursing, Midwifery and Health Visiting (1992) 'Code of Professional Conduct' as a registered nurse, midwife or health visitor we should 'Work in an open and cooperative manner with patients, clients and their families, foster their independence and recognize and respect their involvement in the planning and delivery of care'. This will only be achieved successfully by the use of effective communication. Effective communication will only be gained by understanding issues of increased pressure, with rising dependency on acute medical, surgical and orthopaedic wards. This situation may result in a tendency to see individuals as conditions or illnesses and not as individual people. At times of pressure and great anxiety, which arise while caring for the dependent patient, there is a constant reminder that while you feel anxious, tense or pressurized, the patient, family or carer feels equally, if not more, anxious.

The best support you can offer initially is to be continually aware that 'while it is important to know that all people have common needs, it is equally important to realize that these needs are satisfied by infinitely varied patterns of living, no two of which are alike' (Henderson 1961, p. 7). Henderson's statement reinforces the need for all health professionals to be constantly vigilant about not becoming complacent. Caring for the whole person, physically, mentally, psychologically, culturally, spiritually and socially, requires the development and execution of various and complex ways of communicating. 'Communication' seems to be about an interaction where two or more people send and receive messages, and in the process both present themselves and interpret the other. Communication can be verbal (talking, writing) and non-verbal (the transmission of information through facial expressions, tone of voice and body posture), or both. In essence the nurse's role is that of communicator. Nursing is about assessing, observing, talking to, listening to, liaising with, supporting and responding to the patient, family, carer or other health professionals in an attempt to communicate the patient's expressed or required needs in the hope of providing a positive experience for the patient. Without clear communication, it is impossible to give care effectively, make decisions with clients and families, protect clients from threats to wellbeing, coordinate and manage client care, assist the client in rehabilitation, offer comfort, or teach. In real terms, supporting patients, relatives, carers or significant others will not be achieved effectively and positively, if we fail to explore the ways in which communication is expressed individually and jointly as a multidisciplinary team on any ward or in any high dependency area.

> ### ACTIVITY 9.1
>
> Reflect for a moment and note down all the ways in which you communicate within your clinic area.

VERBAL/WRITTEN COMMUNICATION

- One-to-one with patient, family or even another colleague.
- Interview; admission process.
- Case conference; handover; doctors' ward rounds; group communication.
- Telephone.
- Written; documentation in patient notes; care plans; drug charts.
- Drug rounds.
- Information booklets; leaflets.
- Notice boards.
- Posters.

NON-VERBAL COMMUNICATION

- Listening.
- Body posture/positioning.
- Distance.
- Facial expression.

The points above are all only intended as a guide for reflection, and are not exhaustive lists, which may vary according to your clinical area and specialty. From this first exercise alone, we can clearly see how communication affects every aspect of a health professional's role. The highly dependent patient and clinical area are not static, but constantly change minute by minute, hour by hour and day by day. In the same way the individual(s) (patient, family and carers) with whom you communicate will change. This may be in response to their environment, cultural and spiritual beliefs, age or because of the effects of illness or disease upon them. It is imperative to bear in mind that the perception of a hospital's effectiveness by most patients, families or carers is interdependent on how we communicate as individuals, or within the team. There are compelling human reasons for making sure communication with patients works well. Good communication can transform the patient's experience of hospital care, lessening the impact of what may be painful, difficult or anxiety-provoking situations and decisions. The opposite is also true. Poor communication, with barriers between patients and the people they need to talk to, muddled and contradictory messages and missing information, creates avoidable anxiety and distress. Communication is the most important foundation in providing effective care and support for the patient, carer, family, or significant others.

As identified in Activity 9.1, almost all daily activities and provisions of care are interconnected with how we relay information to or from each other. According to the evidence put forward by Wilson (1996) 'correlation has been demonstrated, through the Health Service Ombudsman Reports, between poor communication/documentation and clinical negligence'. Negligence in this instance refers to a deviation from the acceptable standard of care that a reasonably prudent person would use in a particular set of circumstances. In many instances, negligence in healthcare occurs due to 'malpractice'; a failure to comply with professional standards of care expected from nurses, midwives, general practitioners, etc. A failure to communicate, if it falls short of the required professional standard, can be regarded as negligence and may be actionable if it causes harm to the patient. An example of this was the case between Coles v Reading HMC (1963, 107 SJ 115, cited in Dimond 1990). Mr Coles

had an injury to his finger; he visited a cottage hospital, had the injury cleaned and dressed and was informed by the nurse to attend the proper hospital (i.e. one with accident and emergency with medical cover) for a tetanus injection. Mr Coles never went to the hospital. Several days later he visited his GP who believed that he had had the injection. Mr Coles subsequently died of tetanus. From this case study it was clear that a failure of communication between the patient and professionals had occurred. The nurse should have reinforced the instruction to visit the hospital and perhaps written it down or even contacted the hospital to arrange the visit. The importance of emphasizing vital information or dangers is imperative, and it must never be assumed that the patient is aware without first being told. Poor communication and relationships between patients, carers, family and other healthcare professionals can result in misunderstandings of verbal or written information leading to complaints and subsequent litigation if negligence is proved. 'Litigation claims' according to O'Donovan (1996), 'are increasing to the extent that by 2000, negligence claims could account for 13 per cent of a hospital budget' , reinforcing the need for healthcare and community trusts to look at ways of reducing this trend. The promotion of effective 'communication' seems to be a reasonable starting place.

The communication process

ACTIVITY 9.2: Individual patients and communication

Bill Williams is a retired 75-year-old married man with two daughters who live away from home. He is admitted to the high dependency unit unconscious, with a suspected cerebral vascular accident. *List in chronological order the individuals involved with communication during the acute and rehabilitation phase of care.*

PRE-ADMISSION PHASE

- GP.
- Emergency service: telecommunications operator, ambulance service control.
- Ambulance crew, paramedics.
- Accident and emergency department.

ACUTE CARE PHASE

- Accident and emergency staff:
  - Receiving nurse.
  - Doctors: SHO, consultant.

- Unit staff:
  - Admitting nurse: primary nurse/team leader.
  - Named nurse.
  - Other nurses within the team/ward.
  - Medical staff: HO, SHO, registrar, consultant.
  - Clerical staff/domestic staff.

REHABILITATION PHASE

- Physiotherapist.
- Speech therapist.
- Social worker.
- Occupational therapist.
- Dietitian.
- Support services:
  - Porters.
  - X-ray.
  - Pathology.
  - Pharmacy.
- Family members during all phases of the admission and rehabilitation processes.

Activity 9.2 is aimed at reinforcing the large number of staff involved and considers the potential complexities associated with the communication processes involved with the care of the dependent patient and his or her family. The more dependent and complicated the case, the greater the number of personnel involved, reinforcing the need for effective channels of communication. Note: This again is not an exhaustive list but a guide for reflection and reinforcing the complex nature of communication within healthcare.

The process of communication and reflection from Activity 9.2 is extremely complicated and dependent upon the behaviour and nature of human relationships. Communication theorists like Berlo (1960) and Korzylski (1958) seem to suggest that by labelling communication as a process, we immediately imply that it involves a series of ongoing, changing, continuous steps that are interactive and without end. This concept seems to be confirmed when referring to Activity 9.2, as will be demonstrated. The process of communication occurs when a stimulus or message is given from one individual to another or perhaps several individuals. This may be the case for Mr Williams who through verbal and non-verbal stimulus of blurred vision, slurred speech, and loss of left limb function, conveyed a message to Mrs Williams that he was extremely poorly. This (instigatory message) was transferred to Mrs Williams (the receiver), who (decoded) the message to understand that medical help was needed. Contact was made with the emergency services, where the instigatory message of slurred speech etc. was relayed and positive reassurance received, because help was on its way. Mrs Williams, now the instigator of communication, informs Mr Williams that help is on the way. Mr Williams receives and decodes the information and confirms the feedback by a non-verbal response of squeezing Mrs Williams' hand. From this case illustration it is clear that effective communication is a two-way process of providing and receiving information which is communicated to an individual from verbal/non-verbal cues. The communication can be perceived as either positive, negative or both, but requires interactions to occur. The following illustration attempts to summarize this complex process into a simplified version with reference to Activity 9.2.

The process of communication, as illustrated in Figure 9.1, requires a stimulus that instigates communication to another individual, who decodes the information and gives a response. This may involve an additional person, although it results in feedback to the instigator, for acknowledgement where possible. An important point to remember here is that communication may be enhanced or hindered by the functional abilities of the senses: sight, hearing, touch. For example: Mr Williams may not have been able to relay a verbal response to Mrs Williams' information relating to the contacting of the emergency services, although his ability to squeeze Mrs Williams' hand was a key indicator of understanding the message.

In summary, communication is the link in ensuring the existence and maintenance of an effective and efficient healthcare service. The rising expectations of patient, carers and family, coupled with increased life-expectancy, greater patient dependency and reduced length of stay in hospital, reinforces the need for a more simple, robust and accessible way of communicating with the dependent patient. Communication is an extremely complex system, requiring individual professionals, teams, organizations and structures

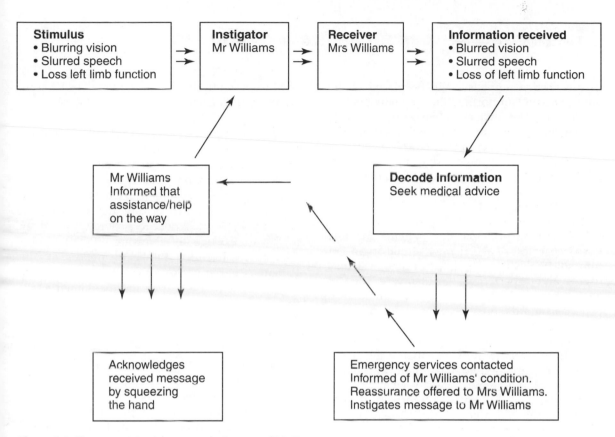

Figure 9.1 The communication process in the case of Mr X

to integrate efficiently and effectively to enhance the quality and standards of patient care. Communication is integral to the daily function of a ward, unit or organization, as demonstrated in Activity 9.1, and involves a variety of health professionals (Activity 9.2). Poor communication can lead to complaints, litigation claims and possible negligence. It is not surprising therefore that communication is usually the underlying theme associated with patient, family and carer dissatisfaction with an individual's stay in hospital. However, while taking into account the physical aspects of caring for the 'dependent' patient as outlined in previous chapters (neurological, respiratory, endocrine, vascular, gastrological and renal), the theoretical, technical and explanatory processes associated with most of these areas are extremely complex and, therefore, difficult for most lay people to understand. It is imperative that as providers of care, we help the patient and family to understand why certain treatments, medication and medical devices are being used, while at the same time taking into account the importance of nursing care in supporting psychological, social, spiritual and cultural needs.

Supporting the dependent patient and family

In this section emphasis will be placed on the importance of 'supporting' the dependent patient and family. This will be achieved by providing reflective questions and case scenarios in relation to caring for dependent patients who have developed the following: myocardial infarction, cerebral vascular accident and newly diagnosed diabetes – scenarios which could occur within the high dependency unit.

The starting point in this section is reinforcing the underlying principle that patients and relatives (regardless of age, gender, ethnic origin, culture, spiritual beliefs, disability or illness) all have 'rights' and 'expectations' for their care. The Citizen's Charter (1992) entitles every individual to expect standards, openness, information, choice, non-discrimination, accessibility and to be able to complain or redress dissatisfactions. In essence, the Citizen's Charter aims to enhance the quality of services provided to the public by offering more choice and an awareness of what to expect from the services, along with informing them of what to do if things go wrong. These rights are transferable within the National Health Service, and as professionals we should strive to meet them or support the patient or family in doing so. In addition, the Patient's Charter (1992) 'Raising the Standard' builds on the Citizen's Charter, highlighting patient rights and expectations as follows:

Key points taken from the Patient's Charter (1992)

- To be treated with care, consideration, and respect
- To receive the right kind of service at the right time
- To be given the opportunity to talk about and to help choose care and treatment
- To have information in English, Welsh and other languages
- That relatives and friends will be informed about progress of treatment subject to the patient's wishes
- To see a consultant, named qualified nurse, to register with a GP etc.

Since the introduction of the Patient's Charter, many hospital community trusts and GP practices have developed their own charter standards which take into account the needs of the local community. Examples include knowing the names of those involved in caring for you, and being treated in clean and comfortable surroundings.

At a glance, the Patient's Charter seems to define exactly the sort of care and services that any of us would expect to provide. However, a Royal College of Nursing (RCN) report 'Uncharted Territory: Public Awareness of The Patient's Charter (1994)' aimed at establishing the effectiveness of the charter and the named qualified nurse, states that: 'while only two-thirds of the population surveyed had heard of The Patient's Charter, only a small minority could actually name any rights or standards it bestowed upon them' (Herriot, 1994, p. 440). The report seems to suggest that patient empowerment is lacking due to ineffective communication between nurses and patients and that 'patients cannot exercise their rights unless they are better informed about the existence of such rights . . . (and must be given explicit information and encouraged to participate in developing services to meet their needs)' (Herriot, 1994, p. 440).

Perhaps the above is not surprising considering the evidence put forward by Shuttleworth (1992), who, after surveying readers of the *Professional Nurse* on how achievable they felt the Patient's Charter was, reported that 71 per cent 'felt that hospitals and health authorities would be unable to achieve the standards of care set out in the Charter' (Shuttleworth, 1992). According to the Secretary of State for Health of the time, the Patient's Charter was extended in October 1994 because the Charter had vastly improved patients' rights, and stated that the 'patient's voice must be heard the loudest when decisions are made on further improvements'. The literature surrounding the Patient's Charter (1992) and (RCN, 1994) seems to indicate a variety of advantages and disadvantages for both patients and staff. My overall opinion favours the introduction of the Charter in empowering patients to become involved with their care. Patients should have a right to privacy, dignity and to be treated with courtesy, although enforceability is dependent upon the hospital or health authority, not the patient. 'The NHS patient has no contractual relationship with the supplier of the services, unlike his counterpart in retail. The protection given in the sale of goods and services legislation is not available to the NHS consumer' (Diamond, 1993). In supporting the patient and family relating to the Patient's Charter, the following key points are recommended.

Points intended to support you in meeting the Patient's Charter

- Greet patients and family in a warm, reassuring and friendly manner
- Always inform the patient, family or carers about the Patient's Charter
- Identify the key parts of the Charter applicable to their stay. For example, introduce the named qualified nurse, inform them of their consultant.
- Provide any ward/unit information booklets to allow the patient and family time to familiarize themselves with the environment and routines.
- Provide information relating to specific care and treatments, reinforcing where necessary with written factual evidence.
- Encourage the medical staff to explain the risks and benefits of specific treatments and interventions along with documenting this in the patient's notes.

It may be argued that the above points are common sense; however, in times of rising patient dependency and expectations, we cannot afford to become complacent in areas of providing support and information. This is reinforced by the recent 'Code on Openness in the NHS' (1997) which reflects the Government's intention to ensure greater access by the public to information about public services. The code aims to ensure that people receive the following:

- *Access* to information about the services provided by the NHS, the costs of those services, quality standards and performance against targets;
- *Explanations* about proposed service changes and the opportunity to influence decisions on such changes;

- *Reasons for decisions and actions* affecting their own treatment;
- *Information about what information is available* and where they can get it.

In summary, the Code of Openness in the NHS (1997) reinforces the need for efficient and effective channels of communication by all members of the multiprofessional healthcare teams. The patient and his or her family (whether the patient is in a high dependency unit, on a ward or in a continuing care setting) have a right to access information about specific medical and nursing care, treatments, equipment or services offered by the hospital. In addition, they should be offered alternatives, and most importantly be provided with the reasons for the specific care or treatment given, along with literature (in the form of leaflets) or the details of where they can obtain the information to enable them to make an informed decision. In essence, the 'codes' reinforce and complement the Patient's Charter (1992) by strengthening the patient's rights to know how to obtain the appropriate information from the correct person at the right level at the right time. The information should be evidence-based in order to promote an informed choice, again reinforcing the need for effective communication.

A template for supporting the patient and their family

Whether an individual is admitted to hospital as a routine patient or an emergency (for example, someone with an acute myocardial infarction, a cerebral vascular accident or newly diagnosed diabetes, or a patient requiring palliative care), the patient and family will undoubtedly require 'support'. The following template offers a guide to assist health professionals caring for the dependent patient and family within the ward, coronary care unit, intensive care unit or high dependency unit in exploring ways of improving the support they give to the patient and his or her family.

Three underlying attributes need to be addressed to establish a platform for the instigation of support to the dependent patient and family. These are based on having the following:

philosophy of care, system of care delivery and a model/documentation for recording, monitoring and evaluating care. From these three attributes many ways of supporting the dependent patient and family can be derived, as the following paragraphs will demonstrate.

Philosophy of care

A starting point in ensuring a supportive environment for patients and their families would be to explore whether your ward or unit achieves its philosophy of care or indeed whether one has been written. Without a clear philosophy of care, health professionals could lack direction when providing care for patients and their families. According to Wright (1986) it is the overall philosophy of the ward that its purpose is to meet the goals of nursing as a functioning unit of the nursing service, as the following activity will illustrate.

ACTIVITY 9.4

Robert is a 35-year-old heavy goods vehicle driver, who is married with three children aged 4 months, 4 years and 7 years. The oldest child has special needs. Robert is admitted onto the high dependency unit for an investigation of a one-day history of chest pain. *By reflecting on this admission, examine how the ward's philosophy may enhance the support given to Robert.*

What are the possible benefits of having a philosophy of care?

A philosophy of care offers an individualistic and holistic approach to caring by encapsulating the following key elements for the patient.

- The philosophy of care offers the patient individuality by the way care is provided to suit their unique needs.
- The patient has a right to be informed of his/her condition in order to be able to make realistic choices about his or her care and treatment.
- The patient has a right to skilled nursing, based upon the most appropriate evidence-based care in order to meet his or her needs.
- The patient, regardless of age, gender, culture, spiritual belief, has a right to receive unique care and treatment in order to promote recovery or even a peaceful death. This should encapsulate the physical, social, psychological, environmental, cultural and spiritual aspects of his or her lifestyle in an attempt to maintain independence (freedom).
- The nurse and patient should develop a partnership that enables the communication processes to be fostered robustly in order to maximize the giving and receiving of information (sharing) within the ward environment.
- The individual nurse and ward/unit must continually strive to improve their educational and clinical skills in order to enhance the quality and standards provided on the ward/unit.

In essence, the ward/unit philosophy is the starting point for Robert's care. If the ward/unit team all share a universal approach to delivering a unique individualized programme of care for their specific ward/unit, this is automatically received by the patient and family. The philosophy sets the environment and climate of the ward and provides direction to those working within that ward. The philosophy is a shared responsibility and cannot be achieved in isolation; decisions about the ward's direction should always be based on mutual cooperation and discussions, and be respectful of all staff regardless of grade or position. It is important to note here that the philosophy is more than a piece of printed paper for staff and the public to read; it is about unifying the unique attributes of nursing with the needs of the patients who come into contact with your specific ward/unit. The philosophy of care is the foundation upon which the individual nurse or the ward/unit team approach the way in which they anticipate the assessment, planning, implementation and evaluation of care and treatment within the clinical specialty. The philosophy of care simply offers the patient and family support by knowing that you as an individual nurse or part of a team/unit aim to offer and maintain a universal and unique approach in the promotion of a patient's independence. This is to be achieved through constantly observing the concepts shown in Figure 9.2.

In summary, it is easy to see why an individual who does not work within the parameters of a given philosophy of care can sometimes lack direction or become disillusioned with working in an environment that does not aim to offer support to patients, family and staff from its principle foundation. A philosophy of care should promote patient independence along with fostering a warm, relaxed environment where freedom of expression exists for patients, family and staff. The philosophy should be the shared responsibility of all the members within that team, and be commu-

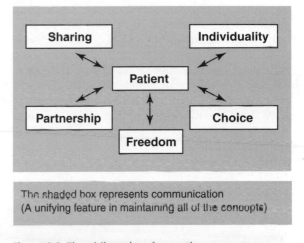

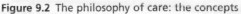
The shaded box represents communication
(A unifying feature in maintaining all of the concepts)

Figure 9.2 The philosophy of care: the concepts

nicated to the patient via the standards and quality of care they provide. Most importantly, the philosophy of care should be relevant, realistic, simple to read and understand, and be achievable for patients, family and staff.

Systems of care delivery

Having discussed the importance of having a ward/unit philosophy of care that sets out the underlying foundations for an individual nurse, or team, to operate within, it is equally important to establish what system of care you practice. The reason for this is that support for the patient and family potentially stems from this. If an individual is a named nurse, team leader or primary nurse operating within the parameters of either team nursing or primary nursing, these approaches to delivering care seem to have a commonality facilitating a system for developing the partnership between the patient and his or her family. The system then takes account of the whole person, recognizing the unique nature of the person. By using a system for care, the relationship between nurses and patients can be prioritized. This is because staffing is divided into smaller functional groups enhancing communication and providing a central person to act as a coordinator for discus-

sion purposes relating to the individual patient's care and treatments etc.

In a hospital ward/unit, it will be clear where the delivery of care is effective. The staff appear to be more relaxed, focus more clearly on the job in hand and share information more easily. The allocation of workload appears to be more evenly distributed and the patient always has the opportunity to talk to their allocated named nurse, team leader or primary nurse. A continuity of care exists where information is passed on and communicated to those who need to know. The support this offers to patients and their families is crucial to fostering and maintaining an open and trusting relationship for the communication of information and the promotion of a therapeutic environment for the patient. This is reinforced by the statement made by the Audit Commission on the two main benefits of improved communication: 'increased compliance with medical instructions and prescribed medications leading to improved functioning in everyday life, particularly for those with chronic pain' (Audit Commission, 1993). There are many well documented systems of care to explore and evaluate. It is essential for you to research and establish the most appropriate system of care delivery to support the ward/unit in achieving its philosophy of care, and most importantly, in the promotion of a holistic and individualized approach to supporting the patient and family.

> 'To be valid, a philosophy of care must reflect the beliefs and values of those nurses who work in the practice situation concerning the nature of their nursing. With this understanding, they are then in a position to consider how best nursing can be organized to facilitate their beliefs' (Johns, 1993, p. 32)

Models of nursing/documentation

In order to provide efficient and effective support to the dependent patient and his/her family, it is important that the individual nurse or health professional works towards providing a unique and universal approach in caring for the patient. This is usually a statement of intent and is a responsibility shared by all members of that ward/unit team. The philosophy is usually achieved through delivering care via an established system of care designed to meet the needs of the ward/unit, such as team or primary nursing. However, for care to be delivered effectively it needs to be based around a recognized framework or model that can communicate to and receive from the patient and family their needs, along with being able to be document clearly what has been said and done relating to the care. Support starts by using the 'nursing process' which offers nurses a systematic approach to planning and delivering care. It is a vehicle by which a model of care is put into practice. There are many 'Models of Care', for example, Roper, Logan and Tierney's 'Activities of Daily Living' (1983); Orems's 'Self-Care Model' (1971); Riehl and Roy's 'Adaptation Model' (1980); and Johnstone's 'Behavior Model' (1984); all of which have been constructed to support the execution of nursing care within a variety of different clinical settings or to meet individual patient's needs. Several models of nursing have been designed with a specific remit of promoting and 'supporting' restoration, maintenance or an

equilibrium of an individual's needs, ranging from the biological, psychological, social and behavioural aspects of a person's life. Models of nursing have a commonality in that they are abstract representations of what nursing is or should be and how nursing care could be provided. Nursing models or frameworks for documenting care delivery provide an opportunity for nurses to use them to understand what they are doing and why. Models of nursing or documentation for providing and recording nursing care are built from a series of words which unite to form a concept. For example, the nursing process has four key parts or phases, all of which contain many attributes that enable the nurse to establish and plan a programme of care for the individual patient. This is clearly identified by the assessment phase which allows the nurse to examine in detail many areas of the patient's lifestyle in order to become informed about their current and previous health status. These range from physical ability, mobility, breathing and sleeping; to social circumstances, housing, employment etc. Similarly to the nursing process, a model for nursing practice may have several parts or phases which is a 'systematically based, and logically related set of concepts which identify the essential components of nursing practice together with the theoretical basis of these concepts and values required for their use by the practitioner' (Aggleton and Chalmers, 1984). It may be argued that models of nursing are complex abstracts of nursing reality and that in their attempt to create a better understanding of what nursing is or should be, the very opposite is occurring. This may be because the staff using them do not have the time, resources and commitment to use them effectively. However, a point to emphasize here is that, without the use of a recognized framework for delivering care, we could potentially be failing our patients by not being able to defend our rationale for providing a continuity of care should a complaint be made against an individual nurse, ward or unit. This is because by using a recognized model for delivering care, a more 'supportive' universal approach to assessing, planning, implementing, evaluating and documenting care is achieved for the patient and carer.

ACTIVITY 9.5 PULLING IT ALTOGETHER?

Claire is a 65-year-old married woman who is admitted to the high dependency unit having been found at home by her husband complaining of chest pain, drowsiness and nausea. Claire is extremely cold, clammy and agitated, and has a history of diabetes (which is currently controlled with oral medication). Claire's husband is disabled, and Claire cares independently for him at home. Her only outside support comes from her strong religious beliefs as a practising Roman Catholic.

Reflect upon the management and support of Claire and her family through the unification of a philosophy of care, system of care delivery and a model of nursing care.

The possible outcomes

The way in which the unification of a ward/unit philosophy of care, system of care delivery and model of nursing/documentation occurs in the provision of support to Claire and her family is summarized in the following simple illustration and a more detailed account.

Figure 9.3 highlights 'communication' as the key foundation upon which the building of a functional supporting environment for the patient, family and staff occurs. It is through the execution of efficient and effective channels of communication that most supporting processes are founded. For example, the philosophy of care outlines what a ward/unit or individuals within a specialty aim to provide in care, allowing the system of care delivery to be used in the 'how' to deliver care where the model of care/documentation enables the 'recording' and 'evaluation' of care to occur. In essence these are the key attributes to the creation of any supporting environment for patients and families. Let us explore this in more detail in relation to Claire's care, where real-life situations and materials have been included relating to philosophy of care, system of care delivery and model of care.

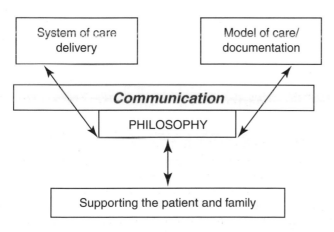

Figure 9.3 Communication as the foundation for patient/family support

> **High dependency unit philosophy of care**
>
> The high dependency unit aims to promote a quiet, relaxed, friendly environment, delivering a professionally high standard of care to those who require intensive care.
>
> The staff will try to increase patients' and carers' understanding and awareness of their condition by providing regular information about their progress whenever possible.
>
> The staff will attempt to take into account the individual physical, social, spiritual and emotional needs of all our patients and carers.
>
> It is our intention that all our staff will be updated and educated in order to maintain and develop our professional standards.

PHILOSOPHY

From this philosophy of care we can automatically depict an appropriate environment for Claire's care. This is the way the unit is trying to encapsulate the key features of a philosophy of care by facilitating freedoms of expression and by promoting individualized programmes of care. Communication is fundamental to providing information in order to increase understanding and allow informed choices to be made. The philosophy is to be achieved by the sharing of information and the establishment of a partnership between the patient, family and staff. Most importantly, the philosophy is realistic, simplistic, understandable and achievable for patients, family and staff.

System of care delivery

The systems of care delivery operational in many wards/units are 'primary' or 'team' nursing, which have many advantages and disadvantages. In relation to Claire's care on the HDU, the system of care delivery used enables the philosophy of care to be achieved by facilitating a holistic and individualized approach to care for the following reasons:

- The similarity of either system of care delivery is in the philosophy, where the patient's right to

be provided with a high standard of care and the carer's right to be given help to produce such standards is ensured. In this way both systems subscribe to humanistic values.

- The fundamental benefit of using either system in aiding Claire's recovery is in the way 'channels of communication' are enhanced, ensuring a more organized and systematic way of providing care and in giving 'supportive' information to, and receiving it from the patient and their family.

- The implementation of the Patient's Charter (1992) and the NHS Code of Openness (1997) is more easily achievable, because the adoption of a system of care delivery allows for the provision of information by identified team leaders, primary nurses or their associate nurses. This type of support, in relation to Claire's care, would hopefully mean that she and her family would become familiar with smaller numbers of staff, and clear, regular information can be given and explained as required.

- Organizational systems to care delivery seem to be built upon a shared and known philosophy, allowing for a holistic and individualized, centred care approach. This is a principle which fosters a collaborative partnership between staff, patient and family, encouraging a continuity of care. This is because information is communicated by fewer individuals, allowing for less misinterpretation of information for Claire and her family.

- The development of a supportive, warm, friendly and relaxed environment facilitates more openness within the ward/unit, where individuals (staff, patients/family included) will express concerns regarding the standards and quality of care. This in turn facilitates a continual review and evaluation of the service.

MODELS OF CARE/DOCUMENTATION

As previously mentioned the model of care/documentation can be seen to be a way of transforming the system of care delivery into a functional tool or model for promoting Claire's recovery. A model/pathway of care (of which there are many) when linked to the 'nursing process' provides a useful framework for assessing, planning, implementing and evaluating care and support for

Claire and her family. In relation to providing 'support' for the dependent patient, a model of care enables an individual's unique lifestyle to be assessed. This may cover physical, psychological, cultural and spiritual needs, so that care can be prioritized in restoring an individual's functional recovery or in some cases the promotion of a peaceful death. In Claire's case it may be useful to explore how the use of the Logan, Roper and Teirney (1983) model of activities of daily living may support her and her family. When using the model in conjunction with the nursing process phase of assessment only (bearing in mind that this could be done for the planning, implementation and evaluation phases), Claire's care can be assessed and categorized into four fundamental areas as shown in Figure 9.4.

From the figure, it would be easy to say that Claire's care and support is dependent upon the nurse's ability to assess and prioritize care into the identified areas of physical, social, psychological and cultural support. However, the effectiveness and outcome of Claire's care is dependent upon the nurse's ability to prioritize and communicate her findings to professional colleagues, Claire and her family. The difficulty often faced by many health professionals is that an individual's physical illness may be exacerbated by overlapping social or psychological factors, as outlined in the illustration. This may be the case relating to some of the 12 activities of daily living identified by Logan, Roper and Teirney.

Assessment relating to Claire's care is illustrated in Figure 9.5. It is clear from the illustration that

Claire's recovery may be promoted by an overlap of several of the identified categories:

1 *Physical*, in resolving the chest pain and nausea.
2 *Psychological*, in providing reassurance to alleviate the fear of dying.
3 *Social concerns* at home regarding care for her disabled husband.
4 *Cultural/spiritual* importance may be the key to resolving this situation by obtaining pastoral care and support for Claire in helping her to come to terms with this admission to the unit.

This illustration, while appearing simple, reinforces the need for effective and efficient channels of communication in the detection and prioritization of care, and in the transmission of information to and from the patient and family in the creation of a supportive environment for Claire and her family.

> Having a philosophy of nursing, system of care delivery and a recognized model of nursing and documentation can be united with the nursing process in providing support to the dependent patient and family

It is within this final section of supporting the dependent patient and his or her family, that the author will attempt to demonstrate how the philosophy of care, system of care delivery and model of care/documentation can be united with the nursing process in communicating a caring,

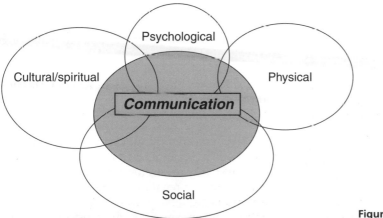

Figure 9.4 Four fundamental areas of care

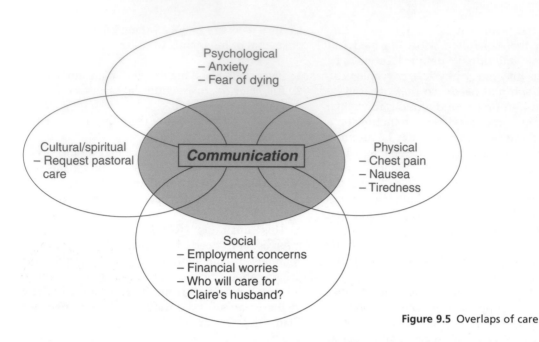

Figure 9.5 Overlaps of care

supportive environment to the patient and family. This is shown in Figure 9.6.

The illustration demonstrates the importance of having a philosophy of care in expressing a statement of intent about how the care is to be provided within that clinical specialty. This in turn will inform the choice of an appropriate system of care, and help the staff to manage and organize care to achieve their philosophy within their clinical specialty. It would be unrealistic for a ward/unit to instigate the implementation of primary nursing without sufficient staffing, appropriate skill mix or having the cooperation and support of their managers. All these variables should be taken into account when planning the philosophy of care. Once the most efficient and effective system of care delivery is agreed upon and operational, the most appropriate model of care/documentation should be adopted, which when combined with the nursing process will facilitate the assessment, planning, implementation and evaluation of care for that clinical area. The model should support the system of care delivery and philosophy. For example, Orem's (1980) self-care model would perhaps be inappropriate for staff working within high dependency or intensive care units, who have to care for unconscious patients. Perhaps in this instance, a systems approach to caring, or activities of daily living models would be more effective.

Once again, 'communication' is the essential component in ensuring a functional and supportive framework for the transfer of information to and from the staff, patient and family. In addition, the illustration can be used to reinforce how the 'evaluation' of care can be obtained from patients and family, and to assess the effectiveness of individual's or ward/unit's philosophy of care, system of care delivery and models of care in achieving these designs. This may become evident from auditing the gratitude shown to and complaints received by the unit, and patterns of length of stay in and readmission to the unit or through the introduction of clinical audit in assessing standards and quality of care. If we pause for a moment and think of all the ways we have of providing support to the patient and family within the various clinical specialties, wards/units in delivering and evaluating care, the application of the 'nursing process' can be used to assess, plan, implement and evaluate the effectiveness of most of the supporting structures we provide to the dependent patient and family, as the following list outlines.

1 *First*, several areas of support emerge for caring for the dependent patient and family, be it for neurological, respiratory, endocrine, cardiac, alimentary or renal conditions, as Figure 9.7 illustrates.

2 *Second*, when applying the principles of the

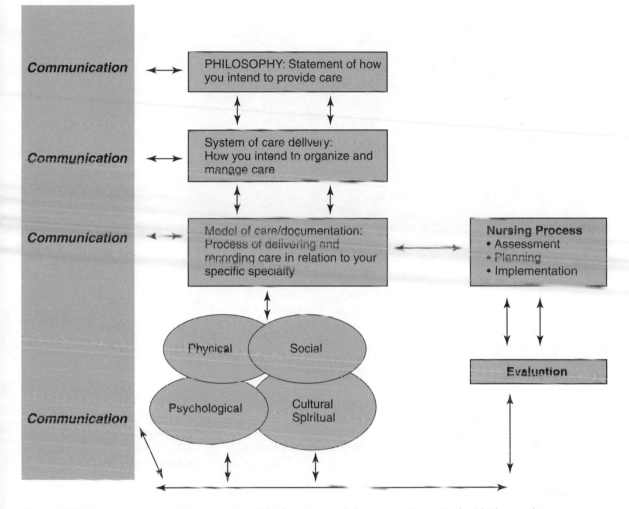

Figure 9.6 Philosophy of care, delivery and model of nursing and documentation united with the nursing process

nursing process, you can work through the following key phases to provide patient and family support:

- *Assessment* will aim to establish if the patient's current illness or condition has affected his or her ability to communicate and receive information. Mr Williams' case (Activity 9.2), for example, may require the information to be written and spoken due to his difficulty with speaking and perhaps because of cognitive dysfunction, his having had a cerebral vascular accident.
- *Planning*: The impairments to communication may mean that both verbal and non-verbal forms of communication are used in the form of explanations, followed up with explanatory leaflets or documentation.
- *Implementation*: The verbal and non-verbal forms of information will be provided to support the patient and his or her family.
- *Evaluation*: The effectiveness of providing information will be evaluated in relation to resolving the patient's problems associated with accessing information. If the problem remains, a new approach will need to be adopted and other health professionals contacted, e.g. the speech and language therapists.

3 *Third*, it is evident from this approach to supporting the patient and family how it can relate

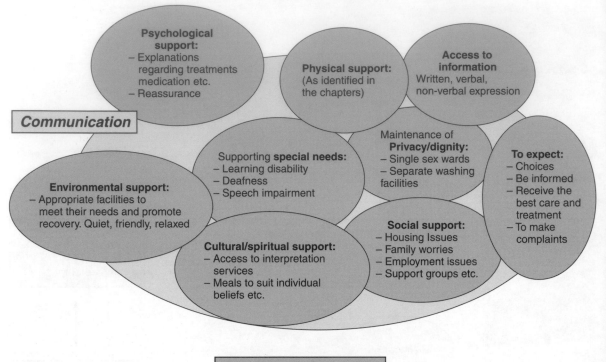

Figure 9.7 Areas of support for the dependent patient and family

to your philosophy of care, system of care delivery and model of care/documentation. For example, you would expect the staff to reassure the patient by providing verbal and non-verbal communication.

The information would be given timely, accessible, understandable, and with documentary evidence in the care-plan to indicate the care provided.

4 *Fourth* and most importantly, while the nursing process appears to offer a framework for identifying key support required by the dependent patient and family, 'communication' is again the key to success. As with any system you operate it is 'only as good as the weakest link' (Rafferty, 1992).

Remember, inaccurate information, poor information flow and blocked communication channels are key barriers to a unified approach to care, as are a lack of time, support and resources.

Before concluding, reflect on the following to see what you have learnt.

Further activity

ACTIVITY 9.6 THE WAY FORWARD: A LETTER

After reading the following fictitious letter of complaint from a patient, and reflecting on this chapter, make a few notes as to how you think the events in the letter may have been avoided.

Points to consider:

- *Communication:* effective or ineffective channels of communication.
- *Philosophy of care*: individualized holistic care, patient choice, freedom, partnership and sharing experiences. Written, realistic, relevant, achievable?
- *System of care delivery*: executed, operational, appropriate?
- *Model of care/documentation*: is there continuity?

Dear . . .

I was admitted to hospital for an emergency operation. The welcome on the ward was good and the doctors and anaesthetist excellent. When I regained consciousness after the op I was cared for by very caring nurses. However, the next day, when I was feeling better, I was transferred to another bay and, whilst accepting I personally didn't require a lot of nursing, the difference in standards was evident. I could not believe I was on the same ward. I have been admitted many times but never seen this happen. There were several elderly ladies around me. One of them waited twenty five minutes for a bed pan and consequently just as it arrived no longer needed it. The lady was upset – her family came later and she insisted that they not complain. Another lady was unable to sit up in bed (she had had a stroke) and required assistance with feeding – her food was always cold by the time somebody came. Her tea was put on a locker where she couldn't reach it.

Another thing that confused patients was if the nurse was in the team that nursed you one day and then for some reason moved to another colour team, they ignored you. I saw an RGN take out a cannula and give the patient a piece of cotton wool to hold onto it because someone else shouted 'tea break girls'. Is this good practice?

I am sorry to have to write to you, but as you are the ward manager I thought that you ought to be aware of what goes on. I am sure that there are only a few bad nurses, but what a shame they spoil such a wonderful ward team. Perhaps it would be possible for you to inform ward managers that these practices do happen.

If you get to this point thank you for sparing the time to read it.

Conclusion

This chapter has provided a guide to help nurses create a truly supportive environment for the high dependency patient and his or her family. Rising patient and family expectations when linked with shorter patient lengths of stay and increased patient dependency reinforce the need for all health professionals to reflect on how efficient and effective their communication skills are. Communication is an extremely complex area and is the key to the nurse's role. Nursing is about assessing, observing, listening to, liaising with, supporting and responding to the dependent patient, family and with other healthcare professionals. Establishing an effective and efficient channel of communication and documentation reduces the chances of developing poor communication and relationships between the patient, family and other health professions within that team, where misunderstandings of verbal or written information may be prevented. Patient satisfaction will then be promoted rather than dissatisfaction and the possible pursuance of litigation claims if a case of negligence were proved. In supporting the patient and family it is essential that you remain aware of the individual rights of your patient through the Patient's Charter (1992). A philosophy of care provides a foundation for the individuals working within that ward/unit to share their beliefs and attitudes in stating how they will care for the patients and their families. It is always important to be mindful of what admission to hospital can mean to an individual and his or her family. If we can put ourselves in the position of the patient and imagine what we would want, we can go a long way in providing a first-class level of support.

Further reading

Aggleton, P. and Chalmers H (1984) Models and Theories. *Nursing Times* September 5, 24–8.

Audit Commission (1992) *What seems to be the matter? Communication between hospitals and patients.* London: Audit Commission.

Berlo, K.D. 1960 *The Process of communication.* New York: Holt, Rinehart and Winston.

Brindle, D. 1995 6000 NHS beds 'blocked' by community care elderly. Reports of National Association of Health Authorities and Trusts survey. *The Guardian.* London.

Burnard, P. 1992 *A communication skills guide for health care workers.* London: Arnold.

Davies, P. 1994 Non-verbal communication with patients. *British Journal of Nursing* **3**(5), 220–23.

Deaux, L.S. 1984 *Social psychology.* Monterey, California: Brookes Cole.

Dimond, B. 1990 *Legal aspects of nursing.* London: Prentice Hall.

Dimond, B. 1993 *Patients' rights, responsibilities and the nurse.* Lancaster: Quay Publishing.

Gardner, K. 1991 A summary of findings of a five-year comparison study of primary and team nursing. *Nursing Research.* **40**(2), 113–17.

DOH 1989 *The White Paper: Working for Patients.* London: HMSO.

DOH 1991 *The Citizen's Charter.* London: HMSO.

DOH 1992 *The Patient's Charter: Raising the Standard.* London: HMSO.

DOH 1993 *Health of the Nation.* London: HMSO.

DOH 1997 *The Code of Openness in the NHS.* London: HMSO.

Henderson, V. 1961 *Basic principles of nursing care.* Geneva: International Council of Nurses.

Johns, C. 1993 Team and primary nursing: a reply. *Senior Nurse* **13**(1), 31–3.

Korzybski, A. 1958 *Science and sanity.* New York: International Non-Aristotelian Library Publishing.

Lidbetter, J. 1990 A better way to learn. *Nursing Times* **86**(29), 61–4.

Morris, M. and Herriott, S. 1994 RCN report highlights the limitations of the Patient's Charter. *British Journal of Nursing* **3**(9), 440–41.

McSherry, R. 1996 Multidisciplinary approach to patient communication. *Nursing Times* **92**(8), 42–3.

Logan, N., Roper, W.W.L. and Tierney, A. 1983 *Using a model for nursing.* London: Churchill Livingstone

O'Donovan, M. 1996 How well do you manage risk? *Medical Interface* March, 75–8.

Orem, D. 1971 *Nursing: concepts of practice.* New York: McGraw Hill.

Potter, A.P. 1993 *Fundamentals of nursing: concepts, process and practice* London: Mosby.

Rafferty, D. 1992 Team and primary nursing. *Senior Nurse* **12**(1), 31–4.

RCN 1994 *Uncharted territory: public awareness of the Patient's Charter.* London: Royal College of Nursing.

Riehl, J.P. and Roy, C. 1980 *Conceptual models for nursing.* Norwalk: Appleton-Century-Crofts.

Shuttleworth, A. 1992 Will the Charter work? Readers' views on the Patient's Charter. *Professional Nurse* April, 439–41.

Smith, V. 1982 *Communication for the health care team.* Cambridge: Harper and Row.

Tierney, A. 1994 Older patients' experience of discharge from hospital. *Nursing Times* **90**(21), 36–9.

Tourish, O.H. 1993 Don't you sometimes wish you were better informed? *Health Service Journal* November, 28–29.

United Kingdom Central Council for Nursing 1992 *Code of Professional Practice.* London: UKCC.

Wilson, J. 1996 Multi-disciplinary pathways of care series: a tool for minimising risk. *Health Care Risk Report* March, 10–12.

Wright, S. 1986 *Building and using a model of nursing* London: Arnold.

Yura, H. and Walsh, B.M. 1900 *The nursing process: assessing, planning, implementation, evaluation,* 4th edn. Connecticut: Appleton-Century-Crofts:

10 Caring for staff

Irene Gilsenan

Introduction

The aim of this chapter is to help prepare the nurse for the huge challenge of caring for the highly dependent and often physically unstable patient. This type of nursing can be extremely rewarding. It demands of the nursing team a very high level of commitment and focused expertise. There are few jobs in nursing that offer the same challenge as that of caring for a seriously ill patient, monitoring their vital signs and preventing their condition from worsening, and supporting the patient's loved ones throughout the acute phase of illness. Unfortunately, however, working in this type of highly emotionally charged area can be very stressful. The chapter will consider the following issues in relation to staff support and introduce the reader to the following topics:

- Stress management.
- Issues concerning managers.
- Preceptorship.
- Clinical supervision.
- Individual performance review.
- Educational needs.
- Working conditions for nurses.
- Career progression.

It is hoped that by exploring these areas of management the care team can remain prepared for the challenges of high dependency nursing.

Stress management

A generally accepted view of stress is that it is something unpleasant and has a negative effect on the individual. This is not necessarily the case as stress, if within acceptable limits, is an essential part of normal life. We need in fact some level of stress present to function normally (Cox, 1975). When stress becomes negative and potentially dangerous, it is because the stress experienced is not managed effectively by the person's internal and external coping mechanisms. These mechanisms can become overwhelmed. The concept of stress must be seen as a personal one; it is possible for two or more nurses working under the same conditions in the same unit to cope quite differently to similar levels of stress. One will thrive and remain well-adjusted; the other will begin to show signs that they are not able to cope. It is true that the way in which an external stressful stimulus is perceived and reacted to is subjective to the individual.

Stress is a subject that has over recent years quite rightly attracted a great deal of scrutiny in nursing.

Theories of stress

There are long-established theories that divide the subject of stress into three models. These look at stress as: a stimulus, a response and thirdly as a transaction between a number of factors including the environment and the person (Cox, 1975).

The stimulus theory explains stress as an external factor which places pressure on a person and causes an impact that can either be dealt with or not dealt with. For example following a change in the weather the outside temperature may be intolerable to some, but comfortable to others.

The response theory considers stress as an intrinsic factor, coming from within the person and being a physical reaction to other external agents. An example of this theory might be the individual interpretation of a situation by one person and their subsequent reactions. Again these

will be different for individuals working in the same situation.

The final theory (the transactional model) looks at how an individual makes sense of a situation and in conjunction with all other factors makes a certain response or set of responses as a result of this.

Because of the conceptual diversity of these theories, it can be difficult to pin down the actual causes of stress.

There are many external factors such as:

- The environment
- Other people
- Life situations (births, deaths, moving jobs, failure, success)
- Personal values

Recognizing signs of stress

The signs that someone may not be adjusting to stressful situations and surroundings are varied and can include many physical signs such as headache, nausea, raised blood pressure, sweating and back pain. These can also be associated with psychological symptoms such as anxiety, anger, mood swings, overwhelming panic and general changes in behaviour. There are of course many more symptoms that may or may not occur; these may occur in isolation or with others. What is certain however is that these symptoms, if allowed to persist, will result in difficulties relating to the maintenance of relationships at work and day-to-day nursing activities. The accumulation of stress and subsequent stress-related symptoms is usually a gradual process, building up until coping mechanisms are stretched to the limit. The recognition that stress is becoming a problem may come from the person themselves, or from others working closely with them. They may notice that the individual's responses are abnormal. Identification of stressful situations and environmental factors is really only the beginning. In the high dependency area, staff must learn to observe their colleagues for signs that stress is becoming intolerable. Nursing teams need to rely upon each other and to care for each other. Those who are suffering severe stress will need help to overcome this problem. The earlier that this is managed the better for all concerned. Decisions will have to be made to deal with future stressful episodes. In some circumstances individuals may have to avoid certain stressful situations altogether.

Exploring situations within the workplace that may cause stress produces common themes that are the same wherever the place of work. There are however many studies that have focused on nursing and they have tried to break down the elements of the job which are considered by all to be stressful.

Nursing and particularly high dependency nursing is a difficult and challenging job. The number and types of situations that have the potential to cause stress are far greater than some other professions. Situations that arise daily in nursing can be categorized to show the diversity of stressful episodes to which nurses are exposed. These include the content and context of the work itself. The nurse knows that life and death situations are being managed and they may question their capability to deal with these situations. Communications issues may arise with both the patients, the relatives and other members of staff, and these can all add to the daily stress total.

The increase in patient turnover and the emergence of high technology care can all affect nurses and their capacity to cope with the ever-present changes. The feeling of not being able to give the best care available due to time restrictions can have a severe effect on the typically busy nurse. Wherever the nurse may work, when there are changes to their working practices or even the environment, then there needs to be a constant element of support for them during the transition period.

There have been a number of studies over the years that have focused on different areas of nursing to try to determine whether certain specialities within nursing are more stressful than others. Some have just focused on one specific area and looked very closely at the responses of the nurses within that area, whilst some have compared the known stressors between a number of areas and drawn conclusions from that. High dependency areas have traditionally been closely monitored for stress levels. This is due to the generally higher mortality rates and higher levels of intervention, the changing technology and the high patient turnover. The identified stressors within these areas have corresponded fairly closely with other clinical areas but at times it is apparent that these levels rise considerably.

What is generally agreed however, is that if an unacceptable level of stress is reached and maintained for a sustained period then the nurses themselves are likely to suffer 'burnout'. This occurs when there are no more facilities available within a person to continue to cope. When this happens there can be a number of different reactions including:

- Taking time off from work.
- Moving to less stressful areas of nursing.
- Leaving the job altogether.
- Breaking down at times of very acute stress.
- Withdrawing from colleagues, patients and relatives.
- General communication difficulties.
- Feelings of everything 'getting on top of them'.
- More serious psychological illnesses.

These symptoms highlight a potentially serious state and one that needs to be addressed promptly. If the nurse continues to expose themselves to the external causes of stress and 'burnout' continues then it can have a deep effect not only on the nurse but on their colleagues also. When looking at the research considering burnout in relation to occupational stressors, Handy (1990) observed that although there were many references to severe occupational stress, the solutions suggested were not always practical. If the generalized occupational stressors are identified and dealt with by the individuals themselves there is a risk that a 'whole organization' approach is lost. This will lead to stress continuing in the organization with other individuals within the system becoming stressed. This is an important point for managers to consider as action should be taken to combat stress from a global approach and not 'piecemeal' which may be easier, but will not improve the overall situation.

As previously discussed, the factors which

affect a person and the creation of stress and stress-related symptoms are very personal. Therefore the methods utilized to try to overcome the stress will probably be specific to that person. Care needs to be taken that the methods used to try to break the circle of stress and reduce suffering do not cause further problems in the future. Positive ways to reduce stress on a personal level can include counselling, both professionally and with friends and family, exercise to keep the body fit and focused, and relaxation techniques such as yoga, meditation and general leisure pursuits. In recent years there have also been a great number of self help groups created that help reduce the harmful effects of stress.

There are unfortunately negative ways of dealing with stress and stressful situations, which can cause further problems in the long run. The use of drugs or alcohol to help relax or just to go to sleep may persist and become a permanent crutch on which to lean. Changes in behaviour can result in problems with family, friends and colleagues. This may add further emotional pressure and compound the problem.

Occupational stress, whilst obviously not good for the individual, can put increased pressure on the workplace itself. If members of staff are taking extra time off sick then further resources have to be found to cover shifts. The recognition by the organization that the area has high levels of stress has to be made and there has to be a strategy set down for such issues as they arise. This theme will be discussed in more detail later in the chapter.

Summary

1 Stress can be caused by a number of factors
2 The relationship between pressure and a person's coping mechanism plays a great part in whether the person will suffer from any aspect of stress.
3 Two people in the same situation may not experience stress or stress-related symptoms
4 Continuing exposure to situations and the environment of stress may cause burnout.
5 The symptoms associated with stress are very diverse
6 In nursing, stress has played a part in staff leaving the job altogether

Management issues

In recent years, studies have been undertaken to see if the rates of nurses leaving can be explained. Once identified, the situation can be examined and dealt with by the profession as a whole, helping retain the staff today and attract future nurses. Lader (1995) undertook a major study to pinpoint reasons for nurses leaving. The mean reasons from the female respondents were related to their family commitments. They felt that they could not successfully juggle the two roles. Number of hours worked, shift patterns and child care provision were all mentioned in this study as reasons why a complete break was made from the job. The male and unmarried younger female groups reasons for leaving were related to poor pay and career enhancement. It is generally accepted that there is no longer the large pool of new staff waiting to come into the profession or return after a break in service. Strategies have to be put in to place that create a balance between the needs of the staff and the needs of the organization. Looking at members of staff currently in post has identified that a lowering of morale generally can push some members of staff into looking critically at their role leading them to consider moving to other areas of work. There are many reasons for low morale and some are shown in Figure 10.1.

How can morale be improved in the high dependency area and staff be retained and recruited?

Staffing shortages have to be addressed both in the short-term and long-term. Staff that come into nursing, either directly from qualifying or returning to practice after a break in service, need to be

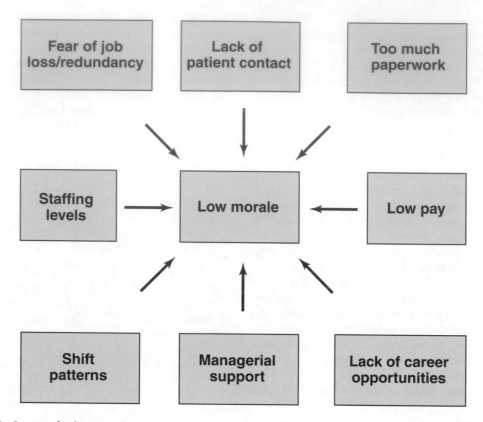

Figure 10.1   Reasons for low morale

welcomed and policies put into place to keep these staff. Managers must be aware that the retention of new and existing staff is a priority.

Using a period of induction when a new member of staff starts work in a specific area will help them settle into their role and be able to ask questions about their job in a non-threatening environment. If the member of staff has not worked in the high dependency area before, then this time can assist them in familiarizing themselves with the role before any expectations are placed upon them. If possible the new member of staff should be used in a supernumerary role assisting them to build up a picture of their new working environment. Putting time and resources into the first period of employment can pay dividends when it comes to retaining staff in post for the future. The induction programme, if well set up may be used as a valuable recruitment tool to encourage staff to join from other areas. If the package is linked with a career plan that includes educational strategies,

then not only will staff wish to come and work there but they will be more likely to stay.

The managerial style that is adopted can also have a great effect on the morale and retention of staff. Managers must allow time for staff needs and keep in regular contact with them so they are aware of what is happening in the unit on a daily basis. Communication is one of the major issues in management and if channels are not maintained negative rumours, gossip and fear may occur.

Effective channels of communication can help in the support systems associated with staff management and aid the implementation of change. This will also help build teams and lead on to provide effective role modelling for staff and managers for the future. Regular team meetings play a great part in the staff feeling that they belong and that their views are valid and worthwhile. Changes to practice or policy can be brought about effectively by a joint staff and management approach which considers all aspects of the situation, deciding what is best for all members of the team and ultimately, of course the patient.

As already briefly mentioned, the work patterns and shift systems can be a deciding point when a job offer is being considered. There are many different shift systems in operation around the country at the present time. These include:

- Twelve hour shifts.
- Three shifts in a 24 hour period.
- Internal rotation onto night duty.
- Regular night and day staff with no interchange.
- On call time to cover unsociable hours.
- Split shifts and twilight shifts.

There can be no doubt that altering the shift patterns can bring about a reduction in costs, but if by bringing about these changes staff are left with family problems or transport difficulties to and from work, then these may create more problems than they solve. Care has to be taken in planning changes in shift patterns to allow for correct skill mix. If the more experienced nurses are used as a resource across the duty rotas and to support the more junior members of staff, then this can create a learning and supportive environment for all staff concerned. If staff are restricted in their shift rotas because of cost then some shifts can be seen as top heavy, whilst others run with very junior staff.

The work environment from the manager's viewpoint has to run smoothly and be efficient in the use of resources such as equipment, staff and general running costs. This viewpoint can vary from the staff's perspective as they see the shortcomings in light of patient care and the reduced ability to deliver an adequate service. There is potential for disagreement between clinical staff and managers if it appears that corners are being cut for financial reasons as the loser is seen to be the patient.

Another management issue concerns that of resources, and more specifically the purchasing of equipment to be used within the clinical area. Specialized medical equipment is now being used in most clinical areas to assist in the most common duties that a nurse now performs. Taking a patient's temperature, in view of current legislation, now involves either tympanic or core thermometers. The monitoring of a patient's blood sugar now uses specialized equipment unheard of perhaps just 10 years ago. This equipment has to be purchased out of general budgets and discussions have to take place as to the suitability of the machine for the place of work. In the area of high dependency care, there is a risk that when specific equipment is introduced or replaced, the most prominent consideration is seen as cost and not necessarily the benefit to patients.

Once equipment has been purchased, managers have to make sure that agreements are made concerning the maintenance and repair so that the staff in the clinical areas are not left without such equipment and having to use other methods or machinery that may be inappropriate.

Preceptorship

The period of time just after qualification can be one of the most stressful episodes in a nurse's career. Other members of staff may look at the qualified nurse's uniform and make assumptions as to their knowledge base, capabilities and skill levels. In the newly qualified nurse, these assumptions can create a great deal of pressure and the nurse may feel that they have to live up to these expectations and gain knowledge rapidly. These feelings can also be felt in members of staff who have been qualified for a length of time, but may have moved to another area or different speciality.

The term 'reality shock' has been applied to the immediate post-registration (Kramer, 1974). It is a period when they may realize their shortcomings in knowledge and experience, and feel that they are not up to the role. The emotions that accompany the transition from student status to a qualified nurse role can be very demanding. If support is not forthcoming at this stage then the chances of that nurse feeling that they fit into the team may be limited.

If these negative feelings continue then there is the risk that the newly qualified nurse may leave the profession altogether in search of a more supportive network.

If the nurse has been qualified for a while and is returning to service or moving from another area, then changes that have happened in nursing in the recent past can reduce their confidence levels. From being a positive practitioner in a clinical area, they can be overwhelmed when returning to work by all the changes that have happened to their role while they have been away. They may feel that their old role is not related to the newer extended role that nurses have undertaken, for instance, to accommodate the reduction in junior doctors' hours.

The United Kingdom Central Council for Nurses, Midwives and Health Visitors (UKCC) has taken this area of uncertainty for these new members of staff and looked at ways to help the settling in period and reduce the stress of such a role (1994). The guidelines that they drew up in association with the Post-Registration Education and Practice (PREP) proposals look at supporting the new staff through this difficult time. The idea of preceptorship, although not an original idea in the United States, is new to nursing in Britain and can be seen as a very different approach in staff management.

Role of the preceptor

- Educator
- Giving information
- Introducing to other team members
- Planning the learning experience
- Work as a link person
- Counsellor
- Confidante
- Evaluating other areas for learning
- Helping to develop the career pathway
- Being a role model
- Assessing knowledge base

The guidelines state that every newly qualified nurse should have a designated person to guide and assist the newly qualified member of staff. There are no direct instructions laid down in the documents that specify who should actually undertake the role of preceptor. There were initial thoughts that it should be the ward sister or charge nurse but others may argue that this would not be appropriate as the role they are helping them into is not strictly their own. Because of these discrepancies there have been reports that the relationships that have built up as part of the preceptorship programme have not been as cohesive and productive as they perhaps should have been. There are of course other issues to be considered when looking at matching people together in a working relationship, especially in an unbalanced power match. Issues of gender, race and culture have to be taken into consideration when looking at who is best suited for the role of preceptor.

Many changes to the way nurses work have in the past been criticized for not allowing for the time that is needed to undertake new roles in the clinical area. There is no doubt that the emergence of preceptorship has added another time burden to nurses working in the clinical area, but it can be argued that the following around of a senior nurse by a junior nurse has in the past taken place under a different guise and a number of positive aspects have come out of it. Personally the newly qualified nurse can gain a great deal from a period of preceptorship. Providing care has been taken in the choosing of an appropriate preceptor, the ground building of a good working relationship can begin. The relationship may at first appear one-sided as the more experienced nurse hands over knowledge and information, but if there is a good communication system set up, then the newly qualified nurse can also give information that will be of benefit to their senior nurse. Information regarding the nurse training programme, the educational frameworks and the types of stresses that are suffered by this group of nurses can be of use to more experienced staff enabling them to communicate, liaise and work on behalf of their staff. It is generally accepted that the formalizing of this preceptorship period will have a very positive effect on nursing and in the future help to retain staff in their clinical posts.

There are some authors who claim that the publicity given to the stresses that newly qualified staff experience have been greatly exaggerated, but conclude that even so, a preceptorship programme can aid a positive outlook within this transition period. In a practical sense it can be assumed that if a newly qualified member of staff has someone whom they can trust, who they can talk freely to and who will show them around and introduce them to others, they will feel better able to cope with the new role and all it entails. There is no set time limit to the preceptorship period and because of this local arrangements have been made in various areas across the country. Because of the individuality of staff these should be tailored to the nurses' needs and their assessment of what they need to learn and how long they think it will take. In the long-term, plans can be made for the career choices that may be necessary for that nurse to progress in that area. For instance, in the high dependency area it may be worthwhile setting a time-span for the preceptorship period and looking into the not too distant future (12 months or so) and consolidating that period with a recognized post-registration qualifi-

cation. These plans have to take into consideration the availability of courses and the relevance to the nurse at that particular stage in their career.

Main points

- Preceptorship can successfuly bridge the gap between being a student nurse and being qualified
- This period can also be used for nurses who are not newly qualified but have moved to another clinical area
- There has to be careful consideration made when allocating staff to a preceptor
- Gender and culture need to be considered
- Time needs to be set aside for the nurse to settle in, visit other areas and meet up regularly with their preceptor
- This period can help form some career plans and help retain staff
- Can enhance staff performance
- It identifies the nurse's individual needs and helps overcome any issues that emerge

Clinical supervision

Supervision is one of those terms that will evoke different responses from many nurses. Some might say it is a management tool that enables senior nurses to monitor the junior staff, making sure they are doing the work they are meant to. Others would say that it entails caring for learners and helping them cope with any problems that may arise.

In nursing 'clinical supervision' tends to be used as a blanket term for a variety of linked strategies that support and maintain the qualified nurses at work. The idea of a preceptorship for newly qualified nurses can be compared to clinical supervision, as would mentorship.

Because the term has a variety of meanings to many people, it is useful to consider its origins and the reasons it was thought necessary for nursing. Butterworth and Faugier (1992) first looked at the idea of support for nurses that were being

discussed and used the term, 'clinical supervision'. They examined the changes that had occurred over the recent years and how the role of the nurse had changed too. The move away from medical domination and the 'handmaiden' image has been well-documented, but in the light of this new independence came a realization that new systems would have to be put into place to support, sustain and help advance nursing.

As nurses have striven to gain an independent position, they have also been building up a body of knowledge that is specific to nursing alone. Without this body of knowledge it might always appear that nurses were still subservient to doctors.

Nurses have been examining their work and the inherent roles and bringing about change through the accepted methods of research, education and self-empowerment. The advent of modern nurse education has brought about a shift in the public's perception of nurses and removed them from the traditional role that has been so prominent in recent times. Learning the lessons from the past, nursing has had to look to other disciplines to gain an insight into how they coped with similar changes. Though the idea of supervision within the clinical setting has not been prominent within nursing, some of the allied professions such as social work, have been practising it for many years.

Some nurses claim that clinical supervision has been carried out for many years, only it has not been called clinical supervision. Informal chatting, reflection upon critical incidents and moral support have, it can be argued, always been present in nursing. What clinical supervision does is that it enables all staff to have access to a support network.

> **Clinical supervision can be seen to encompass:**
>
> - Mentorship
> - Staff support
> - Managerial strategies
> - Work review
> - Preceptorship
> - Relationship building
> - Regular meetings
> - Standards
> - Improve clinical proficiency
> - Recognition of work

Butterworth and Faugier (1992) themselves agree that the term has now become an umbrella for a number of other ideas that are currently emerging in nursing: they are reluctant to put strict definitions on the concept for fear of losing the underlying flexibility that makes it acceptable for varied areas of nursing. The UKCC (1995) however has laid down some guidelines to state what is not considered to be part of the supervision process. They state that a strong managerial element will hinder the process and if the sessions are used instead of formal individual performance reviews, then this may detract from the original supportive concept that it was intended to be. It is generally felt that if supervision was used as a means of 'checking up' on the staff or as a tool for

reprimands this would not be conducive for an open working relationship. They also place emphasis on the effective training of supervisors and state for the system to work well it should not be hierarchical in nature.

Because the concept is multifaceted, there can be no one way to undertake clinical supervision in an area. Many qualified nurses will have some experience of supervision, whether as a student or during a period of orientation.

Across the country there are no formal guidelines for clinical supervision and some or all of the elements described may be used as part of supervision. Hospitals are beginning to recognize that the concept is applicable to all their areas, that it may have a direct link with the recruitment and retention of staff, and are looking at ways of implementation.

There are, as before, arguments as to who is best placed to undertake the role of clinical supervisor within the workplace. Clinical supervision can be seen to cover a number of practices within nursing but all have the common thread of support and development of staff. If the supervision network is set up with unsuitable relationships then the system is likely to fail. Care has to be taken when looking at the attitudes, qualifications and skills required to be a supervisor. There also has to be emphasis placed on the supervisee as their role entails some preparation and work and

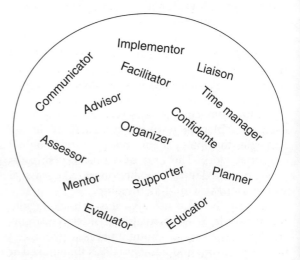

Figure 10.2 Roles of the clinical supervisor

if this is not carried out then success is likely to be limited (Fig. 10.2).

There is some discussion into what occupational group the supervisor should come from and in what format the meetings for supervision should have. In the vast majority of cases a supervisor from the same discipline will be used and the meetings will be one-to-one. However this may not be suitable in some areas, and alternatives may have to be found. It may be that there are staff who work in such a way that someone from another area is better placed to supervise their needs or a one-to-one situation is not applicable, so group supervision can be used. The flexibility must be there to help all members of staff find an arrangement that will work in their clinical area.

The major argument within nursing management against this theory is that of time implications and the increased staffing levels that are required to cover such sessions. It is not always easy to observe the benefits of clinical supervision. However if nurses are being supported within their workplace then there will be benefits such as the reduction of stress and improvement in the standards of care to the patients. These, if proven, will obviously impress managers into supporting clinical supervision. It is important of course that

research is devised into measurement of supervision for the long-term. Perhaps we can reduce staff sickness and increase nurse-led research in these areas, and in so doing will ensure the success of clinical supervision. The practicalities of supervision for the nurses within the clinical areas can be overcome by well-planned off duty and a commitment by ward managers to use time resources to help supervision occur. Once relationships have been established and the meetings are taking place on a regular basis, nurses involved will be happier to examine their own practices and see if they can improve their work. The application of research findings into the clinical area may be helped by other members of staff who are willing to experiment and try out new ideas for the benefit of all their colleagues. Increasing the job satisfaction levels of nursing staff can help them feel more fulfilled and willing to look at their career pathway. Remaining in a particular area or speciality may be related to the amount of support that is available from within. In the high dependency environment, it is important to have all the elements of clinical supervision in place and working to help all the staff within the team to learn, experiment and progress in their work and future.

Individual performance review

The individual performance review (IPR) has undergone many name changes over the recent years; because of this there has developed confusion surrounding it. The terminology of the past gives some indication as to the function of such reviews and perhaps why these misunderstandings have occurred.

In some places of work the review was known as the appraisal system and this was seen rightly or wrongly to indicate an assessment of quality or worth. The feelings was that if the work was not up to a certain level, then at this meeting the truth would come out. Strategies that are developed and used by the managerial system are often seen by the workforce as being threatening and poten-

tially damaging to the individual. In the case of appraisal if you were not seen to fit in with the managerial strategies then you may have been disciplined.

Later the format was adapted along with the title to staff development and performance review (SDPR). This gave the impression that the staff would be involved in the process and the outcome was going to be more positive than negative. In these meetings the work that was being carried out was looked at in relation to the work, courses and study which were discussed as a plan for the future. The emphasis had shifted to underline the value that was being placed on the staff member.

These various systems have been widely used

in all types of industries. In recent years we have seen the advent of performance-related pay. This has added a new factor in assessment of the person before decisions are made towards the person's salary addition. Within the health service, there have been attempts to use these various systems over the years without a great deal of success. Many senior members of staff have had experience of IPRs but when it came to filtering this down to the nurses at ward level there tended to be a breakdown in continuity. The emergence of the IPR system has hopefully been more useful and greater publicity will help enhance the motivation and morale of staff in the future. The health service has particular needs and the use of IPR has to fit in with those needs as well as the requirements of the staff involved. One of the main purposes of IPR in the healthcare setting is to improve the effectiveness of the service as a whole and ultimately of course helping patient care. This is done by general discussion, sharing of information and the agreements and action plans that are brought about by this process.

Individual performance review within the health service has taken on a number of standard elements that can be found across the country. These include:

- A regular meeting between a member of staff and the management.
- An agreement for two-way discussion to take place.
- An agreed action plan at the end of the meeting.
- Discussions about the future aspirations of the member of staff.
- A review of the person's performance over a set time.
- Both strengths and weaknesses to be discussed.
- Jointly agreed areas for developing.
- Confidentiality.

The time scale between meetings can be varied and may depend on the individual's own needs. On a general scale, once a year may be adequate for most members of staff but more often should also be considered in certain cases. For instance if a member of staff is having difficulties within their role, they may need further input and assessment to help them through. In other cases professional circumstances may change, warranting an update or review in between the agreed times. Once the culture of the clinical area accepts IPR as a positive and routine event in the year, then further review and updates will be taken on board and adopted as the norm and the system will gain further credibility with staff. The concept of IPR should, in an ideal world, be used in conjunction with the other strategies explored within this chapter. If the sole contact with a representative from the managerial structure was a once-yearly IPR, then communication levels would be at an unacceptable level. In specialist areas, such as high dependency care, the frequency of contact and communication has to be set at a higher level. Changes in practice and the evolving role of nurses within the high dependency areas can only progress if there is an active discussion network and ideas are allowed to emerge from all the staff involved. Again the recruitment of new staff can be helped by the use of an open and creative management structure.

Although as a concept it fits in with the idea of clinical supervision and preceptorship it would not be used as a short cut to setting up any of the other objectives. If there are already existing support mechanisms in place then extra care is needed to avoid confusion with role boundaries within the care teams.

The use of IPR can be very beneficial to nurses if the strategy is taken and accepted by all members of the team. The communication links have to be established with the management structure that is in place before the first meetings can take place. Once the meetings are happening regularly, then the workforce will start to get a better insight into managerial issues and the managers will be better equipped to help those working for them as key issues will become high on the agenda.

There are some inherent problems with the IPR system; these have been documented in the past. For example the choice of paperwork that is used within the process is important; it has to be developed and tried out in the particular area and any

---

ACTIVITY 10.1

Make a list of the issues surrounding IPR in your area. Consider how you will implement a plan of individual performance review.

amendments made as continual evaluation takes place. If the paperwork is not acceptable or does not allow reflection to take place then the positive aspects of IPR may be lost. Some forms of documentation have been adapted from earlier systems and still have an emphasis on the manager assessing the worker and noting down their comments. More recent examples of IPR documentation have included sections for both people to complete in preparation for the actual meeting and thus setting an informal agenda to structure the agreed meeting. In preparing for the meeting in advance, both parties can gather information and thus gain the most out of the time spent in discussion. Although many may shy away from structuring such a meeting, it is seen as important to follow a set pattern to be consistent and cover all aspects of the review without forgetting important aspects. Some ideas of subject headings may include:

- Performance of the member of staff.
- Personal evaluation of their own performance.
- Perception of their working style.
- Plans for the future.
- Training needs.
- Areas for development.
- Creating a workable action plan.

In the past these sessions could be seen to just revolve around what study days or courses the particular nurse wanted to attend. Now there is more of an emphasis on the role played within the team, a reflection of their work and agreement of feasible plan of action ensuring clarity for both sides. If a manager remains up to date with how the staff are feeling and how they want to develop their careers, then plans can be made to accommodate the aspirations of staff and help keep the staff that are already in post.

Main points summarizing IPR

- IPR can help in the communication between managers and their staff
- The process can help the staff reflect on their practice
- Strengths and weaknesses can be identified in a non-threatening way
- Plans about future career moves can be made
- Agreement must take place to decide on an action plan
- The meetings should be regular and can be updated if needed
- A structure to the meeting will help for preparation and discussion
- Discussion should be open and two way

Educational needs

Nurses, as part of their commitment to Post-Registration Education and Practice are looking for relevant educational study to both bring them up to date and improve the care that they give. This study does not have to take the traditional approach of a formal course with or without an exam at the end. This opens the door to looking at educational experiences both in the clinical areas and in places outside the traditional educational establishments. The needs of nursing staff can be divided into two areas when looking at education and plans for the future. Professionally the nurse needs to extend his or her knowledge and bring themselves up to date, helping them deliver the best possible care. Then on a personal level, nurs-

ing staff need to be able to develop themselves and explore the areas of their role that are not usually taught or covered within a set course.

If the nurse wishes to undertake a traditional post-registration course, there are many available today aimed directly at the specialist area and tailored to the needs of the staff who wish to access them. In the area of critical care there are courses available such as the ENB 100 Intensive Care Nursing Course which contains elements that are relevant to many areas other than the intensive care setting. In more recent times as high dependency care has been identified as a speciality and units have developed and been set up around the country, a specific course has become available.

The ENB A75 High Dependency Nursing Course has been designed to address the educational needs of the nursing staff working in this area and help them develop both professionally and personally. This move by the universities to look at the needs of staff within all clinical areas has brought about an influx of courses aimed at nurses from all specialities. Most nurses can feel that there is a course available for them whatever their speciality.

Outside mainline nursing there are a variety of courses and study opportunities that are open and are now seen as valid within the clinical areas. Conferences, seminars and lectures give the opportunity to get away from the clinical area, meet with others and discuss what happens in their own areas. From this, national and international perspectives can be applied to issues that are raised everyday within the high dependency areas.

As more nurses strive for the graduate status that is expected of them, many staff are finding that they can only achieve this by studying outside their working hours and fitting it in part-time. The universities and further education establishments have tried to cater for this with courses being run in the evenings or on one day a week. Open access and distance learning courses have been developed by organizations such as The Royal College of Nursing to help nurses achieve their PREP requirements and learn at their own pace. From a manager's point of view, if staff are updating themselves by attending courses, then the care that they give when they return is more likely to be more current and research-based. Patients and staff will be more satisfied with the care that is being delivered and this can help raise morale within the area. The cost of sending staff out of the area on a 6-month course for example, can be offset against the likelihood of that member of staff staying within the area and increasing the teaching and knowledge of others. If the funding is not available to send staff on these post-registration courses then other alternatives can be considered. There are other ways in which staff can gain knowledge and update themselves and managers have to utilize other methods if they are trying to balance staff going out of the area to undertake a course and the cost that this involves (*see* Table 10.1).

Table 10.1 Available education opportunities

Within the clinical area	Outside the clinical area
Reflective practice	Lectures
Discussions with colleagues	Specialized courses
Private reading	Conferences – national
Personal clinical projects	and international
Teaching/working with	Seminars
new staff	Forums
Group work	Libraries
Visiting staff from	Journals, magazines,
other areas	books
Videos, leaflets and literature	Contacts
Observation	Workshops

One of the great issues involved in planning for the educational needs of staff is the question, when is the right time to send staff on courses in relation to their career and personal development? Looking at traditional post-registration courses it has been usual for a member of staff to be working within an area for up to 5 years before a place on a course has been made available to them. This is too long. Career planning, when used with IPR, can identify educational needs and help when preparing for courses. A traditional career route may once have been:

- Nurse qualifies.
- Works in a clinical area at lowest level.
- Becomes upgraded after 1–3 years.
- Goes on a post-registration course.
- Further promotion.

The problem occurs when nurses feel that their needs are not being addressed and they are waiting for their turn in a long line. A more acceptable route would be perhaps to send the more junior staff on courses to help them consolidate information and retain them within the staffing complement. If a junior nurse accepted a post with the knowledge that they would be going on a recognized course within a set length of time then they can plan to stay and incorporate this in with their own career plans. Looking at the previous way of sending staff on courses, the question could be asked what benefit will the more senior staff gain from going on a course at a later part of their career? They will have gained a vast amount of experience and knowledge within their clinical field and a specialist course in that field may only repeat this. There is some benefit however of staff being allowed out of the area to look at issues more closely and perhaps research an area close to that speciality without the constraints of rostered practice. This would be more relevant to the senior staff who may have already identified issues within their area that may need some further research and study. When staff return from the course it is important not to allow the information and skills to just remain with that individual or wither and die out if not utilized. The dissemination of information following a course can be a very considerable asset to the clinical area. Using that person as a resource both in day-to-day activities and as a formal teacher can enhance the educational environment of the area and improve the quality of care. Other staff who may be debating whether to undertake a course themselves may use that member of staff as adviser for their concerns and questions. This in the long-term, will encourage others to be more

focused in their career planning and may change the whole approach to courses utilization in the staff. Evaluation of a course may reveal that it may not be relevant for that particular area or the skills that are learnt may not be used or updated enough to warrant attendance.

Many post-registration courses now have taught elements to introduce qualified members of staff to the idea of reflective practice. This is an integral part of the student nurse syllabus. The established qualified nurses within the clinical areas also need to be updated as to its uses and benefits. Reflective practice can assist nurses at all levels and areas in the way they look at and approach their working practices. If they can take a step back and consider the way in which they work, highlighting specific incidents, then they can prepare for future events and help others through similar situations. These events can be recorded and used to teach others or kept in the nurse's personal profile to show learning and recognition in the analysis of the job they are doing.

Reflective practice

This aspect of nursing has become very important in recent years and there has been much written on the subject. As mentioned earlier all formal courses now contain sessions on reflective practice and much can be gained by the individual who includes formal reflection in their practice. There has however arisen a certain mystique surrounding reflection upon practice. The literature abounds with articles on the subject and you are recommended to read around the subject of reflection.

Reflection and you

The first thing one must realize is that reflection is not a new invention: indeed to be a nurse, midwife or health visitor you must constantly be

reflecting upon your practice to remain safe and competent. Perhaps the best way to think about reflection is to divide reflection into two, *simple reflection* and *deep reflection*. The first one we have mentioned, that is using professional knowledge, attitudes and skills to react to the many challenges that we face in our daily practice. The second perhaps more hidden type of reflection could be termed deep reflection when we reflect deeply upon an issue or incident. Let us consider the characteristics of these two types:

SIMPLE REFLECTION

- Occurs at all stages of practice.
- Supports planning, implementing and evaluating care.
- Helps us make safe and timely decisions.

DEEP REFLECTION

- Allows us to consider the more hidden dimensions and issues relating to professional practice
- Helps us challenge the issues relating to how we practice.
- Asks searching questions of the individual.
- Supports deeper exploration of the self, increasing one's awareness of personal strengths and weaknesses.

Issues surrounding reflection

Reflecting might be defined as thinking purposefully about clinical practice to gain new insight, ideas and understanding. There are however several issues currently surrounding reflection (Haddock and Bassett, 1997) the most prominent of which are:

1 Finding the time to formally reflect.
2 How does one reflect in an effective way?

The first issue is particularly worrisome to nurses; workloads are very high and time is precious. One needs to understand that the benefits from structured reflection can be great as it may shed light on alternative approaches to care. In addition to this one does not necessarily need to write a large volume to record reflective insights for the personal professional profile (PPP); short notes will suffice, summarizing clearly the key issues and possible ways forward. It may be that part of one's clinical supervision session could form the basis of a reflective passage for the profile. On the second point you can gain guidance by reading around the subject and your skills will develop gradually over time, just as your nursing skills have developed. An evaluation of recent learning may also provide a valuable insight into practice. As you develop your skills relating to reflection you may wish to keep a reflective diary as an aid to your practice. It should be remembered that there are no absolute rights or wrongs, just what suits you. Very often one can crystallize the key issues of an event on the way home in the car and get key words written down when one gets home. There is always some time that you can find to update your profile and soon it will become a key part of your life.

ACTIVITY 10.2

Consider this case study. What are the potential benefits that can be gained from reflecting on the situation. How will you help your colleagues become more proficient at reflecting upon practice?

Case study

A nurse looking after a particularly poorly patient for a major portion of a shift looks back at the care that was given and uses reflective practice to go over the events. With other members of staff, the care that was given is considered and other alternatives are suggested.

Courses can stimulate nurses into undertaking more in depth research in their own area. By doing this, care can be enhanced by expanding the knowledge base of that clinical speciality. If the other staff become involved in research awareness then it becomes apparent how course attendance can affect the whole of the staff including the managers. Staff should also be encouraged to write to the relevant journals about innovation in the workplace. This will help the process of sharing good practice with other areas.

Main points summarizing reflective practice

- Individual's needs must be addressed
- The balance between cost and benefit has to be made
- Educational input can help in recruitment and retention of staff
- Decisions need to be made regarding when to send people on courses
- Educational input can stimulate further study and research
- Courses have to be relevant to the person and the clinical area
- Better use can be made of resources if information is disseminated after a course of study
- In-service training can address some of nurses' educational needs

Career pathways – working conditions

When looking at what nurses want from their role and how to plan for the future, it is important to take into account what is going on within the clinical area at that time. New policies and legislation affect the work carried out and how the people doing the work are feeling too. The reduction of junior doctors' hours has had a great impact on the role of the nurse and has encouraged the extension to their scope of practice, in some cases to take on several of the previously exclusive roles of medical staff. This whole atmosphere of change within the health service has allowed nurses to see new opportunities within this framework and help them plan for their own progression through the roles. Specialist roles are emerging as a response to need. These new roles are being taken on by nurses to both aid the direct patient care and help the other members of the healthcare team. To plan for such moves and changes within nursing, there must be guidelines created to help with this progression and secure both funding and educational provision. If these are not in place then nurses run the risk of being exploited in positions that may not be beneficial to the nurse or the patient in the long-term. Castledine (1997) warns of nurses achieving senior posts without the necessary qualifications or skills and that removing the clinical link aspect from senior nurses can lead to a distancing from the workforce. He advocates that a common career pathway be introduced into nursing to recognize the route to specialist roles and allow others to follow.

An example of a common career pathway

Castledine (1997) also states that the use of such varied titles in nursing can only lead to confusion and should be halted if nurses are to gain any credibility. The prolific range of titles that are being used by nurses who have undertaken some study or gained experience causes diversion to the progression of nurses as a working group. He suggests that a standardization of the terminology will avoid confusion within nursing, helping all who come into contact with nurses understand why people have these different roles. In the critical care areas of nursing there are some unofficially set pathways to follow for a structured career plan. These include gaining a grounding of knowledge within the area before going on to do a post-registration courses in this area. Promotion or progression into associated roles then follows and further advancement can be made with the right experience and educational input. Career progression must be considered in relation to the pay structure that is in place at the time. Nurses will be more prepared to undertake study and research in the area of critical care if they are rewarded by a pay-scale rise when they return. However since the introduction of the clinical grading structure in Britain it can be said that there have been limitations placed on movements between jobs and specialities. If the option on a move to a different speciality includes a drop in grade and pay, then the nurses involved are more likely to remain where they are. This can lead to the stagnation of staff who would have normally moved into other areas but are now afraid to for fear of losing their grade. In some areas a common pay spine has been introduced and the job that is being done is rewarded at that level. Whichever system is in use, emphasis must be placed on the flexibility for nurses to achieve what is in their personal career goals alongside their role and responsibilities. The extension of roles within the framework has to be supported so nurses do not feel that they are the cheaper option to doctors and that their role is valid and worthwhile. Many nurses within the critical care environment can recognize that by extending their role they give a more holistic and focused care, not having to call a doctor for the things that they are trained to do.

The United Kingdom Central Council (UKCC) has stated that any extension to a nurse's role must be accompanied by training to ensure the standards and competency elements are upheld. If a nurse is not happy to undertake these roles or feels that the training was not adequate, then they are duty bound to report this and not undertake any role that they feel they are not prepared for. The UKCC's document 'Guidelines for Professional Practice' (1996) recognizes that many nurses are taking on other roles from the medical staff and that they need guidance and support to help them in this role. For example, it observes that more nurses are undertaking minor operations and gives direct guidance on consent, legal and ethical issues. It reiterates that nurses must make their concerns known about all aspects of their work including their own ability to undertake these extended roles. There has been some debate surrounding the legality of nurses undertaking the extended roles and some discrepanices have emerged which have worried some nursing writers. Tingle (1997) looks at both the medical and nursing bodies and their opinions of nurses taking on more medical roles. The UKCC assumes that nurses, when undertaking these roles, have a degree of autonomy and power, but this is not reflected in the view from the medical bodies. Nurses when looking at the roles that they are to do must be aware of their position and the support network that is in place to help and guide them if the situation arises. With this atmosphere of change, it can be difficult for nurses to look at

their role and make objective decisions about what they are doing now and what they intend to do in the future. Working conditions and roles are ever changing; care has to be taken to ensure that they are well-prepared for the new role they take on. The elements that shape the decision making process for nurses must include the following factors:

- Nature of the specialist clinical area
- The availability of educational opportunities
- The extended or adjusted roles that come with the change
- The support mechanisms in place
- The pay structure
- Common career pathways
- Future promotion prospects

In the past, nurses would be looking to get a balance of clinical experience before settling to one speciality. Although this may be true to a certain extent today, more nurses appear to be aiming for the speciality that they want and applying themselves to it with the aim of gaining educational and financial rewards later.

Conclusion

The systems that are set up to support staff within the clinical areas must take into account a great many concepts and key issues. Nursing is very different in 2000, with the advent of high dependency care throughout the health service, greater emphasis upon day-care surgery and a steady increase in the medical specialities that are offered by the health service. The role of the nurse has changed with more complex and technical aspects of caring emerging. Many nurses are using these opportunities to expand their roles and develop innovative care for the benefit of their patients. Because of this nurses will require a more structured approach to the way they are developed and supported in the future. The recognition of stress

and stress-related illnesses within nursing has widened the debate on these issues and shown that there is a real need to use clinical supervision to reduce the negative aspects of stress at work. This has in turn helped break the stigma that is associated with stress and shown that it is not a sign of weakness to admit that the job is stressful. Instead it is essential that nurses are proactive at creating systems that support us well into the 21st century. The concepts that are being introduced into nursing now and those in the future have to be relevant and be seen to be adaptable for all nurses. The use of rigid structures when dealing with members of staff in a variety of different clinical areas will be seen to have only a limited success in comparison to a transitional approach to management. Within the frameworks of clinical supervision, preceptorship and individual performance review relationships can be enhanced and built upon to the benefit of all.

References

Butterworth, T. and Faugier, J. 1992 *Clinical supervision and mentorship in nursing*, 1st edn. London: Chapman & Hall

Cox, T. 1975 *Stress*. London: Macmillan Press.

Castledine, G. 1997 Framework for a clinical career structure in nursing. *British Journal of Nursing* 6(5), 264–70.

Haddock, J. and Bassett, C. 1997 Nurses perceptions of reflective practice. *Nursing Standard* 11(32), 39–42.

Handy, J. 1990 *Occupational stress in a caring profession*, 1st edn, pp. 13–26. UK: Avebury.

Kramer, M. 1974 *Reality shock (why nurses leave nursing)*, 1st edn. St Louis: Mosby.

Lader, D. 1995 *Qualified nurses, midwives and health visitors*, 1st edn, pp. 20–26. London: HMSO.

Tingle, J. 1996 Expanded role of the nurse: accountability confusion. *British Journal of Nursing* 6(17), 1011–13.

UKCC 1994 *The future of professional practice*. London: UKCC.

UKCC 1995 *Clinical supervision for nursing and health visiting*. London: UKCC.

UKCC 1996 *Guidelines for professional practice*. London: UKCC.

Further reading

Stress management – recognition – burnout

Bailey, R. and Clarke, M. 1991 *Stress and coping in nursing*, 1st edn. London: Chapman & Hall.

Bond, M. 1986 *Stress and self awareness*, 1st edn, pp. 1–13. London: Heinemann Nursing.

Cole, A. 1992 High anxiety. *Nursing Times* 88(12), 26–30.

Farrington, A. 1995 Stress and nursing. *British Journal of Nursing* 4(10), 574–8.

Farrington, A. 1997 Strategies for reducing stress and burnout in nursing. *British Journal of Nursing* 6(1), 44–50.

Hamilton, P.M. 1996 *Realities of contemporary nursing*, 2nd edn, pp. 335–66. USA: Addison-Wesley.

Jackson, I. 1997 Coping with stress. *Nursing Times* 93(29), 31–2.

Kennedy, P. and Grey, N. 1997. High pressure areas. *Nursing Times* 93(29), 26–8.

Owen, S. 1989 Strategies for stress. *Nursing Times* 85(37), 38–9.

Tschudin, V. 1990 Support yourself. *Nursing Times* 86(12), 40–2.

Wheeler, H.H. 1997 A review of nurse occupational stress research: 1. *British Journal of Nursing* 6(11), 642–5.

Wheeler, H.H. 1997 Nurse occupational stress research 2: definition and conceptualization. *British Journal of Nursing* 6(12), 710–13.

Wheeler, H.H. 1997 Nurse occupational stress research 3: A model of stress for research. *British Journal of Nursing* 6(16), 944–9.

Management issues

Department of Health 1989 *Survey of nurses in high technology care*, 1st edn. London: Department of Health

Dodwell, M. and Lathlean, J. 1989 *Management*

and professional development for nurses, 1st edn, pp. 52–70. London: Harper & Row.

Macleod-Nicol, N. and Walker, S. 1991 *Basic management for staff nurses*, 1st edn, pp. 134–50. London: Chapman & Hall.

Seccombe, I., Patch, A. and Stock, J. 1994 *Workloads, pay and morale of qualified nurses in 1994*, 1st edn. Brighton: Institute of Manpower Studies.

Stewart, R. 1989 *Leading in the NHS*, 1st edn. London: Macmillan.

Traynor, M.G. 1995 Job satisfaction and morale of nurses in NHS trusts. *Nursing Times* **91**(26), 42–5.

Woodroffe, I. 1990 Inhuman terms. *Nursing Times* **86**(23), 52–3.

Preceptorship

Armitage, P. and Burnard, P. 1991 Mentors or preceptors? Narrowing the theory practice gap. *Nurse Education Today* **11**, 225–9.

Bain, L. 1996 Preceptorship: A review of the literature. *Journal of Advanced Nursing* **24**, 104–7.

Brennan, A. 1993 Preceptorship: is it a workable concept? *Nursing Standard* **7**(52), 34–6.

Burke, L.M. 1994 Preceptorship and post registration nurse education. *Nurse Education Today* **14**, 60–6.

Cerinus, M. and Ferguson, C. 1993 A guiding light. *Nursing Times* **89**(29), 40–6.

Cerinus, M. and Ferguson, C. 1994 Preparing nurses for preceptorship. *Nursing Standard* **8**(36), 34–8.

Kennard, J. 1991 A helping hand? *Nursing Times* **87**(49), 39–40.

Lee, S.J. 1991 Guidelines for the role of preceptor. *Nursing Standard* **6**(6), 28–30.

Clinical supervision

Bassett, C.C. 1999 Clinical supervision in perioperative care. *British Journal of Theatre Nursing* **9**, 267–302.

Burrow, S. 1995 Supervision: clinical development or management control? *British Journal of Nursing* **4**(15), 879–82.

Farrington, A. 1995 Models of clinical supervision. *British Journal of Nursing* **4**(15), 876–8.

Faugier, J. and Butterworth, T. 1994 *Clinical supervision: a position paper*. School of Nursing Studies, University of Manchester.

Fowler, J. 1995 Nurses' perceptions of the elements of good supervision. *Nursing Times* **91**(22), 33–7.

Fowler, J. 1996 The organisation of clinical supervision within the nursing profession: A review of the literature. *Journal of Advanced Nursing* **23**(3), 471–8.

Fowler, J. 1996 Clinical supervision: what do you do after saying hello? *British Journal of Nursing* **5**(6), 382–5.

Kohner, N. 1994 *Clinical supervision in practice*, 1st edn. London: King's Fund Centre.

Thomas, B. and Reid, J. 1995 Multidisciplinary clinical supervision. *British Journal of Nursing* **4**(15), 883–5.

Wolsey, P. and Leach, L. 1997 Clinical supervision: a hornet's nest? *Nursing Times* **93**(44), 24–7.

Individual performance review

Atkins, C. and Haigh, C. 1992 Individual performance review – meeting staff needs. *British Journal of Theatre Nursing* **2**(9), 18–20.

Basford, P. and Downie, C. 1991 How to use individual performance review. *Nursing Times* **87**(27), 59.

Dodwell, M. and Lathlean, J. 1989 *Management and professional development for nurses*, 1st edn. London: Harper & Row.

Educational needs

Charles, M. 1982 Continuing education in nursing: whose responsibility? *Nurse Education Today* **2**(1), 5–11.

Chiarella, M. 1991 Developing the credibility of continuing education, *Nursing Education Today* **10**(1), 70–73.

Cormack, D.F.S. 1990 *Developing your career in nursing*, 1st edn. London: Chapman & Hall.

Durgahee, T. 1990 Directions in post-basic education. *Senior Nurse* **10**(7), 15–20.

Hogston, R. 1995 Nurse's perceptions of the impact of continuing professional education on the quality of nursing care. *Journal of Advanced Nursing* **22**(3), 586–93.

James, C. 1995 Professional education – who learns what? *Nurse Education Today* **15**(3), 161–3.

Miller, C. Tomlinson, A. and Jones, M. 1994 *Learning styles and facilitating reflection*, 1st edn. London: E.N.B.

Newall, R. 1995 *Developing your career in nursing*, 1st edn. London: Cassell.

Nugent, A.B. 1990 The need for continuing professional education for nurses. *Journal of Advanced Nursing* 15(4), 471–7.

Perry, L. 1995 Continuing professional education: Luxury or necessity? *Journal of Advanced Nursing* 21(4), 766–71.

Sykes, M. 1985 *Licensed to practice*, 1st edn. London: Baillière Tindall.

Working conditions – career aspects

Andrews, M. 1996 Using reflection to develop clinical expertise. *British Journal of Nursing* 5(8), 508–13.

Bradby, M. and Soothill, K. 1997 Management of leisure time by prospective nurses. *British Journal of Nursing* 6(5), 285–9.

Castledine, G. 1996 UKCC's New Guidelines for Practice. *British Journal of Nursing* 5(13), 824.

Conway, J. 1994 Reflection, the art and science of nursing and the theory–practice gap. *British Journal of Nursing* 3(3), 114–18.

Hallam-Jones, D. 1993 *Career check*, 1st edn. London: Scutari.

Helmer, F. and McKnight, P. 1989 Management strategies to minimise nursing turnover. *Health Care Management Review* 14(1), 73–80.

Hunt, G. and Wainwright, P. 1994 *Expanding the role of the nurse*, 1st edn. Oxford: Blackwell.

11 Ethical issues

Pam Sutherland

Introduction

This chapter will explore some of the ethical dilemmas that the nurse working with seriously ill and injured patients has to deal with in his or her daily work. It will consider theoretical explanations of the differing ethical views but perhaps more importantly it will apply ethics to actual practical problems.

Blackburn (1994) described ethics as 'the study of the concepts involved in practical reasoning: good, right, duty, obligation'. So, when caring for the critically ill patient in an ethical way, this chapter will try to explore ways in which the nurse can demonstrate practical reasoning which brings about good, both for the patient and the worker and which fulfils the professional obligation of duty

of care. Initially it is important to develop a clear understanding of ethical terms, principles and theories. Then the role of the nurse will be considered with respect to obtaining consent, involvement in research and in preserving confidentiality. 'End of life' issues which perhaps cause nurses most difficulty will then be explored. Specifically the topics of euthanasia, resuscitation decisions, withdrawal of treatment, and the value and place for 'living wills' will be examined. These will be illustrated by the use of case studies, around which the specific issues which arise can be discussed.

As nurses we are bound by the professional code of conduct to primarily act always in the best interests of the patient, yet sometimes it seems difficult to know how to act in the best possible manner. The deliberations we make about what action would be the most moral course to take is at times extremely difficult. This is made even more complicated when the potential interventions may cause harm to our patient, although the intended outcome is good. In healthcare, nurses often have to act quickly; there is no choice, because not to act would cause harm, even though to carry out an act may also cause harm. This is called the principle of 'double effect', which will be discussed later. There are a number of theories which would determine our approach to such a problem. These may be called 'the end justifies the means' ethics and 'natural law' ethics (Rumbold, 1983). The first considers the consequences of the proposed action or intervention, the second appeals to the belief that the right course of action is self-evident.

An example of the first theory is called 'consequentialism' which considers that: 'The value of an action derives entirely from the value of its consequences.'

Another way of expressing it is that the proposed action will bring about the most good for the most number of people. A similar theory is 'utilitarianism' in that it achieves the most happiness for the most people and owes its origins to John Stuart Mill (1806–1873), who based his work on the thoughts of Jeremy Bentham (1748–1832).

The second theory is called 'deontology' and is based on the work of Kant (1724–1804). It is concerned with conforming to one's own concept of duty which promotes equality and thus the action is seen to be intrinsically good. The first two theories seek to create a good ending, the final theory seeks to follow self-evident paths in which the object of the interventions is deemed to be an end in itself.

This probably seems complex, but perhaps what will help you differentiate between them is the thought: 'who benefits?'. With consequentialism or utilitarianism, it is necessary that people other than the patient benefit from the intervention: with deontology, others may benefit incidentally but not necessarily. This oversimplifies the issues, but will help clarify the basic concepts.

Some healthcare workers use models to aid decision making and you can do so with ethical issues. Just as with nursing, there are many models. Perhaps the most common model in use is the one based on the work of Beauchamp and Childress (1989). This provides a framework for decision making that is relatively simple and easy to remember in moments of stress and pressure. It has four components:

- Beneficence (the obligation to provide benefits and balance benefits against risks)
- Non-maleficence (the obligation to avoid the causation of harm)
- Respect for autonomy (the obligation to respect the decision making capacities of autonomous persons)
- Justice (obligations of fairness in the distribution of benefits and risks)
Beauchamp (1994: 3)

There are many criticisms of these principles, ranging from the fact that the way they are used could be biased by cultural and social norms, to how they could be used in a ritualistic manner without reflection and consideration and also, perhaps with more reason, that they do not give you definitive courses of action. However, accepting them as useful starting points for discussion but not to be considered as absolutes, can be useful. They can be revised as and when necessary and are useful tools to use when considering ethical interactions or decision making.

The 'ethical' nurse's role

This is a difficult role to define. The Code of Professional Conduct demonstrates the way that the profession, through the UKCC, believes that the nurse should act. But one should ask the question as to whether that is sufficient. The Code expects the nurse to serve the interests of the patient, society, justify public trust and confidence and uphold the good standing of the profession. There would appear to be the possibility of an inherent conflict within these expectations, in that the patient's interests might not be the same as the those of society, nor might acting in the patient's best interests necessarily justify public trust or confidence, and possibly not enhance the reputation of the profession, from some viewpoints. The general tone of the Code would appear to prioritize the patient's needs and interests but not say so specifically. Thus the professional nurse would appear to be eternally juggling these interests. Whatever decisions the nurse comes to, concerning his/her interactions with the patient, there must be a clear demonstration of the processes whereby those decisions were reached and the basis on which they were made. Examples of how these may be reached follow.

CONSENT

ACTIVITY 11.1

Seventeen-year-old Theresa was admitted to your ward following a road traffic accident. She is semi-conscious and confused. She becomes tearful, refusing treatment and wants to go home. How should you act?

There are a number of issues to be considered in this instance, both ethical and legal. These would be issues such as:

- Competence to give consent
- Ability to refuse to give consent
- Informed consent
- Voluntariness and research
- Confidentiality

In an emergency a doctor is allowed to act in a manner she or he considers to be in the patient's best interests to meet an emergency need, without necessarily obtaining consent, but in such a case as this, the initial emergency has been dealt with and the patient has been admitted to the ward for observation. Now Theresa is attempting to carry through a decision which could put her life at risk. How should you act? What does your Code of Professional Conduct say about how you should act?

You are required by the Code of Professional Conduct (UKCC, 1992) to

act always in such a manner as to promote and safeguard the interests and well-being of patients and client.

So you must determine what will promote and safeguard the best interests of this patient. Thus there are a number of questions that you must ask yourself concerning this patient, such as:

ACTIVITY 11.2

What will promote and safeguard the best interests of Theresa?
What would do her the most harm or the most good?
Does she have the knowledge or ability to make such a decision?
Write down your answers to these questions

Competence to give consent

ACTIVITY 11.3

Think back to the four principles model for ethical decision making proposed by Beauchamp and Childress (1989).
  What were they?

- Beneficence
- Non-maleficence
- Respect for autonomy
- Justice

Respect for autonomy is central to the concept of empowering patients to take appropriate responsibility for their own health and wellbeing. But in this instance one must consider whether Theresa is able to understand the potential harm to her own health should she discharge herself and be suffering from an ongoing head injury, such as a subdural haematoma. The nurse's initial role would be one of informing Theresa and her family of the potential risk as well as explaining her general care. Beneficence is generally perceived as the need to do good towards another. In

healthcare workers' terms, in this instance, that means to work in a way which brings about the most good for Theresa. But what does this mean? What would bring about the good for this patient? Would it be to let Theresa discharge herself or would it be to insist that she remain in the hospital? The problem with this would be if she had a head injury which could lead to harm occurring to her at a later time. To deny her autonomy on the basis of her age would be problematic (Harris, 1985), but it would be more reasonable based on the basis of impaired competence to understand the potential risk, due to the injury. The person who could decide this would be the doctor, so the nurse would need to inform the relevant doctor of the situation, and give him or her the data concerning the present neurological, cardiovascular and respiratory status of Theresa. The doctor would consider the health needs of Theresa and decide whether to insist on her continued hospitalization or not. Such a decision would be made on the basis of Theresa's potential health risk and her competence to understand the consequences of leaving the hospital and the potential risk to her continued wellbeing.

Ability to refuse treatment

ACTIVITY 11.4

The Children's Act 1989 allows for a minor, under certain circumstances to give consent for treatment. Does it allow a minor to refuse treatment?

As a 17-year-old and thus still technically a minor, Theresa would not be able to refuse treatment if it was considered in her best interests and necessary, according to the professional in charge of her. Such a decision is always difficult to make. It

becomes easier if Theresa's family are in agreement that she should remain in hospital. However, if they agree with Theresa and wish her to be discharged home, the doctor must once again determine what is in the best interest of the patient, based upon his/her professional assessment of Theresa's health, the potential risk to her health and Theresa's, or her family's, competence to make such a decision. If the doctor is convinced that Theresa's health would be seriously compromised by her discharge, he or she could apply to a magistrate to overrule Theresa and her family's decision on the basis of Theresa's best interests and mental competence to make such a decision in the light of the possible head injury. It might be argued that the doctor has a duty of care towards the patient and would need to consider the foreseeable risk to the patient due to the accident and balance this against the potential hazard of denying Theresa her freedom. Should harm come to the patient through allowing her to discharge herself, the healthcare staff might be considered to be negligent of their duty of care, unless it could be demonstrated, through documentation, that the risks had been fully explained to both Theresa and her family and that they still insisted on Theresa being allowed to leave the hospital. It would be wise for the healthcare staff to ensure that both parents and Theresa sign a form declaring that they have chosen to take such action against medical advice, having had all the potential risks fully explained to them in words that they could understand. Should such forms not be completed, the healthcare worker would be wise to ensure that another healthcare worker was present for all such conversations and fully document these conversations and the actions taken and the rationale for such actions.

The nurse's role is to work with the other healthcare professionals to avoid the causation of harm, i.e. minimize harm (Seedhouse, 1988). Thus, the actions of the nurse would be to continue neurological, cardiovascular and respiratory observations, reporting any significant deviations to the appropriate person, until the time of discharge. The nurse should continue to spend time with the patient and family, explaining what is happening and why and answering their questions to the best of his/her ability. A vital element of the nurse's caring role would be the keeping of appropriate records of actions, conversations and decision making processes, so that future actions of other staff could be based upon appropriate and adequate information. To maintain inadequate records could be considered an act of negligence on the part of the nurse and thus he or she would be failing to comply with clauses 1 and 2 of the Code of Professional Conduct (UKCC, 1992). Such a failure could be seen to be potentially detrimental to patient care, putting them at risk through poor communication, and, should harm come to the patient through such an omission, the nurse could be deemed negligent of their duty of care (Stokes,

1997). Justice would not seem to be a relevant principle to be considered at this moment unless Theresa was seen to be treated in a way that was dissimilar to other cases, for example denied appropriate investigations because of cost, or a bed due to shortages of appropriate beds or staff.

As becomes obvious through discussion of this case, using the four principles as a decision making model means balancing the idea of what constitutes the patient's good with the distribution of risk. To deny Theresa her autonomy must be done on the basis that it was necessary to achieve good (beneficence) and that it would minimize harm (non-maleficence). Deontologists could perhaps consider that to retain Theresa within hospital until the risk had reached an acceptable level was self-evidently the correct course of action, unless the reason for Theresa's desire to discharge herself was overwhelming and intrinsically sufficient to outweigh the potential health risk to Theresa. Alternatively, a deontologist could argue that the concept of autonomy was so important that to deny it would be immoral. Respect for autonomy would then be seen as a categorical imperative, a duty never to be disobeyed (Kant, 1785). Certainly many ethicists place great emphasis on this element in an ethical interaction. Harris (1985) spent considerable time exploring justification for denying autonomy and largely felt that it was a serious step to take, but that under certain circumstances it could be justifiable.

A consequentialist would perhaps consider that it would achieve the most good for the most number of people to deny Theresa her autonomy in this instance and thus would only respect her autonomy when it could be seen that such a course of action achieved the most good for the most number of people. Similarly, a utilitarian would look for the solution which would bring the most happiness to the most number of people. If there was sufficient reason to consider that respecting Theresa's autonomy would have achieved the greatest happiness for the greatest number of people, then the chosen course of action would have been to respect her autonomy and allow her to discharge herself. However, any action which could appear to undermine the concept of duty of care would be perceived as very dubious both by the law and the profession, because both expect more of those regarded as having specialized knowledge and a position of responsibility as a consequence of that knowledge. The very nature of Theresa's condition or injury could be considered sufficient to deny her competence to decide and the law acknowledges that not all parents act in the best interests of their children. Consequently, it would be likely that if reason and discussion failed, the doctor could seek and receive permission from the magistrate to retain Theresa in hospital until such time as it was deemed safe for her to be discharged home, regardless of the wishes of both Theresa and her family.

Informed consent

Another aspect of consent which concerns nurses or healthcare workers is the need for what is called 'informed consent'.

'it is difficult to measure consent, and the degree to which it is really informed'
Tschudin (1989)

How do we know when we have given sufficient information to determine that consent given is informed? It is always difficult to judge the level of understanding of a patient or their family. To assume knowledge or lack of it, denies the patient or significant others the opportunity to demonstrate their understanding or their needs. Kant (1788) based his deontological theories on the hypothetical concept of equality. Thus with patients and their families this means sharing information with them to the level they wish and which enables them to make sound decisions. When working with patients and others it is useful to base information-giving on what is already known and the questions and needs already demonstrated. Naturally, this means finding out what patients and their families know or want to know. This enables you to move them forward from their present level of knowledge, or identify gaps in their understanding which they want or need to be filled. For many nurses this could be difficult if there is not an agreed policy within the organization concerning information-giving, that is, who tells what to whom and where that is recorded. If patients or relatives ask questions not within the domain of the nurse to answer, then it is reasonable to answer that this information is normally given by the sister, doctor or whoever. The nurse's role is then to inform the relevant individual of the desire of the family or patient to know. Such policies then empower both the patient and the information giver to talk together in a meaningful way. However, the absence of such a policy may disempower both patients, their relatives and healthcare workers. The absence of such a policy could lead to the dissatisfaction of both patients and healthcare workers in their attempts to work effectively and consistently together. The presence and knowledge of appropriate policy documents enable healthcare workers to work effectively, consistently, and in a manner which demonstrates coherence in the delivery of healthcare.

Having determined what is necessary for Theresa and her family to know, they must be told in an appropriate way, using language that they understand and in a manner which enables them to ask whatever questions they wish to express and in an environment which does not inhibit them. In other words to be treated as you would wish to be treated.

From time to time patients and/or their families abdicate their responsibilities, asking not to be told the details and giving 'carte blanche' permission. This may be voluntarily chosen but puts the onus on the healthcare worker to ensure that they continue to act in a manner which empowers the patient or the family, never assuming consent, and which continues to attempt to minimize harm and looks for a changing attitude as the individual's stress and defence mechanisms allow. Obviously such decisions need to be clearly recorded, both to ensure appropriate continuity of care and to record such decisions in the event of future disagreement.

Voluntariness and research

In order to include a human being in a research exercise, permission should be sought and gained, so the same rules of consent apply as with all healthcare interventions. The consent should be given voluntarily. If Theresa was judged competent to discharge herself then she is competent to give consent to be involved in research or to refuse to participate in research. However, if her competence to give consent was called into question, due to the nature of her potential head injury, careful consideration would need to be given as to her appropriateness to be included in the research. Competence to give consent has always been a knotty problem in the area of research. It would be useful to consider whether her involvement within the research would do her good and could be demonstrated to be in her best interests. If not, should she be involved? The nurse's code of conduct expects the nurse to act as the patient advocate and thus the role of the nurse in this instance would be as a representative seeking to minimize any harm from the treatment received by Theresa whilst in that nurse's care. There is the possibility of parental permission being given for Theresa to be involved in the research, but when the research involves unproved treatment, there is the possibility that such permission would be invalid. In the event of Theresa's' incompetence to decide, then her family would need to be given sufficient clear and unambiguous information to make a decision as to what they should do to act in the best interests of their daughter. In the absence of a family, then the nurse would have to act as a clear advocate for the patient in his/her care. It could be that if the nurse believed that the family were not being given sufficient information, or had insufficient understanding of that information, to make a safe decision on behalf of Theresa, that he or she would need to consider how to act in Theresa's best interests and discuss these issues further with the appropriate healthcare personnel.

In the event that Theresa's competence is such that she can choose to discharge herself, then her refusal to comply with such a request to be involved with research would need to be respected. Not to do so would cause harm and would be treating her with less than justice. If the reason for Theresa not being allowed to be discharged is linked, not to her healthcare needs, but to the needs of a researcher to incorporate her in an ongoing study, then a deontologist could argue that there is no justification for denial of Theresa's autonomy. If Theresa should fit the profile required to contribute to an ongoing area of research then she may be included if she has given permission, having had a reasonable and clear explanation of the research, its possible effects upon her and any possible side effects that might be experienced and the clear indication that she has the right to say no to participation, or withdraw from the study at any time. Having been presented with this information in such a manner as will allow her to make an unpressurized and clear decision, based on all the facts, then Theresa can elect to remain in the hospital and participate in the research programme or follow through with her discharge plans. This would not only respect her autonomy, it would act to promote her wellbeing, minimizing harm and treating her with justice.

The nature of the research format could be of considerable importance, as could the nature of the research. For example, some forms of research take the form of a randomized clinical trial (RCT). This means that those directly involved in giving the care do not know the exact form of treatment that will being given to which patient. Naturally healthcare professionals have preferred forms of treatment for specific patient needs, but in the event of an RCT it should not be possible to identify if such preferred treatment is to be given or not. It could be that Theresa received a placebo, a drug with no effect, for good or evil, in other words to receive no active intervention at all. This means that the healthcare professional cannot be sure, nor assume, that Theresa is receiving the care which, in the professional's opinion, is the very best to achieve her full recovery. In the light of this, Kennedy (1991) advised that patients should be given sufficient information to make an informed choice. They should be told that they are to be involved in a randomized control trial. The risks and alternatives must be made clear and the fact that they are not obliged to take part must also be stated. Most importantly they must know.

- that they can withdraw at any time;
- that the doctor may give treatment running counter to his/her preferences;

- that the doctor might ignore trends indicating that a certain treatment is preferable;
- that the patient might be exposed to procedures in addition to the normal which they might not like;
- that the patient's stay in hospital might be extended beyond the normal;
- that the patient might only receive a placebo, i.e. no treatment at all.

In the light of this it could be possible that no patient in their right mind would be involved in such a trial, unless they are uncommonly altruistic.

Sometimes the research is testing one theoretical approach to achieve recovery against another, perhaps less highly favoured or even controversial approach. Surely if the healthcare professional is acting in the best interests of the patient, attempting to achieve the most good, then they should be giving the very best of care, rather than one less demonstrably effective. A consequentialist might argue that Theresa's participation in the trial would be of the highest good in that it would bring about the increase of the total knowledge of mankind, benefiting humanity, even though it might be detrimental to her recovery.

Confidentiality

ACTIVITY 11.6

In such a case as Theresa, with whom would it be appropriate to share information?
Write these down and compare them with the ensuing discussion.

Confidentiality is defined as: 'To trust another with private and personal information about yourself'. Confidentiality is a significant matter. If the person to whom that information is given is a nurse, midwife or health visitor, the patient or client has a right to believe that this information given in confidence, will only be used for the purpose for which it was given and will not be

released to others without their permission. (UKCC, 1996).

The original Hippocratic oath, to which doctors in this country ascribe, can be translated:

Whatsoever I see or hear in the course of my practice, or outside my practice in social intercourse, that ought never to be published abroad. Emson (1988: 87)

This indicates that information given with the understanding of the protection of confidentiality should be available to no one without the express permission of the individual themselves. In more recent years the understanding has been expanded to include the idea that any information given to the healthcare worker by the patient or family is divulged only to those involved directly in the patient's care and the information given should be sufficient to ensure appropriate care and no more, unless the patient gives permission for other information to be shared. This is an interesting expansion and one which be will referred to later.

ACTIVITY 11.7

How do you store and convey information about patients in your care?
How could others gain access to this information:

- legitimately
- illegitimately?

Write these down and consider them in the light of the ensuing discussion.

Staff should ensure that information remains confidential, whether in writing, in the patient's notes, on computer, or by word of mouth. One of the commonest problems is telephone communications. Healthcare workers receive telephone inquiries every day concerning patients and it is easy to forget that you do not know the identity of the enquirer or even whether they are being honest. Again, appropriate records enable effective identification. The patient or family could clearly indicate who should be informed and to what extent, and this be recorded in the patient's notes. Routine hospital policies usually give appropriate ways to deal with requests for information from the media, with enquirers being put through to designated personnel. Should Theresa or her family wish to notify the media for any reason, then that is their privilege. If they are to be treated with justice and their autonomy respected, then they have the right to tell whatever they wish to whomever they will. However, healthcare workers should be aware of hospital policies concerning the presence of media on hospital grounds and of talking with them. Few trusts condone staff interviews with the media unless they have already given permission for this to occur and

have carefully considered the content of the interview prior to it taking place. It is unlikely that even Theresa or her parents would be allowed to conduct an interview with the media on hospital grounds, on the basis that it could cause distress to other patients, or lead to problems in patient care.

Many cases of breaches of confidentiality occur through thoughtlessness. Conversations about work in public places can lead to such breaches, so nurses must remember clause 10 of their Code of Professional Conduct (1992) which says they must:

Protect all confidential information concerning patients and clients obtained in the course of professional practice and make disclosures only with consent where required by the order of a court or where you can justify disclosure in the wider public interest;

Gossiping on a bus or in a bar would be perceived to be an abuse of your privileged position (clause 9) and if harm should come to the patient as a direct result of your breaching confidentiality then you could be held negligent of your duty of care.

Some authors would argue that confidentiality is a fading concept in the real world. Emson (1988) argued that within societies who derive their law from English origins, there is a decreasing emphasis on the absoluteness of the concept of confidentiality. Some information has to be given to appropriate healthcare workers for them to give optimum care, but he argued that the more who knew, the more easily confidential information reaches those that it shouldn't.

The information concerning Theresa, her condition and healthcare needs is relevant only to the healthcare staff, except when it is necessary and in the patient's best interests to pass it to another, for example, the court to whom the doctor applied for an order to ensure that Theresa remained in hospital.

In the environment where Theresa is prepared to put her life at risk and discharge herself from the hospital, others have to be told. The hospital solicitor would be the first person informed as the healthcare workers approached the law for help. Should the help of the courts be advised then the judge would be informed, so the private information concerning Theresa would gradually spread from officials and decision-makers to secretaries and/or clerks.

There are some laws which require the doctor to inform appropriate bodies, such as those concerning communicable diseases. However, such information is not for public consumption, nor even for other close family members to know, unless it is required for them to know. Information concerning such infections as measles and chicken pox are usually notified to individuals if they are considered to be at risk of infection, but in the case of sexually transmitted diseases this rarely occurs. In fact, if the disease is diagnosed within a genitourinary clinic, the diagnosis may not be passed on to another without the patient giving express consent. The Venereal Disease Act (1974) requires every health authority to ensure that all information which makes it possible to identify such a disorder must be removed or disguised in such a way as to ensure patient anonymity.

Perhaps the onset of acquired immune deficiency syndrome (AIDS) has brought this issue to greater media attention. Certainly in the case where a healthcare worker attempted to inform a local newspaper that two doctors were HIV-positive because they felt that it was in the best interest of the public, it was found that the law did not agree and the information was not allowed to be released by the newspaper which was fined £10 000 for contempt of a court order (X v Y and another 1988 2 All ER 648). The court felt that AIDS should be covered by the Venereal Disease Act.

There are six exceptions to maintaining confidentiality (Dimond, 1995):

- If the patient gave consent
- If it could be demonstrated to be in the best interests of the patient
- If a court ordered the release of information
- If there was a statutory duty to release the information
- If it was in the interests of the public
- police

Protecting the confidentiality of a patient is perhaps not as easy to do as at first might be thought. It is however essential that the nurse caring for the highly dependent patient maintains as much as possible confidentiality. This must be so upon the basis of respect for the patient's autonomy, promoting patient/doctor contact, and of benefit to society as a whole. It can be argued that an agreed degree of confidentiality is necessary for the development of a therapeutic relationship, but the level should be agreed between both parties rather than presumed. There is always the opportunity for a patient to retain some information, because they did not wish it to be disclosed. It is their right, and giving the patient the opportunity to make the decision would be a more ethical approach. The risk to their health would be explained and then it would be a risk that they would choose or not.

To interact in an ethical manner with the patient, the nurse must consider how their interactions will minimize harm towards the patient and be seen to do good for the patient. The nurse must also act in a way that would preserve justice, especially if the patient could not have given permission for information to be released. Warwick (1989) argued that the approach whereby the patient determined what could or should be released would 'increase personal privacy and personal autonomy', and argued against the social and legal undermining of confidentiality

END OF LIFE ISSUES

Mr James, aged 87, was admitted to the high dependency unit complaining of severe abdominal pain, haematemesis and jaundice. It was clear from his records and the history he gave that he had cancer of the stomach with secondary spread to the liver and peritoneum. He was accompanied by his daughter and son-in-law, with whom he now lived, since the death of his wife, 3 years ago.

End of life issues are very difficult for us to deal with. It is often difficult to talk with patients about their death. It seems as if all efforts are aimed towards sending the patient home, fit and well, yet so often our best efforts are to no avail. Patients sometimes are untreatable. Henderson (1966) recognized this element in her famous definition of the role of the nurse, when she said:

> The unique function of the nurse is to assist the individual sick or well in the performance of those activities contributing to health or its recovery (or to a peaceful death) that he would perform unaided if he had the necessary strength, will, or knowledge. And do this in such a way as to help him gain independence as rapidly as possible.

Discussion concerning end of life decisions and the role of the nurse within these decisions is widespread. Due to the enormous developments in treatment that are now available we can keep patients alive for much longer, sometimes when any hope of recovery has passed. This situation is increasingly common in the high dependency/critical care areas.

Euthanasia

We talk about respecting the autonomy of the patient. At times the patient may ask us to commit an illegal act, such as end their life prematurely, or aid them in suicide; it is then we find ourselves in a dilemma. Such an act could be considered to be voluntary euthanasia. The literal meaning of the word 'euthanasia' means good death, that is a death which may be more desirable than to undergo possibly futile or painful treatment. This is often thought to mean a peaceful, painless, quiet death, and at a time of their own choosing. Voluntary euthanasia can be described as being administered to people who have requested it or given their informed consent (Nowell-Smith, 1994).

It is possible to distinguish between active euthanasia, which is when death is brought about by an action, such as an injection of a lethal dose, and passive euthanasia, which is when death is brought about by inaction, such as non-resuscitation after cardiac arrest. From these it is clear that involuntary euthanasia occurs when death is brought about when there is no patient request or informed consent.

Euthanasia has been discussed by parliamentary committees, the British Medical Association, the media and is even the subject of debates in nursing classrooms. Dimond (1995) wrote:

> It would be illegal, however, for the doctors to prescribe, either intentionally or recklessly, a substance to bring about the patient's death.

It is against the law to deliberately take a life. It is also against the law to aid suicide, although it is not against the law to commit suicide. The Suicide Act (1961) clearly states in section 1,

> The rule of law whereby it is a crime for a person to commit suicide is hereby abrogated

but it goes on in Section 2 to say:

> A person who aids, abets, counsels or procures the suicide of another or an attempt by another to commit suicide, shall be liable on conviction to an indictment to imprisonment.

It would be right to not give life saving treatment such as antibiotics, as long as the patient was both competent to give or refuse consent and had chosen to refuse treatment; it would be wrong to withhold treatment in the event that a patient was not in a fit state to give consent or refuse. However, in recent years the law appears to be moving towards the withdrawal of treatment to be considered as legal omission rather than commission, even if death is the outcome. It is not necessarily seen to be euthanasia. The case of Airedale NHS Trust v Bland was just such a case. The withdrawal of artificial nutrition and hydration was seen, in this instance, as an act of omission rather than commission. Johnson (1993) described the doctrine of acts and omissions saying:

> The failure to perform an act that would prevent negative consequences is morally better than to perform an act that would result in identical consequences, i.e. it is worse to kill someone than to allow them to die, or, passive euthanasia is less reprehensible than active euthanasia.

Henderson (1966) when defining the role of the nurse as: 'Assisting the individual to a peaceful death' did not mean that an intrinsic part of the nurse's role was to deliberately administer the agent which brought the patient to their, perhaps untimely, death, but it could be seen as to comply with the idea of omitting treatment, which by its very omission, brings about death. Clauses 1, 2 and 7 in the Code of Professional Conduct could all be interpreted in such a manner as to be used to justify such an act. What could be seen as the overriding clauses, would be the ongoing part of the opening statement that nurses shall act at all times, in such a manner as to:

- serve the interests of society;
- justify public trust and confidence;
- uphold and enhance the good standing and reputation of the professions.

Once again, an element of compromise is introduced, in that there is an expectation to act in the best interests of the patient, but not perhaps as interpreted by the patient.

> ### ACTIVITY 11.8 Case study
>
> If Mr James should ask you to end his life, what would be the most ethical approach to adopt?
> Would it be to agree to his wishes, recognizing that it is against the law, and might not be deemed to justify public trust and confidence?
> Consider how you should act in the most ethical way in the light of such a request?
> Reconsider your conclusions in the light of the following discussion.

The law would argue that it was not appropriate for a nurse to comply with such a patient's request, and in several recent cases has made it clear that nurses who do so are considered to have committed murder. The professional body, the UKCC, takes a similar view. However, the question remains, what is the most ethical approach towards a patient making such a request, or who asks for the means to terminate their own life? When considering the issue of autonomy, Harris (1985) considered the patient's potential to change their mind as being a valid and reasonable human characteristic, regardless of age. Although Harris considered the possibility of changing one's mind as an insufficient reason for failing to respect a patient's autonomy, he did recognize that when life would be lost as a result of respecting autonomy, then further considerations should be made, such as considering mental competence to make such a decision. If all other pathways had been explored, only then could one begin to consider complying with such a request. However, as a nurse you have certain rights to be recognized. Edwards (1996), when considering the issue of 'whistleblowing', thought that nurses had rights and responsibilities which should be considered when taking such risky actions. He argued that it was only ethical that healthcare workers should also consider their responsibilities as providers, parents, carers within their own homes, which could be weighed against the need of the patient whose treatment has given rise to the desire to expose poor practices or provision of care. A consequentialist would argue that if the 'whistle-blower' was sacked, the care they would have given to many patients in the future would outweigh the good done for the one patient. Similarly, the happiness of more people might be achieved by keeping quiet, rather than exposing a failure within the system. So, in the case of a patient begging for release from an intolerable life, the healthcare worker could form an argument which would outweigh the patient's desire for an early end to their life.

A deontological viewpoint would look more carefully at the patient as being an end in themselves, a person with a right to be involved in the decision making process, not a legislative right perhaps. Campbell (1995) would appear to indicate that such an approach could be acceptable, saying:

> A human being is a member of the biological species *Homo sapiens*; a person is a moral agent who has plans and purposes and the capacity for free choice. From the point of view of personhood, all persons are morally equal in as much as there is no adherent reason for preferring one's plans and purposes to another's.

He then went on to consider that to disregard another's decision concerning consent or refusal of treatment might be interpreted as valuing that individual as less than your equal, or having less 'moral importance' than yourself. It may be that there is psychological value to the patient in being involved in decision making. It enables the patient to be autonomous, that is 'a free moral agent'. If the patient has a greater vested interest in what happens to their own life than any other, least of all the healthcare professional's, then they would be most committed to making the right decision about their own life.

Perhaps a more ethical approach could be gained by identifying why the patient would make such a request. If the reason was uncontrolled pain, or unpleasant symptoms, or uncontrolled fear, there may be options available to control these symptoms which would alter their desire to die. If you consider the model, beneficence, non-maleficence and justice are elements to

be considered in ethical decision making, as well as respect of autonomy. What would be the route to take to maximize good, minimize harm and act with justice towards this patient? Surely it would be to ensure that all had been done to improve the quality of life being experienced by that individual. In fact, not to have already done so might be a major contributory factor in this patient's expressed wish to die. There is abundant evidence to indicate that healthcare professionals consistently underestimate patients' pain and thus undertreat pain (Hunt *et al.*, 1977; Marks and Sacher, 1973; Seers, 1987). Poor pain management is a major factor concerning end of life issues. To be in chronic uncontrolled pain causes depression, leading to a loss of interest in life activities. Effective pain control reduces the likelihood of depression and thus encourages continued interest in participation in life activities. Castledine (1997: 895) wrote: 'A patient request for euthanasia will usually be due to fear of pain, helplessness, and loss of control'. Campbell (1995: 228) agreed with this and concluded that: 'once in control of their pain, patients are often able to control their lives and prepare for their deaths'.

The healthcare professional is bound by law, professional guidelines and their own personal beliefs and values when faced with such a dilemma as a patient requesting active euthanasia. They have the clear legal rule that they are not allowed to assist in suicide. Before making any steps which could lead to professional isolation, they must have demonstrated that there is nothing further to be done to make that life tenable, and that all other alternatives have been exhausted. The case of Regina v Cox (1993) where a consultant administered an injection with the intent to kill a patient whose pain from severe arthritis was uncontrollable, clearly indicated the law's beliefs. Had he administered another death inducing drug that had analgesic properties, which potassium chloride has not, he would have been considered to have carried out a legal act. As it was, by using potassium chloride, he became guilty of the crime of murder. The family indicated that they were grateful to the doctor for his actions. The patient had asked to die, but his actions were seen to be active euthanasia and thus illegal. Had a nurse administered the injection, he or she would have been held personally accountable for acting in such a manner, both by the law and by the ruling body. The action was illegal, whether it was moral is another issue entirely. The theoretical argument which differentiates between the act of Dr Cox and that of the doctors caring for Tony Bland is that which is called the principle of double effect and was mentioned earlier. It is one favoured by the Roman Catholic church. It can be seen perhaps as a guide rather than a rule for moral decision making. Every action we take has both good and bad effects and what must be considered is whether the good that we do is justified in the light of the inevitable evil. Hoose (1994) states

> that the evil effect might be justified if all four of the following conditions are fulfilled:
>
> 1 The act performed is good in itself.
> 2 The good effect does not result from the evil effect.
> 3 The person acting intends only the good effect.
> 4 There is a proportionate reason for causing the harm.

So as far as the case of Dr Cox was concerned, his intention was to bring about the death of the patient. He could perceive of no other way to relieve the pain that she was in, so his desire might have been to relieve her pain, which in itself would have been a good act, but it could only have been achieved by bringing about her death. There was no other possible outcome to administering a large 'bolus' dose of potassium chloride than death by cardiac arrest, so there was no possible way that he could be said to be trying only to ease her pain. Potassium chloride has no analgesic properties nor does it potentiate analgesic properties in other drugs and the potential for her death was equal to that of her achieving pain release through death. So there was no way in which Dr Cox could be seen to be working within the principles of double effect. However, the doctors caring for Tony Bland, who was diagnosed as being in a persistent vegetative state, in that he could neither see, hear, taste, smell, speak nor communicate, wished to withdraw treatment. The continuing of treatment would be of no benefit to the patient. They believed that it was immoral to continue ineffective treatment, even though its withdrawal could bring about his death. Shortly after the treatment was discontinued Tony Bland did die, but his death was imminent and only held at bay by the treatment which could do nothing to improve his chance of recovery. The argument is one of deliberate intent, does one actively kill or allow death to occur naturally? It is a difficult question.

Do not resuscitate orders and withdrawal of treatment

There are many philosophers and ethicists who would argue that the distinction between the act of omission or commission which brings about death is a spurious one. Nurses have a recognized duty of care towards their patients. They also have a duty not to kill others. The patient's perspective of life and their perception of quality of life must be of considered in any decisions made which might shorten that life. Moreland and Geisler (1994) believed that an act which was agreed to be in everyone's best interests could be considered to be morally acceptable. Letting the patient die could be interpreted as an act of charity which is an overriding duty and therefore justifies the failure to perform duties correlative to the right to life (Johnson, 1993). In other words, there should be consideration given to the degree of benefit achieved by treatment as opposed to the harm, discomfort or pain that that same treatment might bring about. If such benefit achieved outweighed the harm it might also cause, then it would be reasonable and ethical to continue, with the patient's consent. However, if the benefit was so limited that it did not justify the potential harm, then it should not continue. Thus the principles of beneficence, non-maleficence and justice would be brought into play. The duty of care to a patient would not allow the nurse to consider attempting to prolong life should the owner of that life no longer value it or desire to prolong it. In many hospitals today there are clear policies concerning decisions not to resuscitate patients. Within many such policies is the requirement for multidisciplinary discussion to take place, rationale for decision making made clear and a requirement for such decisions to be updated on a frequent basis, according to the changes in the patient's condition.

The problem is that cardiopulmonary resuscitation treatment can be harmful in its outcomes, even if it is successful in restarting heart function. To carry out cardiopulmonary resuscitation in the presence of advanced illness from other causes or extreme old age may be inappropriate. Using the four principles approach, Hilberman *et al.* (1997) argued that the most recent research concerning cardiopulmonary resuscitation indicated that it was not necessarily beneficent to the patient, even if they arrested in a coronary care unit, with skilled staff present. Nor was it non-maleficent, in that frequently brain damage accompanied apparent successes. However, in justice, it may be reasonable to administer such an intervention, if it could be seen through research to be beneficial to that group of patients or clients. Their recommendations are useful. The one major difference in their approach is their recognition of the legal need to seek a patient's consent as to whether resuscitation should take place. Unlike the USA, in this country it is not a legal requirement, but certainly would appear to be a moral one, in that the patient should be seen to be treated ethically and professionally. In deontological terms, not to involve the patient in the decision making process would be to deny their autonomy, possibly fail to treat them with beneficence, and maleficence and certainly fail to administer justice. The patient would be considered as less than an equal, thus not a person, but as a means to an end. For the consequentialist and the utilitarian, not to consult the patient could perhaps be justified as reasonable, because it would only distress the patient. Thus the decisions would be better made by those professionals who understood the possible risks, costs and benefits. The British Medical Association appear to back this approach, believing that a non-medical person could not easily maintain an objective and rational approach to their own illness, even if the patient had the knowledge and understanding to make such a decision. Schutz (1994) criticized the combined BMA/RCN (1993) statement concerning resuscitation orders, in that she felt that they failed to go beyond seeing the patient's involvement in such decision making as 'valuable' or 'important'. She indicated that possibly the reason patients were not consulted was the healthcare workers' unease with the topic rather than the fact that it was harmful to patients. There is no doubt that if a nurse is to act in a moral way towards her clients she would need to perceive them as individuals, with individual needs and wants. Therefore, to work to maximize their healthcare outcomes she must identify the individual's priorities and wishes to develop appropriate care plans. Not to spend time identifying the patient's short and long-term goals, beliefs and values would be to fail in the duty of care, especially in an area as important to the individual as to how they wish to die. Nurses spend more time with their patients, get to know them better than any doctor or consultant who is responsible for final decision making in the event of resuscitation decisions. Although the research to support this affirmation is thin, it is certainly true that it is required by the Code of Professional Conduct (1992) for the nurse to take into account the cultural and religious beliefs and values of their patients. Thus not to do so could be seen to be failing in their duty of care. Not to involve a patient in the decision making process, especially in relation to end of life decisions, could be seen to be negligent care, and unethical unless there were mitigating circumstances such as inability to give consent, on the basis of physical or mental incompetence. In which case, the advice of those closest to the patient must be sought. Although the family have no legal right to refuse consent to any life-saving treatment (Dimond, 1995), they may have the role of knowledgeable informer. In the absence of such an individual, ethical decision making should be made following discussion by all healthcare staff involved with the care of the patient prior to any proposed actions.

Advanced directives or living wills

Legislation on advanced directives or 'living wills', as they are sometimes known, would clarify their use in practice. Such documents could provide an indication of a patient's beliefs, values and will. However the case involving Dr Cox indicated that to actively participate in hastening death is still unacceptable in our society, whereas in the case of Tony Bland, such a document would have indicated his ideas concerning end of life issues. The value of such documents would be in such situations where an individual is unable to indicate their preference or wishes regarding the end of their life. The Select Committee on Medical Ethics Report (1994) looked very seriously at the legalization of advanced directives or living wills. They concluded that legislation was not necessary, but recognized the need for a code of practice to be developed. They felt that doctors increasingly recognized the ethical need to respect patients' wishes. There appears to be little evidence to substantiate this. Unfortunately there is often little discussion between healthcare workers and patients to clarify what patients want. This is especially true in the case of end of life issues. A solicitor was once asked if it was appropriate to ask a patient at an admission interview about their end of life wishes or if they had made an advanced directive.

The solicitor was not happy at such an approach feeling that it would cause undue fear and anxiety at an already stressful time. Although this was a perfectly valid view, one wonders when else one could approach patients, without causing them stress and anxiety. Death is still a very sensitive topic. Although increasingly people do tell their families their beliefs and wishes, they rarely tell their doctor or nurses. Dimond (1995), quite rightly, indicated the legal invalidity of patients' relatives giving consent, either for treatment or its withdrawal, because of their potentially suspect motives. But if they are the only knowledgeable persons, can we afford to ignore their statements? It becomes obvious that we should encourage patients to make their wishes known in writing, or at least to have discussed their wishes with their nurse, who can make written records of such discussions to enable consistent and ethical ongoing care. Obviously, these views should be considered to be dynamic, in that they could change at different times and in different circumstances. Nurses need to determine the extent to which previously written documents or records are still valid. At least there would be an already established precedent to discuss the patient's present wishes and thoughts.

Conclusion

It is obvious that an ethical approach to healthcare provision is dependent upon an understanding of the patient, their goals, beliefs, values and wishes, as well as a knowledge of the relevant law. An appropriate ethical decision making model to consider the patient and their needs enables the nurse to consider alternative ethical options and give rationale for the chosen course of action. In an increasingly litigious society this is essential for the worker, but it should also ensure that the patient is always involved in the decision making process, except when it could be seen as detrimental to their care and justified on that basis. The decision making process concerning the patient should be clearly demonstrated beyond a shadow of doubt. The processes employed to achieve a partnership in care between both the high dependency patient and nurse must be transparent. This transparency should engender and substantiate a truly trusting relationship.

Further reading

Beauchamp, T. L. 1994 The 'four-principles' approach. In: Gillon, R. (ed.) *Principles of healthcare ethics,* Chichester: John Wiley.

Beauchamp, T. L. and Childress, J. F. 1989 *Principles of biomedical ethics,* 3rd edn. Oxford: Oxford University Press,

Blackburn, S. 1994 *The Oxford dictionary of philosophy.* Oxford: Oxford University Press.

BMA/RCN. 1993 *Statement on cardiopulmonary resuscitation.* London: BMA/RCN.

Brahams, D. 1995 The critically ill patient: the legal perspective. In: Tingle, J. and Cribb, A (eds) *Nursing law and ethics.* Oxford: Blackwell Science.

Campbell, R. 1995 An ethical perspective – declining and withdrawing treatment. In: Tingle, J. and Cribb, A. (eds) *Nursing law and ethics.* Oxford: Blackwell Science.

Castledine, G. 1997 Is euthanasia a 'quick-fix' to the dying process? *British Journal of Nursing* **6**(5), 895.

Clough, A. 1860 The latest decalogue. In: Nicholson, R. (1975) Should the patient be allowed to die? *Journal of Medical Ethics* **1**(1), 4–9.

Dimond, B. 1995 *Legal aspects of nursing,* 2nd edn. London: Prentice Hall,

Edwards, S.D. 1996 What are the limits to the obligation of the nurse. *Journal of Medical Ethics* **22**, 90–4.

Emson, H.E. 1988 Confidentiality: a modified value. *Journal of Medical Ethics* **14**, 87–90.

Gillon, R. (ed.) 1994 *Principles of healthcare ethics.* Chichester: John Wiley

Harris, J. 1985 *The value of life: an introduction to medical ethics.* London: Routledge

Henderson, V. 1966 *The nature of nursing: a definition and its implications for practice, research and Education.* New York: Macmillan.

Hilberman, M. 1997 Marginally effective medical care: ethical analysis of issues. In: Kutner. Cardiopulmonary resuscitation. *Journal of Medical Ethics* **23**, 361–7.

Hoose, B. 1994 Theology and the four principles: a roman catholic view. In: Gillon, R. (ed.), *Principles of healthcare ethics.* Chichester: John Wiley.

Hunt, J.M., Stollar, T.D., Littlejohns, D.W., *et al.* 1977 Patients with protracted pain: A survey conducted at The London Hospital. *Journal of Medical Ethics* **3**, 61–73.

Johnson, K. 1993 A moral dilemma: killing and letting die. *British Journal of Nursing* **2**(12), 635–40.

Kant 1788 Critique of practical reason. In: Blackburn, S. (1994) *The Oxford dictionary of philosophy.* Oxford: OUP.

Kennedy, I. 1991 *Treat me right.* Oxford: Clarendon Press.

Marks, R.M. and Sacher, E.J. 1973 Under treatment of medical inpatients with narcotic analgesics. *Annals of Internal Medicine* **78**, 173–181.

Moreland, J. and Geisler, N. 1994 *The life-death debate.* New York: Greenwood Press.

Nowell-Smith, P. 1994 In favour of voluntary euthanasia. In: Gillon, R. (ed.) *Principles of healthcare ethics.* Chichester: John Wiley.

Rumbold, G. 1993 *Ethics in nursing practice.* Ballière London: Tindall.

Schutz, S. 1994 Patient involvement in resuscitation decisions. *British Journal of Nursing* **3**(20), 1075–9.

Seedhouse, D. 1988 *Ethics: the heart of healthcare.* Chichester: John Wiley.

Seers, C.J. 1987 *Pain, anxiety and recovery in patients undergoing surgery,* unpublished PhD Thesis, King's College, University of London.

Select Committee on Medical Ethics 1994 *Report of the Select Comittee on Medical Ethics* (House of Lords: Session 1993–94: HL Paper 21–1), 1, 38–44, 58. London: HMSO.

Stokes, B. 1997 Setting the record straight. *Nursing Standard* **11**(41), 14.

Tingle, J. 1995 *Nursing law and ethics.* Oxford: Blackwell Science,

Tschudin, V. 1989 Ethics, morality and nursing. In: Hinchliff, S.M., Norman, S. and Schober, J. E. *Nursing practice and healthcare.* London: Arnold.

UKCC 1992 *Code of Professional Conduct.* London: UKCC.

UKCC 1996 *Guidelines to Professional Conduct.* London: UKCC.

Warwick, S.J. 1989 A vote for no confidence. *Journal of Medical Ethics* **15**, 183–5.

Index

Note: the abbreviation ARDS stands for adult respiratory distress syndrome.